Surgical Anatomy
of the Ear
and Temporal Bone

Surgical Anatomy
of the Ear
and Temporal Bone

Bruce Proctor, M.D., F.A.C.S.

Clinical Professor
Department of Otolaryngology—Head and Neck Surgery
School of Medicine
University of Michigan

Research Associate
Kresge Hearing Research Institute
University of Michigan

Clinical Professor
Department of Otolaryngology—Head and Neck Surgery
School of Medicine
Wayne State University

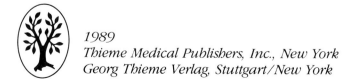

1989
Thieme Medical Publishers, Inc., New York
Georg Thieme Verlag, Stuttgart/New York

Thieme Medical Publishers, Inc.
381 Park Avenue South
New York, New York 10016

SURGICAL ANATOMY OF THE
EAR AND TEMPORAL BONE
Bruce Proctor

Library of Congress Cataloging-in-Publication Data

Proctor, Bruce.
    Surgical anatomy of the ear and temporal bone / Bruce Proctor.
        p.   cm.
    ISBN 0-86577-295-9
    1. Ear—Anatomy. 2. Temporal bone—Anatomy. 3. Anatomy. Surgical
and topographical. I. Title.
    [DNLM: 1. Ear—anatomy & histology. 2. Temporal Bone—anatomy &
histology. WV 201 P964sJ
QM507.S87   1989
611.85—dc19
DNLM/DLC
for Library of Congress   89-4392
                                                               CIP

Important note: Medicine is an ever-changing science. Research and clinical experience are continually broadening our knowledge, in particular our knowledge of proper treatment and drug therapy. Insofar as this book mentions any dosage or application, readers may rest assured that the authors, editors, and publishers have made every effort to ensure that such references are strictly in accordance with the state of knowledge at the time of production of the book. Nevertheless, every user is requested to carefully examine the manufacturers' leaflets accompanying each drug to check on his own responsibility whether the dosage schedules recommended therein or the contraindications stated by the manufacturers differ from the statements made in the present book. Such examination is particularly important with drugs that are either rarely used or have been newly released on the market.

Some of the product names, patents, and registered designs referred to in this book are in fact registered trademarks or proprietary names even though specific reference to this fact is not always made in the text. Therefore, the appearance of a name without designation as proprietary is not to be construed as a representation by the publisher that it is in the public domain.

Printed in the United States of America.

5 4 3 2 1

TMP ISBN 0-86577-295-9
GTV ISBN 3-13-730001-0

Contents

vi   Contents

Preface

The temporal bone and ear present a very complex anatomy. Minute details of its structure are studied in depth, and are carefully illustrated in this text. The purpose of this text is to provide a guide for obtaining access to the various regions of the temporal bone. This is particularly of value to the otologic surgeon.

Osteology of the temporal bone is presented for the intact temporal bone and its constituent bones: the petrosa, the squama, the tympanic bone, and the styloid. Sutures between these constituents are reviewed in great detail. Cavities are studied individually: the external auditory canal, the middle ear as a whole, the attic, the hypotympanum, the eustachian tube, and the air cell system of the mastoid and petrosa.

The development of the middle ear spaces, their compartments, and the significance of the tympanic diaphragm are discussed with particular reference to their importance in the development of middle ear diseases.

The facial canal is presented in considerable detail, with special emphasis on its variations and anomalies. Also included is a description of the petromastoid canal. Its clinical significance is reviewed.

Minute details of the vestibule, semicircular canals, and cochlea are presented with numerous detailed drawings. Included are the vestibular and cochlear aqueducts and the internal auditory canal. Great emphasis is placed on describing the relations of these structures to their adjacent bony environment.

The blood supply to the ear is described in considerable detail, with emphasis on the effects of various disease states on circulation. Disorders of the blood flow in the dural sinuses are of particular interest to the otologist.

At intervals throughout the text, and when appropriate, a discussion of practical considerations has been inserted to correlate anatomic details with their application to clinical problems.

The detailed anatomy of the round window niche was translated from the Hungarian text of Dr. Bela Bolobas of Budapest, and is presented in a discussion in Chapter 9. This is important to those surgeons performing cochlear implant surgery for alleviation of profound deafness. Minute details of anatomy, variants, and embryology of this very complicated area of the temporal bone are presented in English for the first time.

This author was impressed a half-century ago with the paucity and unavailability of anatomic information on the ear as new procedures were developed for the treatment of various ear disorders. A careful search of the literature combined with appropriate dissections of human temporal bones resulted in a slow, steady accumulation of the anatomic information produced in this text.

Various methods of study were employed. Cadaver material was used for soft tissue studies of the eustachian tube and its musculature, fascia, vasculature, and innervation, as well as for dissections of the extratemporal portion of the facial nerve. Fresh temporal bones obtained from autopsy specimens were dissected immediately, or at least after preservation via deep-freeze methods. This was particularly useful for study of the viscera in the middle ear.

Most useful for studying the osteology of the interior of a temporal bone is the motor-driven diamond saw which can cut the temporal bone in various planes. A large number of dry temporal bones cut in this way, in various planes and in a variety of temporal bones, will demonstrate the anatomy of bony structures and their relationship to adjacent structures.

For final interpretation of structures, one can resort to a temporal bone bank where bones are decalcified, embedded, sectioned, and stained for careful microscopic study.

Further information can be obtained by observation during otologic surgery, using the operating microscope.

Most of the drawings in this text were done by experienced medical illustrators. Their drawings far surpass the use of photography because of their three-dimensional effects. With temporal bone sections, however, illustrations are best shown via photomicrography performed by a photographer experienced in this type of work.

Earlier encouragement for this book was given by Dr. A.C. Furstenberg and Dr. James Maxwell of the Department of Otolaryngology at the University of Michigan. In recent years, support was rendered by Dr. Charles Krause and Dr. Josef Miller of the same department. The material on the variations and anomalies of the facial nerve and canal was provided, for the most part, by Dr.George Nager from the Temporal Bone Histological Laboratory of Johns Hopkins University. I am very grateful to him for his support.

Aiding in some of the dissections were my son, Dr. Conrad Proctor, and Dr. Eric Nielsen, Dr. Ping Chang (Taipei), Dr. Alan El Seifi (Cairo), and, most recently, Dr. John Niparko of Ann Arbor. The medical illustrators were William Loechelle, Grant Lashbrook, Evelyn Sullivan, Ellen Jacobs, Edgar Yaeger, and Pat Banks.

Photomicrographs were prepared by Arthur Boden of Henry Ford Hospital in Detroit.

Special attention was paid by this author to certain subjects in the text: detailed descriptive osteology, the petrosquamosal suture and lamina,[1] the eustachian tube,[2,3] the middle ear cleft with its contents, folds and compartments,[4] the origin and development of the posterior tympanum,[5] the facial canal with a presentation of its variations and anomalies,[6] the internal auditory meatus, and, finally, a series of original drawings on structures of the cochlea and vestibule.

Bruce Proctor, M.D., F.A.C.S.

1   The Intact Temporal Bone

Extracranial Surface of the Temporal Bone

The extracranial surface presents the four components of the temporal bone: the squamosa, the petrosa, the tympanic bone, and the styloid bone. The temporal bone forms a portion of the lateral and inferior walls of the skull.

External Surface of the Temporal Bone

Squamosa

The zygoma is found at the union of the horizontal and vertical portions of the squama (Fig. 1).

The Zygoma. The zygoma (Figs. 2–6) arises from a narrow and long base. It is flattened from above downward, curves laterally (Fig. 2), and then extends directly forward.

The *base of the zygoma* is large in front and narrow behind. The superior surface is irregular. It is thickened posteriorly on its inferior aspect to form the *posterior zygomatic tubercle.* In front of the posterior zygomatic tubercle, the bone is thinner with an upward concavity forming the external zygomatic portion of the *glenoid cavity* of the temporal bone. In front of this cavity, the zygoma thickens considerably to form the *anterior zygomatic tubercle,* which lies at the external extremity of the *temporal condyle.* Thus, the base of the zygoma has an articulating inferior surface. Its superior surface serves as the point of attachment for the posterior fibers of the powerful temporal muscle.

Behind the posterior zygomatic tubercle, the base of the zygoma extends as a crest posteriorly and slightly upward —the *supramastoid crest* or *linea temporalis.* It marks the level of the floor of the middle cranial fossa.

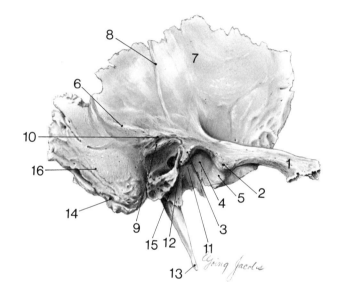

Figure 1. External view of the right temporal bone. 1, Zygomatic process. 2, Anterior zygomatic tubercle. 3, Posterior zygomatic tubercle. 4, Glenoid (mandibular fossa). 5, Temporal condyle. 6, Supramastoid crest (linea temporalis). 7, Vertical portion of squama. 8, Groove for posterior deep temporal artery. 9, Spine of Henle (suprameatal spine) with retromeatal cribriform zone above it. 10, Suprameatal triangle. 11, Glenoid fossa posterior to petrotympanic fissure (Glaserian). 12, Tympanic crest. 13, Styloid process. 14, Digastric groove. 15, Vaginal process tympanic bone. 16, External petrosquamosal suture and mastoid process.

The *free part of the zygoma* presents two smooth surfaces. The internal one is muscular; the external one is cutaneous and readily palpable through the skin. Of the two edges, the superior is thin and straight, while the inferior is thick and concave. In front, the zygoma ends by a narrow serrated zone, oblique anteriorly and superiorly, to articulate with the maxillary bone.

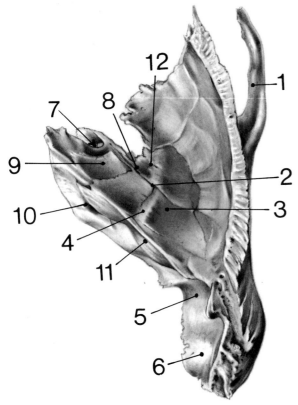

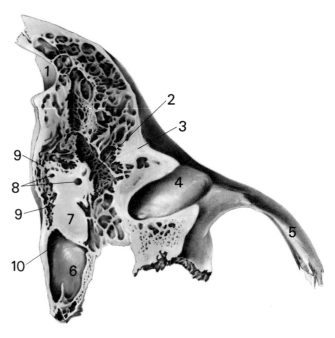

Figure 3. A view of the top half of a horizontal cut. 1, Groove for sigmoid sinus. 2, Mastoid antrum. 3, Roof of external auditory meatus. 4, Mandibular condyle. 5, Zygoma. 6, Large cell in petrous apex. 7, Top of cochlear capsule. 8, Superior semicircular canal. 9, Superior cell tract leading to petrous apex.

Figure 2. Superior view of right temporal bone. 1, Zygomatic process. 2, Hiatus for canal of the greater superficial petrosal nerve. 3, Arcuate eminence. 4, Prominence of superior semicircular canal. 5, Sigmoid sinus groove. 6, Mastoid portion. 7, Anterior orifice carotid canal. 8, Canal for greater superficial petrosal nerve. 9, Meckel's cave. 10, Orifice of internal auditory meatus. 11, Groove for superior petrosal sinus. 12, Angle formed by the squama laterally and the petrosal medially marks the internal extremity of the internal petrosquamosal suture.

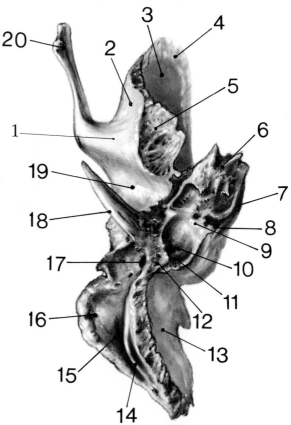

Figure 4. Inferior view of right temporal bone. 1, Temporal condyle. 2, Subtemporal plane. 3, Vertical portion of squama. 4, Superior edge of squama. 5, Anterior edge of horizontal portion of squama. 6, Anterior orifice of carotid canal. 7, Groove for inferior petrosal sinus. 8, Orifice of cochlear aqueduct in jugular facette. 9, Orifice of Jacobson's canal. 10, Jugular fossa. 11, Foramen for Arnold's nerve. 12, Jugular facette. 13, Sigmoid sinus. 14, Groove for occipital artery. 15, Digastric groove. 16, Mastoid process. 17, Stylomastoid foramen. 18, Styloid process, 19, Glenoid fossa. 20, Zygomatic process.

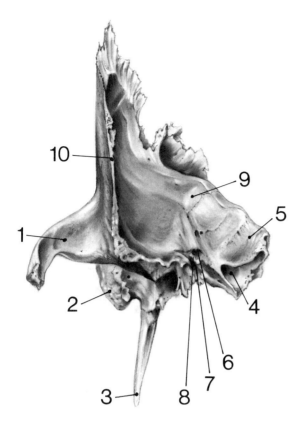

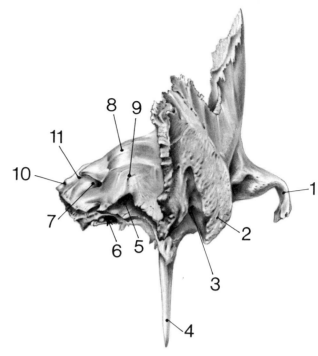

Figure 5.   Anterior view right temporal bone. 1, Zygomatic process. 2, Mastoid process. 3, Styloid process. 4, Anterior orifice of carotid canal. 5, Meckel's cave. 6, Semicanal for tensor tympani muscle. 7, Semicanal for auditory tube with septum canalis musculotubarii above (8). 9, Arcuate eminence. 10, Vertical portion of squama.

Figure 6.   Posterior view of intact right temporal bone. 1, Zygomatic process. 2, Mastoid process. 3, Digastric groove. 4, Styloid process. 5, Jugular fossa. 6, Internal carotid canal. 7, Internal auditory meatus. 8, Arcuate eminence. 9, Orifice of vestibular aqueduct. 10, Meckel's cave. 11, Groove for superior petrosal sinus.

Vertical and Horizontal Portions of the Squama.   The base of the zygoma separates the vertical from the horizontal portions of the squama (Figs. 1–8).

The vertical portion is smooth. An almost vertical groove is seen posteriorly for the *posterior deep temporal artery.*

The horizontal portion is more complex. Beginning anteriorly, the following are presented:

1. The *subtemporal plane* is a small triangular surface with an anterior apex. It is separated externally from the vertical portion by a ridge—the *temporal crest.*
2. The *temporal condyle* is horizontal, but slightly inclined inferiorly and posteriorly. Its external part corresponds to the base of the zygoma.
3. The *glenoid cavity,* which is large and deep, is formed externally by the base of the zygoma. It occupies the larger part of this horizontal portion of the squama, and may be separated from the intracranial cavity by a very thin wall of bone. This area is susceptible to fractures.
4. The *tympanic crest* is a projection running transverse and medial to the posterior zygomatic tubercle. It does not extend as far medially as the glenoid fossa.

5. A narrower and smaller surface forms the roof of the *external auditory canal.* It is partly hidden by the tympanic bone, which is in contact with the posterior surface of the tympanic crest.

Retromeatal Portion of the Squama   The horizontal portion of the squama stops at the level of the roof of the external auditory canal. Immediately behind it, the squama spreads out to form the posterior wall of the external auditory canal and the somewhat transversely flattened outer portion of the mastoid process.

This portion of the squama (Fig. 9) situated below the supramastoid crest and behind the external auditory canal continues in the plane of the vertical portion of the squama. It is not classified with the latter, because it is not seen on the intracranial surface of the temporal bone and its inner surface is in contact with the petrosa.

On the posterosuperior circumference of the external auditory canal orifice is a variable-sized projection called the *spine of Henle* or *suprameatal spine.* A small recess may exist above it. This spine develops from the squama and is not of tympanic bone origin. Behind this spine, one may

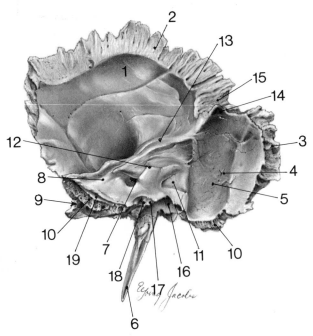

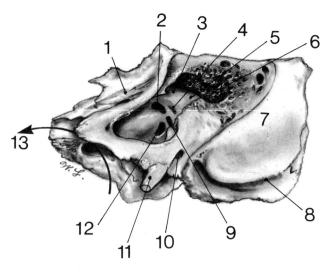

Figure 7. Internal view of the right temporal bone. 1, Vertical portion of squama. 2, Beveled superior border of the squama. 3, Parietal articular surface. 4, Mastoid foramen. 5, Sigmoid sinus groove. 6, Styloid process. 7, Internal auditory meatus. 8, Groove of superior petrosal sinus. 9, Anterior orifice of carotid canal. 10, Articular edge with the occipital bone. 11, Unguinal fossa. 12, Arcuate eminence. 13, Groove for superior petrosal sinus. 14, Orifice of petrosquamosal sinus. 15, Parietal notch. 16, Pyramidal fossa. 17, Stylomastoid foramen. 18, Jugular dome. 19, Groove for inferior petrosal sinus.

Figure 9. External view of left temporal bone after removal of the tympanic bone and squama. 1, Canal for tensor tympani muscle. 2, Oval window. 3, and 5, Horizontal semicircular canal. 4, Facial canal (dehiscent). 6, Mastoid antrum. 7, Petrosal portion of mastoid. 8, Digastric groove. 9, Sinus tympani. 10, Opened descending facial canal. 11, Styloid process. 12, Round window niche. 13, Carotid canal.

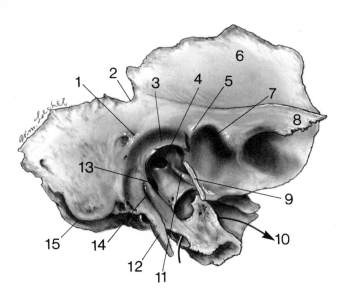

Figure 8. External view of the right temporal bone in which the tympanic bone has been removed. 1, Spine of Henle. 2, Incisura parietale. 3, Roof of external auditory canal. 4, Oval window. 5, Posterior zygomatic tubercle. 6, Squama. 7, Mandibular fossa. 8, Zygoma. 9, Petrosal hernia. 10, Carotid canal. 11, Tensor canal. 12, Styloid process. 13, Round window niche. 14, Facial canal. 15, Digastric groove.

occasionally see a group of small orifices called the *retro-meatal cribriform zone.* In an infant, vessels pass through to the mucosa of the underlying antrum.

Summary. The external surface of the squama is divided into two zones by the zygoma and the supramastoid crest, which prolongs it posteriorly.

1. The superior zone corresponds to the vertical portion of the squama and possesses both a deep cerebral surface and a superficial muscular surface in contact with the temporal muscle.

2. The inferior zone is, in turn, divided by the external auditory canal into two parts: (a) The anterior part constitutes the horizontal part of the squama and makes the roofs of the external auditory canal, the glenoid cavity, the condyles and a portion of the infratemporal fossa. (b) The posterior part corresponds to the retromeatal portion of the squama. The horizontal portion of the squama spreads out immediately behind the external auditory canal, and its deeper surface is in contact with the petrosa as the petro-squamosal lamina, which can sometimes be a persistent and complete bony partition in the substance of the mastoid.

Petrosa

The retromeatal portion of the squama fuses behind the petrosa to form the mastoid region. The *external petro-squamosal suture* indicates this point of contact on the external surface of the mastoid (Fig. 1). This suture leads upward to the parietal incisura. It continues forward rather indistinctly with the internal petrosquamosal fissure.

The mastoid process is roughened behind and below to give insertion to the powerful sternomastoid and splenius capitis muscles. A little above the posterior border of the mastoid process, one often sees a variable-sized foramen (*mastoid foramen* or *canal*) for the mastoid emissary vein, which leads inward to the groove for the lateral sinus. The position of the mastoid foramen varies, and may be at the level of the occipitotemporal suture or petrooccipital suture.

Tympanic Bone

The external auditory canal is formed only in part by the squama. It is completed in front, below, and in great part posteriorly by the tympanic bone (Figs. 10-13). This bone is in the form of a gutter. From its inferior convex aspect, a thin plate of bone extends anteroinferiorly to abut on the styloid process.

1. The external extremity of the tympanic bone is rough and irregular due to the attachment of the cartilage of the external ear.

2. Its anterior surface, the *tympanic plate,* is made up by both the anterior wall of the gutter and the inferior prolongation of the tympanic bone. The lower edge of the tympanic plate ends free. A part covering the base of the styloid process is the vaginal process, which sometimes splits to enclose it. The tympanic plate is separated from both the mandibular fossa and the thick anterior edge of the squama by the petrotympanic fissure, which opens into the tympanic cavity. The outer end of the fissure is closed, the inner part is double, since a thin piece of the

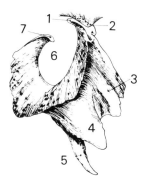

Figure 11.   Tympanic bone—right side. Superficial surface. 1, Anterior tympanic crest. 2, Posterior zygomatic tubercle. 3, Tubal process. 4, Vaginal process. 5, Styloid process. 6, External auditory canal. 7, Posterior tympanic crest.

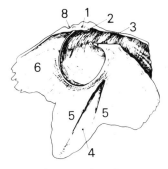

Figure 12.   Tympanic bone—right side. Deep surface. 1, Crista spinarum. 2, Anterior tympanic crest. 3, Posterior tympanic crest. 4, Styloid groove. 5, Vaginal process. 6, Tubal process. 7, External auditory canal (anterior wall). 8, Malleus sulcus.

petrosa, the *tegmen tympani,* bends down between the squamous and tympanic portions.

3. The posterior surface formed by both the posterior slope of the tympanic gutter and the inferior prolongation of the tympanic bone contacts the squama first, and then the petrosa. Found externally is the posterior *tympanosquamosal suture* and internally the posterior *tympanopetrosal suture.*

4. The tympanic gutter is limited by two slopes of unequal length: (a) the posterior slope is short. Its height increases as it extends inward. Externally, it forms the inferior part of the posterior wall of the external auditory canal, but at its medial end, it constitutes the entire height of this wall. The edge that limits this slope superiorly and externally is easily seen. Curving inward with an inferior concavity, it climbs obliquely upward and inward (the *tympanosquamosal fissure* or posterior *tympanosquamosal fissure*). Midway in its course is a tiny *perforation for the passage of Arnold's nerve.* (b) the anterior slope is more developed. At first, it forms the anterior wall of the external auditory canal, then in its inner half, it forms the lateral wall of the protympanum.

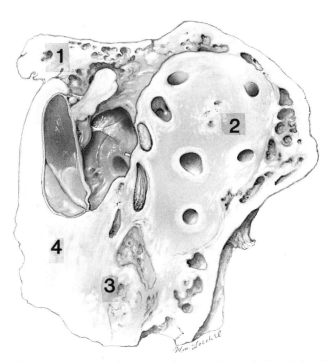

Figure 10.   A vertical cut across the petrosal axis, which includes all constituent bones of the intact temporal bone. 1, Squamous base. 2, Petrosal bone. 3, Styloid bone. 4, Tympanic bone.

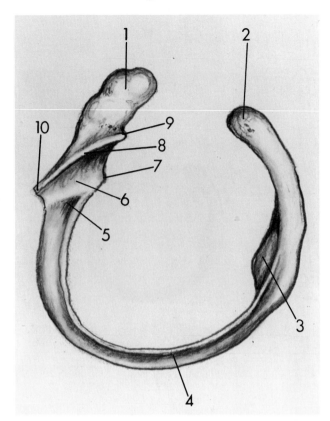

Figure 13.   Tympanic bone at birth looking laterally at its medial surface. 1, Anterior horn. 2, Posterior horn. 3, Posterior tympanic tuberosity. 4, Sulcus tympanicus. 5, Tympanic crest of Gruber. 6, Mallear gutter. 7, Anterior tympanic tuberosity. 8, Crista spinarum of Henle. 9, Posterior tympanic spine. 10, Anterior tympanic spine of Henle.

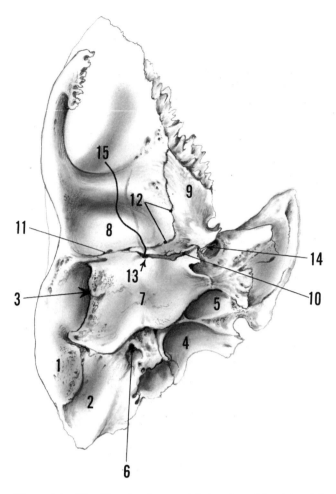

Figure 14.   The Glaserian fissure—inferior view of the right adult temporal bone. The petrosquamosal sinus may persist and pass through the external limit of the anterior external petrosquamosal suture (12). Note the lateral extension of the petrosa to inset between the squamosa and tympanic bone. 1, Mastoid tip. 2, Digastric groove. 3, External auditory canal. 4, Jugular dome. 5, Carotid canal. 6, Stylomastoid foramen. 7, Vaginal plate. 8, Glenoid fossa. 9, Crista tegmentalis (petrosa). 10, Anterior tympanopetrosal suture. 11, Anterior tympanosquamosal suture. 12, Anterior external petrosquamosal suture. 13, Arrow points to the foramen for the anterior tympanic artery. 14, Arrow points to the orifice of the canal of Huguier (chorda tympani nerve). 15, Wire enters the tympanum.

5. The anterosuperior edge of the tympanic bone is applied onto the horizontal part of the squama against the tympanic crest. It crosses the horizontal portion of the squama transversely, reaches its internal border, and separates progressively. The tegmen tympani of the petrosa appears in the angle thus formed. It forms a sort of herniation, which is not always readily apparent (*petrosal hernia*).

This superior border forms the Glaserian fissure. Laterally, this is the *anterior tympanosquamosal suture*. It divides to enclose the tegmen tympani. One arm is the *anterior tympanopetrosal suture*, which opposes the posterior tympanopetrosal suture. This is the more medial of the two arms. The other arm, which is more lateral, is the *anterior petrosquamosal suture* (Figs. 14, 15).

In the tympanopetrosal suture, there are two orifices leading into the tympanum. The external orifice is larger and permits the passage of an artery (*anterior tympanic artery*) and a ligament (*anterior mallear ligament*). The smaller internal orifice is the *canal of Huguier*, which transmits the chorda tympani nerve (Figs. 14, 16).

6. Medially, the anterosuperior edge of the tympanic bone leads to the internal extremity of this bone. This internal edge is free only in its superior part. It is adherent below to the petrosa and styloid, and forms the internal extremity of the *posterior tympanopetrosal suture*. The free part of this internal border of the tympanic bone corresponds to the anterior slope of the gutter formed by this bone. The adherent part of this same border appears as an inferior prolongation of the tympanic bone (Fig. 17).

7. The inferior prolongation ends below by a free edge—the inferior edge of the tympanic bone. It presents

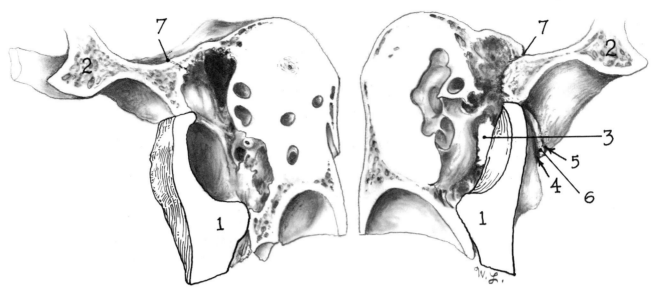

Figure 15.   Vertical section of an adult temporal bone. The petrosal tympanic roof is thin. The lateral wall of the protympanum is constituted by the tympanic plate of the tympanic portion of the temporal bone. Its upper edge is separated from the squamosa by a thin piece of the petrosa—the tegmen tympani, which projects through the petrotympanic fissure as the intertympanosquamosal crest. 1, Tympanic bone. 2, Squamosa. 3, Tubal isthmus. 4, Glaserian or petrotympanic fissure. 5, Anterior external petrosquamosal suture. 6, Intertympanosquamosal crest or crista tegmentalis of the petrosa. 7, Internal petrosquamosal suture.

a large expansion in its mid portion, the *vaginal process*, which partly sheathes the styloid process.

In viewing the tympanic bone as a whole (Figs. 11, 12, 13) it is compared to a curtain whose narrow superior border crosses the horizontal portion of the squama (perpendicular to its great axis), later placing itself almost parallel to its internal border.

The inferior part of this curtain (inferior prolongation of the tympanic bone) is largely adherent and gives rise exter-

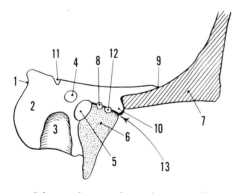

Figure 16.   Schema of a vertical cut of a temporal bone at the level of the vertical carotid canal to show the anterior chordal canal (Huguier) (8), the anterior mallear foramen for transmitting the anterior mallear ligament and anterior tympanic artery and veins (12), and the intertympanosquamosal crest (crista tegmentalis of the petrosa) (10). 1, Internal auditory meatus. 2, Petrosa. 3, Carotid canal. 4, Tensor tympani canal. 5, Protympanum. 6, Tympanic bone. 7, Horizontal plate of the squamosa. 9, Internal petrosquamosal suture. 11, Facial hiatus. 13, Glaserian fissure.

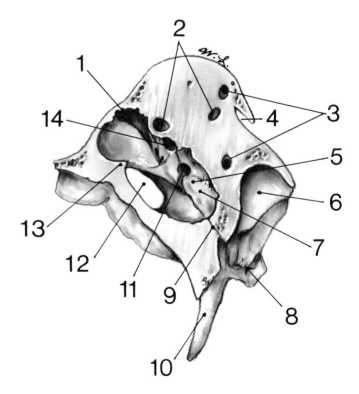

Figure 17.   Vertical cut across the petrosa. 1, Antrum. 2, Horizontal semicircular canal. 3, Posterior semicircular canal. 4, Slit for saccus endolymphaticus. 5, Styloid eminence and subiculum. 6, Jugular dome. 7, Styloid complex giving off the fustis. 8, Stylomastoid foramen. 9, Petrotympanic suture. 10, Styloid process. 11, Sinus tympani. 12, External auditory canal. 13, Scutum. 14, Facial canal.

nally to a well-developed bony process, which transforms the external part of the tympanic bone into a gutter. This bony process is the posterior slope of the tympanic gutter. The free part of this curtain covers a portion of the external auditory canal and middle ear.

Intracranial Surface of the Temporal Bone

The intracranial surface of the petrosal portion of the temporal bone forms a portion of the bony floor of the middle cranial fossa (Fig. 7). This surface is directed diagonally and slopes anteriorly and downward. A vertical portion of the petrosa also helps in the formation of the anterior wall of the posterior fossa. This wall slopes anteromedially.

Laterally, one can distinguish an oblique groove directed anteriorly, which marks the junction of the medially positioned petrosa with the laterally placed squamosal portion of the temporal bone. This groove is the *internal petrosquamosal suture.*

Squamosa

The squamosa is irregularly concave due to the adjacent cerebral convolutions. Its vertical portion is large and flat. Its horizontal portion is smaller and has a triangular form that is thickest in its midportion, fading out quickly as it extends posteriorly. On the intracranial surface, one can see grooves for the middle meningeal artery and its branches. It is easily traced laterally from the foramen spinosum.

The squamosa has a large, flat dentate border that articulates anteriorly with the great wing of the sphenoid bone and superiorly and posteriorly with the inferior border of the parietal bone.

Petrosa

Superior Edge

It is oblique in a posterior and external direction. Near the petrosal apex, it is indented by the passage of the large trigeminal nerve. Along the superior edge extending posteriorly and externally is found the *groove of the superior petrosal sinus.* In the midportion of this edge, and usually a little below it, is found an irregular depression that is the vestige of a very large excavation in the newborn called the *subarcuate fossa* (Fig. 18). The external portion of this edge becomes more pronounced, and often overhangs the underlying bony surface.

Anterior and Posterior Intracranial Surfaces

1. The anterior intracranial surface increases from within outwards and looks forward and upward. Medially,

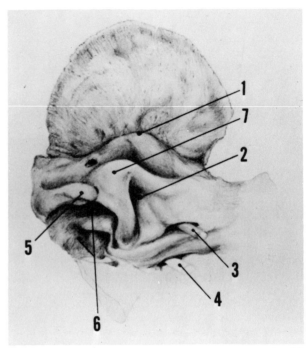

Figure 18.   Six-month-old fetus, showing the posterior and middle fossa aspects of the temporal bone. Note the petrosquamosal suture, where the petrosa and squamosa meet. 1, Petrosquamosal suture. 2, Subarcuate fossa. 3, Auditory nerve. 4, Hypoglossal nerve. 5, Posterior semicircular canal. 6, Posterior lacerated foramen. 7, Superior semicircular canal.

near the apex, it presents a depression corresponding to the Gasserian (trigeminal or semilunar) ganglion—*Meckel's cave.* Lateral to this depression, there are two small, slit-like orifices—the *Fallopian hiatus* above and the *accessory hiatus* below. Further laterally can be seen the *arcuate eminence,* which varies in shape and size (see Fig. 2).

2. The posterior intracranial surface is almost vertical and expands laterally. At about the junction of its inner third and outer two thirds is found the orifice of the *internal auditory canal,* with a length of 6 to 9 mm. Laterally and above the orifice of the canal lies the vestige of the subarcuate fossa (see Fig. 7).

External to the internal auditory canal is the site of origin of a narrow canal called the *vestibular aqueduct.* Its orifice, usually in the form of a cleft, has a very variable configuration. Immediately lateral to the cleft is a variable-sized depression called the *unguinal (L-finger nail) fossa.* This orifice, generally situated at the level of the midportion of the posterior surface of the petrosa, varies in its position relative to the internal auditory meatus and *sigmoid sinus groove* (see Fig. 7). This groove is variable and may be absent. It is grooved to carry the lateral, or transverse, sinus. Medially, at the posterior surface of the petrous apex and running inferiorly is the small groove of the *inferior petrosal sinus.*

Anterior, Posterior, and External Edges

The intracranial surface of the petrosa borders anteriorly with the sphenoid, posteriorly with the occipital, and externally with the parietal bones.

1. The anterior border presents medially (see Figs. 2, 7) a large irregular orifice inferiorly and externally—*the anterior orifice of the carotid canal.* The circumference of this orifice is usually incomplete laterally, because the anterior wall of the carotid canal is lacking for a variable distance. This breach, which drops in to the carotid canal, corresponds to the anterointernal part of the anterosuperior wall of the petrosa.

The superior segment of this anterior orifice of the carotid canal is short and smooth. The internal carotid artery is deflected against it to become vertical, and to enter the cranial cavity. This cranial orifice, partially formed by this superior segment of the anterior orifice of carotid canal,is completed medially, anteriorly, and laterally by the sphenoid bone.

The cavernous sinus groove on the body of the sphenoid bone is prolonged posteriorly and laterally by a thin lamella of bone called the *lingula.* This does not normally reach the petrosa. The lingula lies at the junction of the body and great wing of the sphenoid. Almost all of the anterior edge of the lingula is in contact with the great wing of the sphenoid. Between it and the great wing lies an irregular, narrow cleft that enlarges medially—the *anterior lacerated foramen.* Lateral to the foramen lacerum, the edges of the petrosa and the squamosa form an acute angle in which is lodged the posterior extremity of the great wing of the sphenoid.

2. The posterior edge of the petrosa is much more extensive than the anterior edge. It articulates, in its medial portion, with the body of the occipital bone. Lateral to this suture is a large opening—the *jugular foramen*—which together with a corresponding foramen of the occipital bone forms a *posterior lacerated foramen* (Figs. 19, 20).

This jugular foramen is divided by a spine—the *jugular spine*—into two parts: the posterior part is venous and receives the lower end of the lateral or sigmoid sinus, the anterior part permits passage for the IX to XI cranial nerves. (Fig. 21). In this anterior compartment is a small crater-like fossa—the *pyramidal fossa,*—at the bottom of which is found the small opening of the *cochlear aqueduct* (Fig. 4). This lies 4 to 7 mm below the lateral lip of the internal auditory meatus.

Anteriorly, the jugular foramen receives the termination of the groove for the inferior petrosal sinus. At this level, one may find a small spine separating the inferior petrosal sinus from the rest of the jugular foramen. Thus, the posterior-lacerated foramen is divided into three parts (see Fig. 21):

1. A larger posterior part for the lateral sinus.
2. A smaller anterior part for the inferior petrosal sinus.
3. A middle compartment for the IX to XI cranial nerves.

External to the jugular foramen, the posterior border of the

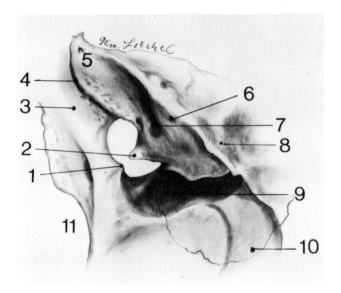

Figure 19.   Superior view of posterior lacerated foramen. 1, Jugular spine of occipital bone. 2, Jugular spine of temporal bone. 3, Basilar process. 4, Groove for inferior petrosal sinus. 5, Petrosal tip. 6, Orifice of petromastoid canal. 7, Orifice of internal auditory canal. 8, Groove of superior petrosal sinus. 9, Groove for sigmoid sinus. 10, Groove for lateral sinus. 11, Foramen magnum.

petrosa presents a rough surface called the *jugular facette* (see Fig. 4), which articulates with the prominent jugular process of the occipital bone. If the jugular facette is large, the inferior part of the lateral sinus passes entirely on the superior surface of the jugular process of the occipital bone. If, however, the surface of this facette is small, the groove of the lateral sinus in its terminal segment will include part of the petrosa. The remainder of the posterior edge of the petrosa is large, dentated, and strongly convex, with a portion horizontal at first and then vertical. It articulates with a corresponding notch of the occipital bone.

3. The external edge of the petrosa is very rough. Anteriorly, this edge and the free edge of the squama form a deep incisura that articulates with the parietal bone (*the parietal incisura*); (see Fig. 7). Posteriorly, the external edge turns downward as the edge of the posterior border of the petrosa. This is the posterior angle of the petrosa. At this point, three bones make contact: the temporal, parietal, and occipital bones.

Petrous Apex

The free edge of the squama forms two incisuras with that of the petrous, one is anterior (sphenoidal) and the other is posterior (parietal) (see Fig. 7). The posterior and anterior edges of the petrosa converge medially to form the petrous apex. This apex reaches the junction of the occipital bone and the body of the spenoid bone.

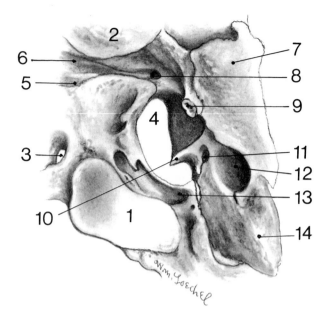

Figure 20. Inferior view of posterior lacerated foramen. 1, Occipital condyle. 2, mastoid tip. 3, Posterior condylar canal. 4, Jugular foramen. 5, Groove for occipital artery. 6, Digastric groove. 7, Anterior wall of external auditory canal and vaginal process. 8, Stylomastoid foramen. 9, Styloid process. 10, Jugular spine of temporal bone. 11, Orifice of Jacobson's canal. 12, Carotid canal. 13, Anterior condyloid foramen. 14, Petrous apex.

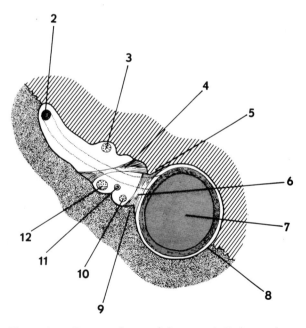

Figure 21. Posterior lacerated foramen. 1, Endocranial view—right side schematic. The temporal bone is indicated by diagonal lines, and the occipital bone by dots. 2, Inferior petrosal sinus. 3, Glossopharyngeal nerve. 4, Jugular ligament. 5, Jugular spine of temporal bone. 6, Jugular ligament. 7, Internal jugular vein. 8, Foramen jugulare. 9, Jugular spine of occipital bone. 10, Spinal accessory nerve. 11, Posterior meningeal artery. 12, Vagus nerve.

Inferior Surface of the Temporal Bone

On viewing the inferior surface of the temporal bone, (see Fig. 4), one sees the squama externally and anteriorly, the petrosa medially and posteriorly, the tympanic bone between the two, and the styloid bone between the tympanic bone and the petrosa.

Squamosa

The squamosa is limited to the anterior segment of its horizontal portion (mandibular fossa, condyle, and subtemporal plane). The large, serrated free edge limits it in front and develops at the expense of its extracranial surface.

A small part of the vertical portion of the squama can be seen anteriorly and externally from the horizontal portion. Posteriorly, the inferior view of the squama in the intact temporal bone is limited by the supramastoid crest—the posterior prolongation of the zygoma.

Tympanic Bone

Its inferior edge and the vaginal process are seen, as well as the half-cover that this process forms with the styloid process. Internally and externally, one sees the two extremities of the tympanic bone from the orifice of the external auditory meatus to the isthmus of the eustachian tube.

Petrosa

This inferior view exposes a series of morphologic structures that we have not yet had the occasion to observe.

Externally lies the tip of the mastoid process and its internal surface. On this surface, lies a variable-shaped groove that is unusually well marked—the *digastric groove*. The posterior extremity of this groove frequently appears on a lateral or external view of the temporal bone, and it can be palpated on a live patient.

Behind and medial to the digastric groove is a small *vascular groove for the occipital artery.*

The stylomastoid foramen is always readily identifiable. The digastric groove points to its position. It is the termination of the *facial canal (Fallopian aqueduct)*, which transmits the facial nerve.

One often finds in front of and external to the stylomastoid foramen a small orifice through which passes the chorda tympani nerve—the *posterior canal of the chorda tympani.* If it is not seen in this location, one will find it at a higher level in the anterior wall of the facial canal.

The *styloid process* is encountered medially and a little forward. The styloid is not of temporal origin. It is derived from Reichert's cartilage of the second branchial arch. It does extend into the temporal bone, making up the posterior wall of the tympanum as high as the fossa incudis. It separates the bony labyrinth from the tympanic bone. The facial nerve is the nerve of the second branchial arch, and extends along the posteromedial aspect of the styloid complex in the facial canal to emerge at the stylomastoid foramen.

Behind the styloid process lies the *jugular facet* (jugum petrosum, facette jugulaire), which continues for 1 cm or so posteriorly and externally to the posterior edge of the petrosa.

Immediately medial to the jugular facet appears the *jugular fossa*. Its size varies considerably, depending on the size of the transverse sinus. The size may vary considerably from side to side. The posterior border of this fossa forms the anterior wall of the jugular foramen. The jugular fossa is clearly outlined externally when the jugular facet is large and well developed. On the contrary, when the jugular facet is small, the jugular fossa includes a part of the lateral sinus groove.

In the interior of the jugular fossa and on its external or anteroexterior wall, one finds a small foramen through which passes the auricular branch of the vagus nerve (*Arnold's nerve*).

The jugular fossa is a venous depression for the *jugular bulb*. In front of it and medially is found the inferior orifice of a large anterior canal called the *carotid canal*. This orifice and the initial part of this canal are immediately behind and medial to the tympanic bone. On the anteroexternal wall of the initial portion of this canal are usually found several small foramina for passage of the *caroticotympanic vessels and nerves* into the tympanum. It may be one large foramen and, on occasion, a large dehiscence, so that the carotid artery may be exposed on the medial wall of the anterior tympanum. It may also be the route for air to pass into the cranial cavity (air embolism) when air is forcefully blown up the eustachian tube.

Behind the inferior orifice of the carotid canal and medial to the jugular dome, we again find the anterior nerves (IX to XI) containing part of the jugular foramen within the corresponding *pyramidal fossa* (see Fig. 19). This fossa is especially well seen from the intracranial surface of the petrosa.

Between the jugular fossa and the carotid canal lies the inferior orifice of *Jacobson's canal* (see Fig. 20) for passage of the inferior tympanic nerve, which is a branch of the glossopharyngeal nerve. This canal is not always easy to find, because its position varies according to its relation to the carotid canal and jugular fossa. The carotid canal and jugular fossa are in close proximity. They are separated by a prominent crest that is either blunt or sharp. The inferior orifice of Jacobson's canal varies in position:

1. On the crest separating canal and fossa.
2. On the jugular slope of the crest.
3. On the carotid slope of the crest.

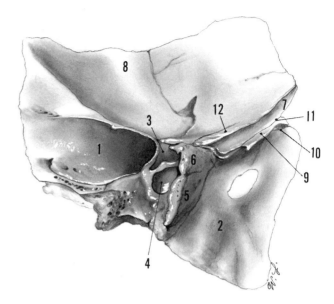

Figure 22.   Left adult temporal bone. Inferior view showing details of the Glaserian fissure and tubal isthmus. Note how the petrosal shelf (9) goes laterally between the squama (7) and tympanic bone (2) to form the Glaserian fissure (10). The upper part of the double-armed fissure goes into the cranial cavity as the anterior internal petrosquamosal suture (11). The lower arm goes into the tympanum (10) and transmits the anterior tympanic vessels, chorda tympani nerve, and anterior mallear ligament. At the isthmus of the eustachian tube, the bone walls are made entirely from the petrosa (lateral wall—downward projection) from the tegmen (6) and upward projection from the carotid wall (5). 1, Carotid canal. 2, Vaginal plate of the tympanic bone. 3, Semicanal for tensor tympani muscle. 4, Isthmus of bony eustachian tube. 5, Petrosa forming the inferior shelf of the lateral wall of the bony eustachian tube isthmus. 6, Petrosa forming the superior shelf of the lateral wall of the bony eustachian tube isthmus. 7, Lower edge of the vertical segment of the squamosa. 8, Petrosal middle fossa. 9, Petrosal hernia or shelf. 10, Glaserian fissure. 11, Anterior petrosquamosal suture. 12, Anterior internal petrosquamosal suture.

4. A little behind the point where the canal and fossa are closest together.
5. On the large zone interposed between canal and fossa when present.

The inferior aspect of the petrosa is very rough, especially posterior. Its anterior part is directed forward and forms the bed for the cartilaginous portion of the eustachian tube (*sulcus tubaris*).

The tympanic bone, in its internal part, forms the anterolateral wall of the bony eustachian tube; by the free part of its internal edge, it constitutes the anterior periphery of the bony tubal orifice as it emerges from the base of the skull (Fig. 22).

This tubal orifice is completed behind and above by the petrosa (See Fig. 22). Posteriorly, the petrosa may present a little crest that appears to prolong the free edge of the tympanic bone. Above, one sees a lamina detaching from the petrosa, which extends forward and continues with the herniation of the tegmen tympani (see Fig. 22). This lamina, whose free edge completes the tubal orifice circumference, is the *tegmen tympani*. It extends along the entire length of the petrosa and forms, in its anterior part, this herniation of the petrosa into the interval between the squama and the tympanic bone (see Fig. 16).

Above the protympanum, in the interval betwen the petrosa and squama and under the tegmen tympani, we have another bony canal running parallel to it—the *canal for the tensor tympani muscle*.

The smooth bony surface of the petrosa in contact with the cartilaginous portion of the eustachian tube (sulcus tubaris) is separated from the carotid canal, lying immediately posterior to it, by a roughened bone. Adjacent to the orifice of the eustachian tube, this bone is thickened to afford the site of origin of the levator veli palatini muscle. From the inferior carotid orifice to the petrous apex, the petrosa underlies the horizontal segment of the carotid canal.

The most distant portion of the internal segment of the petrosa presents thick, deep suture lines between the temporal and occipital bones.

The *groove of the inferior petrosal sinus* is seen behind the very rough bone on the inferior aspect of the petrous apex (see Fig. 19). It leads extracranially to the jugular at its anterior limit. It disappears towards the internal part of the petrosa. It is best seen from the intracranial aspect of the temporal bone.

The landmarks on the inferior aspect of the petrous tip are not all visible on an articulated skull. One can see only those that appear anterior to the articulation with the occipital bone. As for the groove of the inferior petrosal sinus, it is best seen and studied from the interior of the cranial cavity.

2 Connections of the Four Temporal Bone Constituents

Many previous studies have given us a very imperfect notion of the connections that exist between the four constituents of the temporal bone. On the intact temporal bone, it is difficult to understand the continuity of certain sutures. This very complex bone can be better understood by reconstructing it in space so that we get an exact idea of its constitution and of the relations of different cavities in the temporal bone.

These connections of the petrosa, squama, tympanic bone, and styloid complex can be best studied on examination of sections. To facilitate this study, we will first disarticulate the components of the temporal bone.

Departing from the external view of the temporal bone, we first lift out the tympanic bone, then the squama, and finally the styloid complex. We then have ideal preparations that are impossible to realize in the adult. A concept of design is then made possible after studying sutures in the newborn, the infant, and the adult.

External View of the Temporal Bone After Removal of the Tympanic Bone

On removal of the tympanic bone, we see the zone of contact with the squamosa below the posterior zygomatic tubercle, above the semi canal for the tensor tympani, and anterior to the oval window (see Fig. 8). Also seen are its narrow zone of contact with the squamosa from immediately behind the oval window down to near the point where the chorda tympani leaves the facial nerve (styloid complex). Internally and inferiorly, we see the zone of contact with the petrosa, which is more extensive than the contact with the squamosa. This petrosal zone is notched at the level of the carotid canal. The tympanic bone intervenes at this point in order to complete the anterior wall of the carotid canal.

Anteriorly, the superior border of the tympanic bone is hidden by the petrosal hernia. Beneath, it is adherent to the squama.

Removal of the tympanic bone has thus uncovered parts of the squama and petrosa that have not been seen until now.

Squamosa

The horizontal part of the squama is now visible in its entire extent. One follows its internal border (see Fig. 8) the length of the roof of the auditory canal up to the tympanic crest, behind which it hides before continuing the length of the glenoid cavity.

Removal of the tympanic bone also permits a better understanding of the segment of the retromeatal part of the squamosa that is normally hidden by this tympanic bone.

This infero internal portion of the squama offers a large surface for contact with the tympanic bone, and presents a sulcus for passage of the chorda tympani. A corresponding sulcus is present on the tympanic bone.

This canal can be considered as the persistence, at the level of the chorda tympani, of the posterior tympano-squamosal suture.

Petrosa

The parts of the petrosa beyond the zone of contact with the tympanic bone (see Fig. 8) belong to one of the most important cavities of the temporal bone. This large *middle ear* cavity is visible only on this figure in its internal part. Its external part is still concealed by the squamosa.

The visible part of this middle ear is composed of two parts: one is large and externally placed, representing the greater part of the *tympanum*, the other is narrow and situated internally constituting the bony part of the eustachian tube.

One notes at the level of the tympanum, the projection of the promontory with the *canal of the tensor tympani muscle* above it. This conduit, usually incomplete in the part we see, turns up slightly externally to form the *processus cochleariformis*. Behind and above the promontory,

13

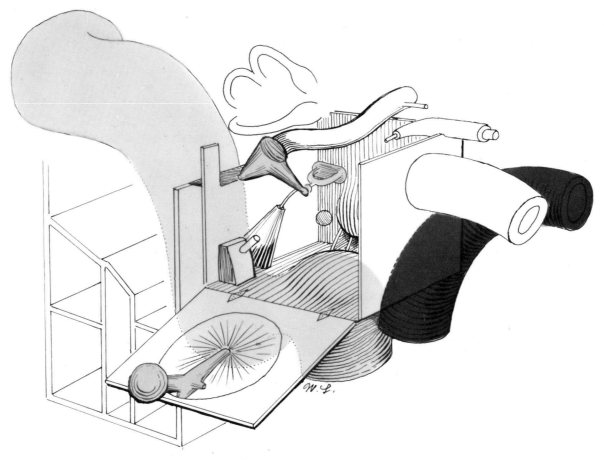

Figure 23.   Schema emphasizing relations of the jugular dome and carotid artery to the hypotympanum.

one sees the greatest part of the *oval window*; behind and below this same projection, one distinguishes the *round window*. On the inferior part of this tympanum exists an inconstant projection (Figs. 7, 23, 24) the jugular dome (Fig. 25). To this vascular prominence is added what is determined by the internal carotid artery and the carotid canal. At times concealed by trabeculae or bony tissue, this prominence occupies the internal part of the tympanum.

The *bony eustachian tube* represents the narrow part by which the middle ear opens internally—at the level of the angle formed by the squama and petrosa (Fig. 22). Its development appears bound to that of the internal carotid artery, which is placed medial to it. Large and very short in the newborn, this eustachian tube stretches out, in proportion to the growth of the internal carotid artery and the carotid canal.

External View of the Temporal Bone After Removal of the Tympanic Bone and Squama

If we remove the squama on the preceding preparation (Fig. 9) we see the zone of contact betwen petrosa and squamosa, and we also uncover the parts of the middle ear hidden until now.

Contact Zone Between Petrosa and Squamosa

Internally, there is above and in front of the petrosal hernia an excavated surface with anterior concavity. It articulates with the internal border of the horizontal part of the squama at the level of glenoid portion of this border. This excavated surface corresponds above to the internal petrosquamosal fissure and below to the anterior petrosquamosal branch of the Glaserian fissure. Therefore, these two fissures are only the visible parts of the same petrosquamosal suture.

More externally, the zone of contact, in general smaller than the preceding one, looks more inferiorly; This is why Figure 8 shows only its anterior border. The latter still corresponds to the internal petrosquamosal fissure (see Fig. 1).

This fissure leads us to the level of the parietal incisura and continues there with the external petrosquamosal fissure.

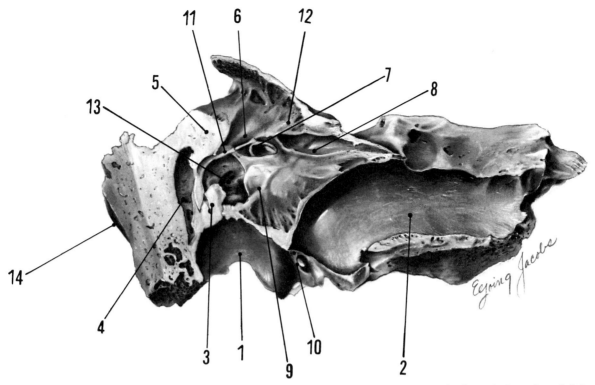

Figure 24. View of medial tympanic wall with high jugular dome and high stylomastoid foramen. 1, Jugular dome. 2, Carotid canal. 3, Lateral tympanic sinus. 4, Third part of facial canal. 5, Posterior buttress. 6, Facial canal (second part). 7, Stapes. 8, Tensor tympani canal. 9, Promontory. 10, Opening of cochlear aqueduct. 11, Ponticulus. 12, Geniculate cells. 13, Subiculum. 14, Lateral sinus groove.

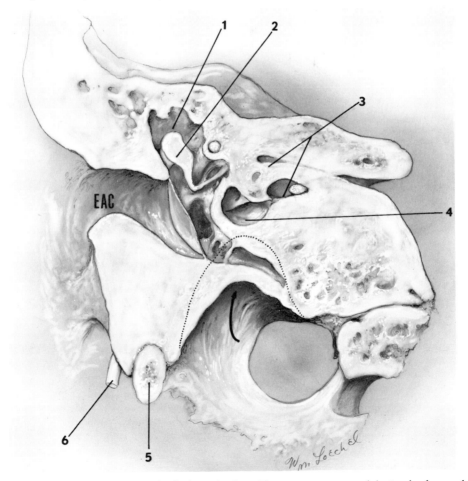

Figure 25. Sagittal cut through a temporal bone with a high jugular fossa. The arrow points toward the jugular dome, which rose 8 mm above the cut edge of the bone. 1, Antrum. 2, Incus. 3, Internal auditory meatus. 4, Cochlea. 5, Styloid process. 6, Emerging facial nerve.

The petrosa, in this external part is in contact with the squamosa by a large surface. It is occupied either by spongy tissue called diploic at the level of the cranial bones, or by cellular bone—pneumatic cavities that invade this diploic tissue secondarily.

Petrosal Antrum

This surface partly encircles a cavity of the middle ear—the *petrosal antrum* (See Fig. 1).

The latter is not visible in its entire extent, its superior segment is hidden by a prolongation of the petrosa protruding from the roof, which proceeds below and forward. It is the *tegmen tympani*, which on the endocranial view of the petrosa (see Fig. 7) corresponds to the anterior segment of the cerebral surface (or anterior endocranial surface) of this bone. Well developed on the greater part of its extent, it ends medially at the level of the orifices of the eustachian tube, and of the canal for the tensor tympani muscle; then it disappears externally at the level of the external part of the petrosa. It corresponds by its anterior border almost entirely to the internal petrosquamosal fissure, and produces the surface by which the petrosa contacts the squamosa at this spot.

The petrosal antrum is joined to the tympanum by a type of narrows called the *aditus ad antrum*. The internal wall of the aditus is elevated by a projection with a smooth surface (See Fig. 9) that corresponds to the underlying *external semicircular canal*.

A more or less marked groove separates this projection from an underlying prominence that is still more important to recognize than the projection of the external semicircular canal. This projection is due to the *facial nerve* contained in a canal—the *Fallopian aqueduct* with external walls that are always thin and sometimes dehiscent.

The facial nerve and the superior portion (in part hidden by the tegmen tympani) of the external semicircular canal belong topographically to the tympanun. The latter is now fully visible. One sees the oval window below the facial nerve, and behind it a conical projection called the *pyramid*. Above, the tegmen always conceals a bit of the tympanum.

If we now examine the whole of this surface by which the petrosa contacts the squama, it appears possible to divide it into two very different portions. The internal one includes a great deal of the tegmen tympani; the external one corresponds to the external part of this tegmen and to all the large external and inferior articular surfaces of the petrosa.

The first reaches the horizontal part of the squama and extends nearly up to the level of the aditus ad antrum.

The second represents the zone of contact of the petrosa with the retromeatal part of the squama. Defined above by the external segment of the internal petrosquamosal fissure, this zone reaches the deep surface of this retromeatal part of the squama; but it is not in contact with it along its entire extent. Between the two bones is insinuated a prolongation of the middle ear—the *petrosal antrum*—which diminishes the surface of this extensive petrosquamosal suture.

The posterior tympanum, derived from the second branchial arch, separates the tympanic bone from the petrosa at the level of the stylomastoid foramen up to the fossa incudis—the *styloid complex*. This includes the descending facial canal with its contained facial nerve.

Sutures

The junction of the petrosal and squamosal portions of the temporal bone has important relationships of interest to the otologist. The resultant suture extends from the Glaserian fissure across the top of the middle ear cleft into the mastoid portion of the temporal bone. It may permit quick passage of infection from the middle ear to the middle cranial fossa. The petrosa may override the squama, forcing it down into the tympanum, where it could cause malleus fixation and a conductive-type hearing loss.

In the mastoid, the suture is identifiable on the surface; but in the interior, it is represented by the petrosquamosal lamina. The deeper portion in the petrosal portion of the mastoid may be easily overlooked in mastoid surgery, and may lead to facial nerve injury.

The Petrosquamosal Suture

In the course of development of the temporal bone, the two larger components—the petrosa and the squama—embrace the first branchial pouch and cleft. The third component of the temporal bone—the tympanic bone—develops around the closing membrane (tympanic membrane), dividing branchial pouch (eustachian tube, middle ear, and ultimate mastoid air cell system) and branchial cleft (external auditory canal). The fourth component is the styloid complex, which develops from Reichert's cartilage.

The petrosa originates from cartilage. The ultimate osseous capsule surrounding the inner ear structures arises from 14 ossification centers beginning at about the 16th week of intrauterine life, when the inner ear has attained its adult dimensions. By the 23rd week, all centers have fused to form a complete bony capsule in which "suture lines" have been obliterated.[1] The styloid complex also originates from cartilage (Reichert's cartilage).

The squamous and tympanic parts of the temporal bone develop in membrane. The squama is formed from one center of ossification, which appears in the eighth week. The center for the tympanic part appears from the 9th to 10th fetal week.

Upon examining the the interior of the skull in a newborn, one can discern the petrosquamosal suture lying externally in the middle cranial fossa (see Fig.18). It points anteromedially. It is where the thin edge of the overlapping tegmen contacts the underlying projection from the

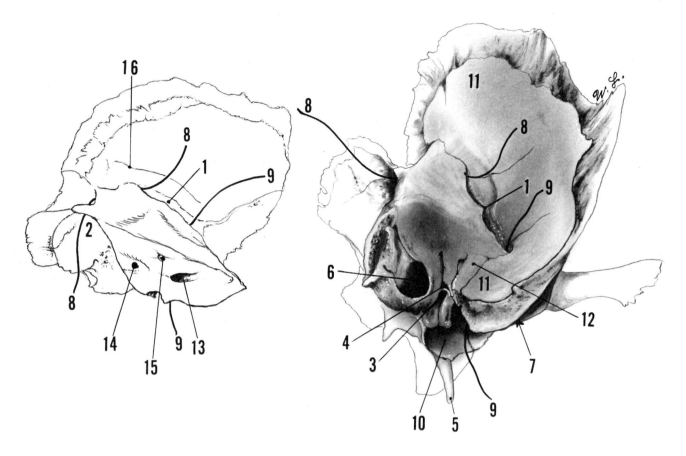

Figure 26. Adult temporal bone, showing details and relations of the internal petrosquamosal groove. 1, The petrosquamosal sinus. The sinus communicates posteriorly with the sigmoid sinus (8); anteriorly, it is in communication with the deep temporal veins after passing through the Glaserian fissure (9). 2, Sigmoid sinus groove. 3, Eustachian tube. 4, Tensor tympani canal. 5, Styloid process. 6, Carotid canal. 7, Mandibular fossa. 10, Vaginal plate. 11, Squama. 12, Petrosa. 13, Internal auditory meatus. 14, Unguinal fossa. 15, Subarcuate fossa. 16, Groove for middle meningeal artery.

squama to form the roof of the eustachian tube, the attic, and the antrum (Figs. 27-29).

Under the free edge of the tegmen, (Figs. 27-29) a portion of the dura mater extends, sometimes containing persistent remnants of the *petrosquamosal sinus of Lushka* (Fig. 26). This sinus is a venous channel affording communication between the veins of meninges and those of the middle ear. These veins emerge at an opening in front of the meatus. In the fetus, it carries away most of the blood from the brain via numerous meningeal tributaries before development of the jugular and vertebral venous systems.

In infancy and early childhood, the petrosquamosal sinus is sometimes seen grooving and canalizing the bone in the immediate course of the suture and lying partly under the overlapping tegmen.

This sinus is important clinically, since it maintains a connection between the middle ear and meninges. This is especially true in infancy, when the suture is wide and unclosed. Meningitis may develop during an attack of otitis media without perforation of the tympanic membrane.

The petrosquamosal sinus (see Fig. 26) is not constant and is extremely variable in its course. When present, it

more commonly lies in a sulcus in the middle cranial fossa between the petrosal tegmen and the squama, and empties into the sigmoid sinus (Fig. 30) near its juncture with the transverse sinus at a point below and external to the superior petrosal sinus by a valve-like opening. It passes under a bridge of bone in doing so. At other times, it communicates anteriorly, passing through near the most external part of the Glaserian fissure. Its foramen of exit lies between the mandibular fossa and the external auditory meatus. It empties into the deep temporal vein.[1]

The external opening of the petrosquamosal sinus (see Fig. 14) is usually obliterated by six months of age, but its remains may often be seen in the usual position in front of the external auditory meatus and just external to the Glaserian fissure.[1,7] Sometimes a fine groove may be seen running outwards in the glenoid cavity, the zygomatic process, or the base of the zygoma—or it may even be bridged over by the junction of the postglenoid tubercle with the bony meatus. These veins drain the tympanum, the meninges, and even the overlying temporosphenoidal lobe of the brain.

The petrosquamosal sinus is of clinical significance,

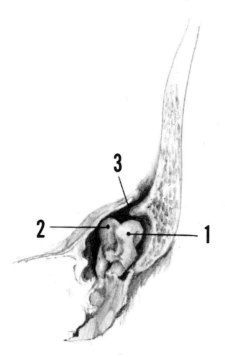

Figure 27. Frontal section through the left temporal bone of a six-month-old fetus. Note the overlap of the petrous tegmen over the squamous tegmen. The latter may fix the malleus head. 1, Malleus. 2, Incus. 3, Petrosquamosal suture.

since infection from the middle ear can spread to the cranial cavity without macroscopic erosion of bone. Retrograde septic thrombosis from the middle ear to the cranial cavity can also occur by way of the internal auditory vein, the veins of the aqueduct to the inferior petrosal sinus, and the mastoid emissary vein to the sigmoid sinus.

A branch from the middle meningeal artery passes through the petrosquamosal suture and into the tympanum as the *superior tympanic artery.*[8]

Politzer[9] pointed out that the tegmen tympani above the malleus head is usually 5 to 6 mm thick, and contains many small cellular spaces (Fig. 31). In other cases, it is extremely thin and may present one or more irregular dehiscences, or it may be defective for a considerable distance. Politzer[9] thought this was due to an arrest in development or atrophy, and also observed that these dehiscences are closed by a thin membrane in which long osseous spines that have a sagittal direction are sometimes enclosed. This may represent widening of the middle ear cleft, with lateral movement of the tympanic ring and squama as the middle ear becomes pneumatized.[5]

Anson and Bast,[10] in an exhaustive study of fetal and infant temporal bones, found masses of residual cartilages in seven different regions:

1. Fissula ante fenestram.
2. Fossula poste fenestram.
3. The posteroinferior portion of the cochlear capsule or infracochlear region.

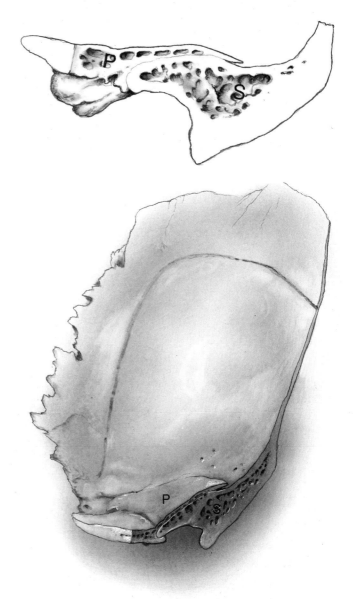

Figures 28, 29. The petrosal tegmen. *P* overrides the horizontal portion of the squama. *S*, leaving a distinct suture, is seen in this seven-month-old fetus.

4. Basal portion of the styloid process.
5. The petrosquamosal suture and in the capsule, beneath the suture.
6. The canalicular region.
7. The region of the cochlear (round) window.

This would tend to indicate that the petrosquamosal suture plays an important role in the development of the temporal bone.

The inferior portion of the squama widens to form its horizontal portion, which extends from the anterior edge of the temporomandibular joint to the base of the petrosa, ending at the angle of the *parieto-squamo-mastoid suture.*

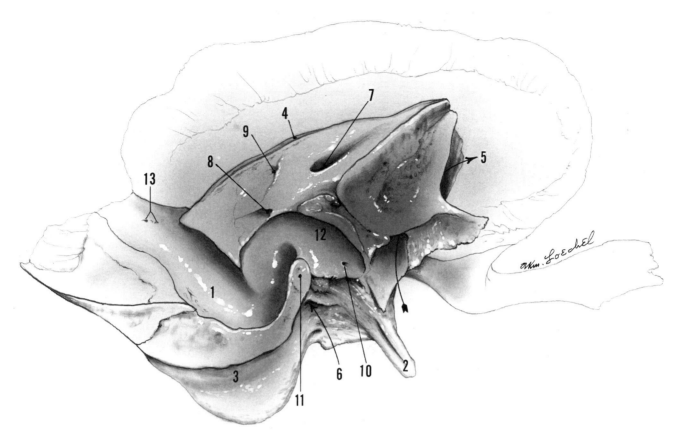

Figure 30.   Intracranial view of an adult temporal bone looking laterally from an inferior aspect. This shows point where the petrosquamosal sinus enters the sigmoid sinus (13). 1, Sigmoid sinus groove. 2, Styloid process. 3, Digastric groove. 4, Superior petrosal sinus groove. 5, Arrow emerging from the carotid canal. 6, Arrow pointing to the stylomastoid foramen. 7, Internal auditory meatus. 8, Unguinal fossa (orifice of vestibular aqueduct). 9, Subarcuate fossa. 10, Canal for Arnold's nerve. 11, Jugular facette. 12, Jugular fossa.

The horizontal portion of the squama can be divided into three segments:

1. The anterior or temporomandibular segment. This forms the roof of the temporomandibular joint.
2. The middle or tympanic segment, which forms the roof of the external auditory canal and the external half of the attic.
3. The posterior or mastoid segment, which overlays a great part of the base of the petrous bone.

The internal or intracranial lamina of the squama (the tympanosquamosal lamina) extends medially above the tympanum to join an identical lamina, which arises from the external edge of the petrous bone (the petrotympanic lamina). These two laminae form the roof of the middle ear. At first, these laminae are not in contact; through the fissure between them, they pass connective tissue and vessels from tympanum to dura. The suture is usually closed by one year of age, but dehiscenses often remain.

The tympanosquamosal lamina (*squamosal tegmen*) may grow excessively and be deflected beneath the petrotympanic lamina (*petrosal tegmen*). It can extend inferiorly

to engage the head of the malleus and prevent its normal vibration in response to sound waves transmitted from the tympanic membranne (see Fig. 31).

If one examines the intracranial surface of the petrosa in the middle fossa of an adult skull, an oblique groove can be detected that runs anteriorly and medially. This is the *internal petrosquamosal suture* (see Fig. 26). It has an anterior segment corresponding to the temporomandibular portion of the squama.

The *anterior petrosquamosal suture* is best studied in a vertical cut through the temporal bone just anterior to the sulcus tympanicus (see Figs. 15, 16, 22). The *intertympanosquamosal crest* of the petrosa or *crista tegmentalis* can be seen to form a small portion of the anterior tegmen. It is an extension of the petrotympanic lamina, which divides the Glaserian fissure into two fissures in its posterior half (Figs. 15, 16, 22). Its inferior surface limits the canal for the tensor tympani muscle above. The anterior tegmen tympani, along with the anteromedial surface of the intertympanosquamosal crest, forms a concave surface that articulates with the internal surface of the horizontal part of the squama. This suture appears in the interior of

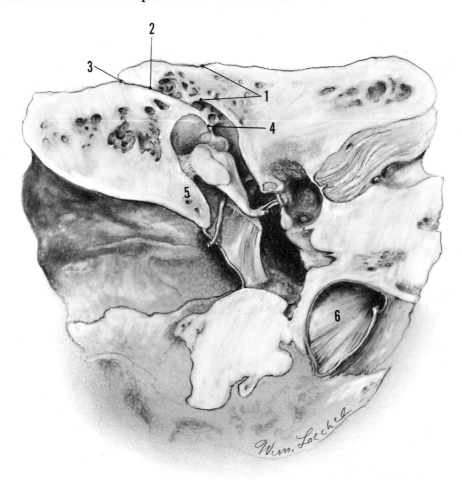

Figure 31. Frontal section of the left adult temporal bone looking anteriorly. 1, Thick tympanic roof. 2, The direction of the petrosquamosal suture. 3, Fixation of the malleus head by the squamosal tegmen (4). 5, Scutum. 6, Jugular dome.

the cranium as the internal petrosquamosal suture. This suture appears externally as the anterosuperior arm of the Glaserian fissure. This should be termed the *external anterior petrosquamosal fissure*, as suggested by Bellocq.[11] It does not lead into the eustachian tube, but rather into the cranial cavity. The fissure appearing below the intertympano squamosal crest of the petrosa is the true Glaserian fissure, which leads from the tympanum to the glenoid fossa.

The term external petrosquamosal suture is also applied to the suture between the *squamomastoid ala* and the base of the petrosa. A more descriptive name would be *external posterior petrosquamosal suture* (see Fig. 26).

On the posterior portion of the bony eustachian tube (*protympanum*), we find that the walls of the eustachian tube are made up of:

1. The superior portion of the petrosa.
2. The internal edge of the temporomandibular segment of the base of the squamous bone.
3. The superior part of the anterior half of the tympanic bone.

As we approach the isthmus of the eustachian tube, we find sudden dramatic changes. The anterior protympanum becomes completely intrapetrous by the interposition of two lamina, which join on the external side of the eustachian tube (see Fig. 22). One lamina descends from the superior edge of the petrous bone; and the other lamina ascends from the carotid canal, separating the tubal lumen from the tympanic and squamosal bones. The Glaserian fissure transmits the anterior tympanic artery and veins and the anterior mallear (sphenomandibular) ligament. This fissure may be a route for the spread of infection from the anterior tympanum to the extracranial aspect of the base of the skull (infratemporal fossa).

The *anterior tympanopetrosal suture* is located between the superior border of the tympanic bone and the crista tegmentalis of the petrosa. It corresponds to the posterior branch of the Glaserian fissure.

Internally, at the eustachian tube level, the tympanic bone applies its anterior surface against the posterior surface of the crista tegmentalis. The superior border of the tympanic bone ascends posterior to the crista tegmentalis,

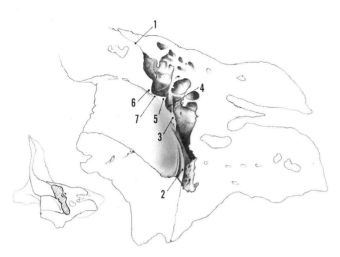

Figure 32. Vertical section of the left adult temporal bone showing details as one approaches the Glaserian fissure anteriorly. 1, Internal petrosquamosal suture. 2, Sulcus tympanicus. 3, Tympanic crest of Gruber. 4, Mallear groove. 5, Anterior tympanic spine of Henle. 6, Posterior tympanic spine of Henle. 7, Crista spinarum.

and may reach as far as the canal of the tensor tympani without contributing to any portion of this wall.

The tympanic surface of the tympanic bone is smooth, but at the level of the Glaserian fissure, it has a groove (*sulcus mallearis* or *mallear groove*) along which the anterior mallear ligament passes. The upper ridge of this groove is called the *crista spinarum* (Henle)or *mallear crest* (Bellocq),[11] and the lower ridge of the groove is called the *tympanic crest of Gruber* (Fig. 32). The anterior end of the crista spinarum is prominent and is termed the *anterior tympanic spine of Henle.* The posterior end of the crista spinarum is referred to as the posterior tympanic spine.

External to the mallear crest, the superior border of the tympanic bone curves inward until a portion of the anterior surface of the tympanic bone is seen in the tympanum. It is covered externally by the squama.

The tegmen tympani over the protympanum dips down to contact the upper border of the tympanic bone. At times, the bones do not meet completely, instead, there is a cleft of variable length extending the Glaserian fissure. As the inferior projection of the tegmen tympani approaches the isthmus of the bony eustachian tube (protympanum), it gradually displaces the tympanic bone laterally and, instead, contacts the upward projection from the petrosa of the carotid canal to completely surround the bony eustachian isthmus with petrosal bone (see Fig. 22).

The tegmen tympani at the level of the mallear crest may contact the crista spinarum so that there is an enclosed mallear gutter, as well as a parallel groove external to the point of contact. The mallear gutter is always present. It transmits the tympanic artery and veins, the anterior mallear ligament, and the chorda tympani nerve.

The corda tympani nerve does not follow the entire course through the mallear groove, but, instead, im-

mediately upon entering the groove, it leaves and extends obliquely downward and inward, crossing between the downward prolongation of the tegmen tympani and the upper border of the tympanic bone. Thus, the canal containing the chorda tympani nerve is made up of two semi grooves—the petrosal and tympanic. The posterior orifice of this canal is the *canal of the chorda tympani* or *canal of Huguier*. Running parallel to the inferior margin of the tegmen, it emerges by a small opening on the anterior surface of the tympanic bone. At times, the anterior canal of the chorda tympani extends deep into the inferior prolongation of the tegmen tympani (Bellocq).

External posterior Petrosquamosal Suture

This suture (see Fig. 26) is large and represents the contact of the deep aspect of the retromeatal portion of the squama with the petrosa. It ends posteriorly at the parietal incisura, where it meets the posterior termination of the internal petrosquamosal suture (see Figs. 18, 26). It appears externally on the surface of the mastoid process as the external petrosquamosal suture. Anteriorly, it extends under the tympanic bone. It then extends posteriorly on the floor of the aditus ad antrum, and then onto the inferior and posterior walls of the petrosal antrum. It then meets again at the level of the superior wall of this antrum with the inferior part of the suture between the tegmen tympani and squama. This suture is difficult to observe. Its study requires examination of the temporal bones in the newborn —in infants as well as adults.

The external lamina of the squama is extracranial and overlays the external aspect of the temporal bone. It can be divided into three segments: the temporomandibular segment (which we have already discussed), the tympanic segment, and the mastoid segment.

At the level of the tympanic segment, the extracranial lamina of the base of the squama folds back on itself, following the direction of the intracranial lamina. Thus, the two laminae join to form the roof of the external auditory canal. In the depth of the meatus, the two laminae again separate; the intracranial continues above the attic as far as the internal petrosquamosal fissure, while the extracranial curves inferiorly to form the external wall of the attic (scutum of Leidy) (Figs. 31, 33).

At the level of the mastoid segment, the extracranial lamina of the base of the squama descends vertically on the largest part of the external surface of the base of the petrous bone, forming a wide, long bony plaque (the *squamomastoid ala*) (Figs. 34, 35). Between this squamosal lamina and the petrous surface, which it covers, is found a wide fissure that opens externally on the mastoid as well as internally at the level of the antrum—the *external petrosquamosal fissure* (posterolateral petrosquamosal fissure) (see Fig. 35). Usually, this fissure also closes, but it may persist in part with connective tissue and vessels of the

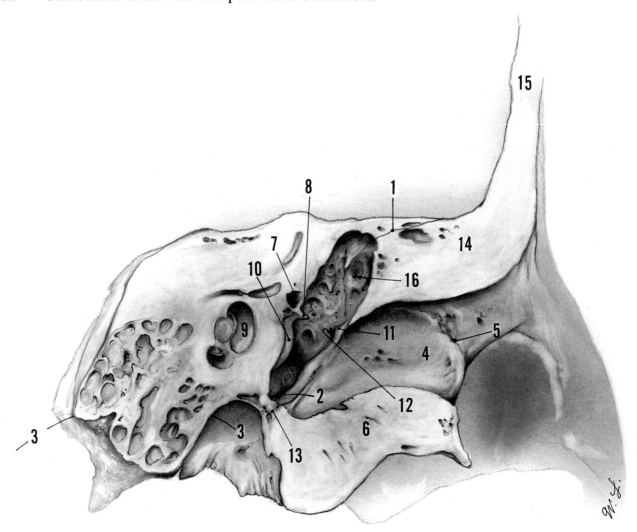

Figure 33. Frontal view of the right adult temporal bone looking anteriorly. The mallear foramen transmits the anterior mallear ligament and anterior tympanic blood vessels. 1, Petrosquamosal suture. 2, Eustachian tube isthmus. 3, Carotid canal. 4, External auditory meatus. 5, Anterior tympanosquamosal suture. 6, Tympanic bone. 7, Facial canal. 8, Processus cochleariformis. 9, Cochlea. 10, Canal for the tensor tympani muscle. 11, Anterior tympanic spine. 12, Mallear foramen. 13, Posterior tympanopetrosal suture. 14, Horizontal portion of squama. 15, Vertical portion of squama. 16, Pretympanic recess.

antrum, communicating with the periosteum of the mastoid region (see Fig. 35). This would account for some of the subperiosteal abscesses seen on the mastoid process of young children early in the course of an acute suppurative otitis media.

The juncture of the petrosa and squama extends across the mastoid portion of the temporal bone (Figs. 36-42). It is directed medially, superiorly, and anteriorly. Their contact in this portion of the temporal bone may persist as a bony septum or lamina (*petrosquamosal lamina* or *Körner's septum*). When this bony septum is present, it divides the mastoid process into a superficial squamosal portion and a deep petrosal portion. Both portions open separately into the antrum (Fig. 43).

However, if the squamosal portion is not pneumatized (but sclerotic instead), there may be serious difficulty in finding the mastoid antrum at surgery, unless the operator is aware that a petrosquamosal lamina is present and must be penetrated to reach the air cells in the deeper portion of the temporal bone.

A well-developed septum may be mistaken for the bony covering of the lateral sinus, as pointed out by Schulman and Rock.[12] They stressed that a Körner's septum (*petrosquamosal lamina*) should be considered: (1) if there is difficulty in approaching the antrum, (2) if the antrum is small and constricted, and (3) if it is felt that it is an anomalous position. Whenever a persistent, dense petrosquamosal lamina is found, it can and should have the

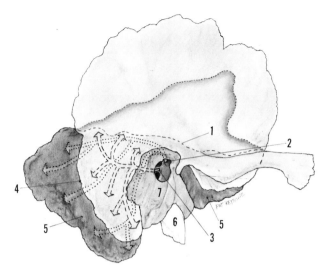

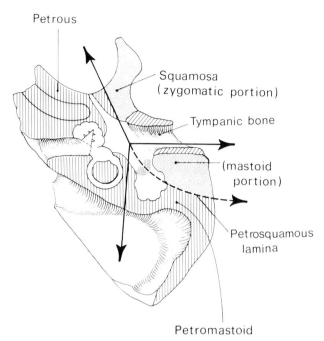

Figure 34. The squamosa is in direct contact with the petrosa except for the structures that originate from the first branchial cleft (tympanic bone), the first branchial pouch (eustachian tube, tympanum and mastoid air cell system), and the styloid complex. The squama forms the anterior, superficial portion of the mastoid, which is pneumatized by the saccus superior extending into the squamosal mastoid via the posterior tympanic isthmus (dashed arrows). The petrosa forms the deeper, posterior portion of the mastoid, which is pneumatized by the saccus medius extending into the petrosal mastoid via the anterior tympanic isthmus (dotted arrows). Where the petrosa and squama are in direct contact in the mastoid, there is a bony partition of varying thickness, which may even be membranous in places. This is the petrosquamosal lamina or Körner's septum. 1, Internal petrosquamosal suture. 2, Course of saccus medius as it pneumatizes the petromastoid. 3, Course of saccus superior as it pneumatizes the squamomastoid. 4, External posterior petrosquamosal suture. 5, Petrosa. 6, Styloid process. 7, Tympanic bone.

Figure 36. Schematic horizontal section showing the relationship of the squamosa and the petrosa. The point of contact in the mastoid forms the bony petrosquamosal lamina, or Körner's septum. The mastoid portion of the squama is pneumatized by the saccus superior, which leaves the tympanum via the posterior tympanic isthmus. The mastoid portion of the petrosa is pneumatized by the saccus medius, which leaves the mesotympanum via the anterior tympanic isthmus. The adult temporal bone is divided into its four portions: tympanic (meatus), petrosal (including the petromastoid), squamosal (zygomatic and mastoid portions), and styloid (separating mesotympanum from the antrum).[11]

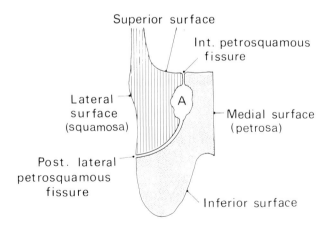

Figure 35. Schematic verticofrontal section, showing the position of the bony petrosquamosal laminal or fibrous tract extending from the antrum (A) to the posterior external or posterior lateral petrosquamosal suture. The lined segment is squamosal bone, and the dotted segment is petrosal bone.

party wall removed as much as feasible to eliminate a dual pneumatic system into the mastoid segment of the temporal bone.

Failure to recognize the presence of a petrosquamosal lamina may lead the surgeon to seek the antrum at a more external level—where upon dissecting inferiorly at this level, one may expose the facial nerve to injury. The safest approach, if in doubt, would be to dissect along the middle fossa dural plate until the antrum is identified.

Mastoid cells develop in the petrosa and also in the squama. They originate from the saccus medius (which pneumatizes into the pars petrosa by way of the attic) and from the saccus superior (which pnematizes into the pars squamosa by way of the posterior tympanic isthmus).[4] Air propelled into these sacs during swallowing and with forceful respirations, plus the pull of the muscles attached to the mastoid tip (sternocleidomastoid and splenius capitis muscles) with growth of the neck, gradually forces these sacs into the middle ear spaces.

Initially, the two groups of mastoid cells are separated from each other by the interosseous fissures and walls (ex-

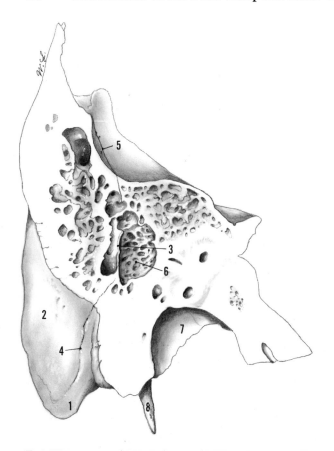

Figure 37. Vertical section through the right adult temporal bone. The cut is directed medially and slightly posteriorly. The petrosquamosal lamina (Körner's septum) is well preserved (3). Note the petromastoid cells lying internally or medially to it. The squamomastoid cells are all superficial to the petrosquamosal suture system. 1, Petromastoid. 2, Squamomastoid. 3, Petrosquamosal lamina. 4, Posterior external petrosquamosal suture. 5, Internal petrosquamosal suture. 6, Antrum. 7, Jugular dome. 8, Styloid.

ternal and internal petrosquamosal laminae). There is a constant relationship of the two groups of cells to the antrum.

The squamal cells lie superiorly and externally. The petrosal cells are medial, posterior, and tend to extend further inferiorly. Between them is the petrosquamosal lamina or Körner's septum. When the septum is complete, both groups open separately into the antrum. One group may be poorly pneumatized so that its portion of the mastoid may consist of compact bone. If the squamous portion is made of compact bone, access to the deeper petrosal portion may be difficult; nonetheless, however, the otologic surgeon must reach the deep pneumatic portion of the petrosa if it is infected. In such an anatomic situation, the deeper petrosal infection is more likely to extend intracranially and may not be manifest with postaural swelling and tenderness.

During the course of normal development, however, the interpetrous-squamosal walls are usually absorbed, and the two types of cells communicate with each other.

The roof (tegmen) of the attic and antrum is usually extremely thin and translucent throughout life. When the roof of the tympanum is examined from below (Fig. 44), the free border of the squamosal tegmen is seen to pass beneath the petrosal tegmen, forming a distinct ridge (*crista transversa*) all along the roof of the middle ear cleft (Figs. 44,45). This ridge is often seen at surgery and must be removed to properly clean out the long, narrow space lying medial to it. This ridge may also be very prominent and extend down to the malleus head or anterior mallear process, where it may cause fixation of the malleus and prevent its normal vibration with sound waves.

Internal to the roof of the attic is the hiatus Fallopii, where the facial nerve lies against the dura mater. It is possible for infection to pass from the middle ear to the middle fossa by this route. Behind the hiatus is the anterior crus of the superior semicircular canal. Internal to the hiatus lies the smooth, compact bone covering the cochlea anteriorly and a mass of diploetic bone posteromedially. Anteriorly, between the cochlear capsule and the compartment of the tensor tympani muscle, and immediatley below the anteriormost portion of the tegmen, lies the *epitympanic sinus* recently described by Wigand and Trillsch.[13]

The Tympanopetrosal and Tympanosquamosal Sutures

The anterosuperior border of the tympanic bone is applied to the horizontal part of the squama at its tympanic crest. The tympanic bone crosses the horizontal portion of the squama transversely, running parallel to the tympanic crest for 6 to 7 mm until it reaches the medial end of the horizontal portion of the squama. At this point, the tympanic bone terminates at the anterior tympanic spine. This forms the *anterior tympanosquamosal suture*. The two bones are then separated by a lateral extension of the petrosal tegmen called the *intertympanosquamosal crest* or *crista tegmentalis*. Although constant, the crista tegmentalis is not always apparent on simple examination; but its presence produces a double fissure (Glaserian fissure), which courses anteriorly, medially, and inferiorly, paralleling the course of the eustachian tube. The anterior portion of this double fissure is the *anterior petrosquamosal fissure*. It is smaller than its accompanying, posteriorly placed *anterior tympanopetrosal fissure*.

Two foramina can be found in the anterior tympanopetrosal fissure. The external are easily seen. The internal are smaller. Both lead ot the tympanum and give passage—the first to the anterior tympanic artery and veins and the anterior mallear ligament; the second to the chorda tympani nerve (canal of Huguier).

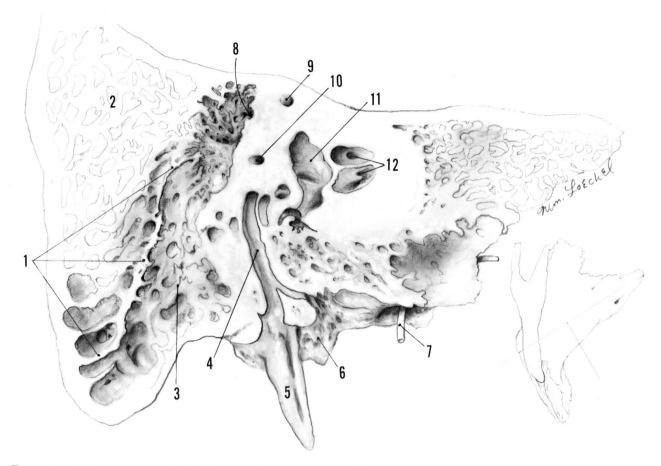

Figure 38.   Vertical section of the left adult temporal bone looking anteriorly. The cut is directed anteromedially at a 45° angle. The position of the petrosquamosal lamina is well shown. As it approaches the antrum, it terminates. 1, Petrosquamosal lamina. 2, Squamomastoid cells. 3, Petromastoid cells. 4, Facial canal. 5, Styloid. 6, Vaginal plate. 7, Carotid canal. 8, Arrow pointing to aditus. 9, Superior semicircular canal. 10, Horizontal semicircular canal. 11, Vestibule. 12, Cochlea.

Tympanopetrosal Suture

The tympanic bone is attached by its superior border to the petrosa from the anterior tympanic spine to the beginning of the Glaserian fissure (anterior tympanopetrosal suture). It has a much larger attachment where its posterior surface contacts the petrosa to form the *posterior tympanopetrosal suture.*

Posterior Tympanopetrosal Suture.   This suture is usually not very distinct in the adult, but it is found where the inferior portion of the tympanic bone contacts the petrosa below and lateral to the hypotympanum. In making this contact, it includes the styloid complex, which lies between the petrosa and tympanic bone at this level. Most of the posterior half of the tympanic bone is in contact with the petrosa on the posterior wall of the external auditory meatus.

The superior extremity of this suture is usually seen as a groove along the floor of the eustachian tube and tympanum (see Fig. 17). Sometimes a fissure appears at the external and posterior extremity of this groove (the *posterior tympanopetrosal fissure*). This fissure again joins the inferior part of the squama and continues posteriorly with the anterior petrosquamosal fissure. It terminates at the lateral aspect of the posterior chordal canal.

Anterior Tympanopetrosal Suture   This suture is located between the superior border of the tympanic bone and the crista tegmentalis of the petrosa. It corresponds to the posterior branch of the Glaserian fissure (Fig. 14).

Internally at the eustachian tube level, the tympanic bone applies its anterior surface against the posterior surface of the crista tegmentalis.

The superior border of the tympanic bone ascends posterior to the crista tegmentalis, and may reach as far as the canal of the tensor tympani without contributing to any portion of this wall.

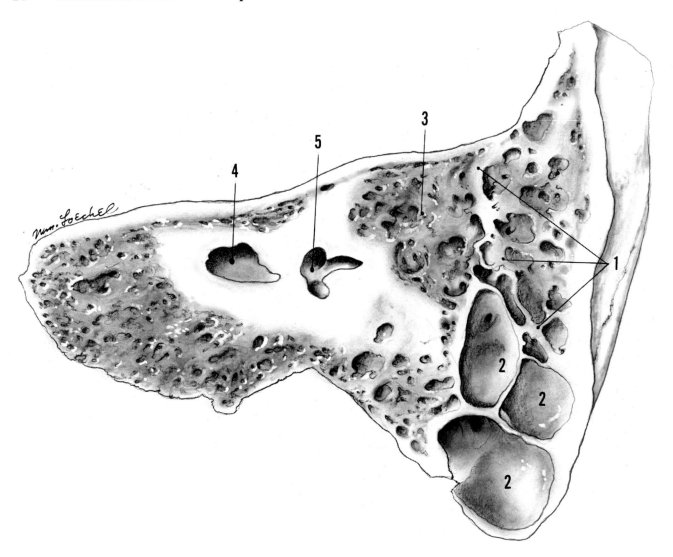

Figure 39.   Vertical section of the same left adult temporal bone looking posteriorly. This is the posterior half of the bone shown in Figure 38. 1, Note the large cells of the petrosa below the petrosquamosal lamina. 2, Petromastoid cells. 3, Antrum. 4, Internal auditory meatus. 5, Vestibule.

The tympanic surface of the tympanic bone is smooth; but in the level of the Glaserian fissure, it has a groove (sulcus mallearis, or *mallear groove*) along which the anterior mallear ligament passes: (1) the upper ridge of the groove is called the crista spinarum (Henle), or *mallear crest* (Bellocq); and (2) the lower ridge of the groove is called the *tympanic crest of Gruber* (Figs. 13,32).

The anterior end of the crista spinarum is prominent and is termed the *anterior tympanic spine* of Henle. The anterior tympanic spine, often poorly developed, is sometimes visible at the level of the Glaserian fissure (see Fig. 14). It limits a groove externally (see Fig. 13) which proceeds along the entire length of the mallear crest and leads from the tympanum to the posterior branch of the Glaserian fissure. It is the mallear groove or sulcus mallearis

(see Fig. 13). The posterior end of the crista spinarum is referred to as the *posterior tympanic spine of Henle*. It is more developed and easily seen (see Fig. 13).

External to the mallear crest, the superior border of the tympanic bone curves inward until a portion of the anterior surface of the tympanic bone is seen in the tympanum. It is covered externally by the squama.

The tegmen tympani over the protympanum dips down to contact the upper border of the tympanic bone. At times, the bones do not meet completely; instead, there is a cleft of variable length extending along the Glaserian fissure. As the inferior projection of the tegmen tympani approaches the isthmus of the bony eustachian tube (protympanum), it gradually displaces the tympanic bone laterally; it contacts the upward projection from the petrosa of the carotid canal to completely surround the bony eustachian isthmus with petrosal bone (Figs. 14, 22).

The tegmen tympani at the level of the mallear crest may contact the crista spinarum so that there is an enclosed mallear gutter, as well as a parallel groove external to the point of contact. The mallear gutter is always present. It transmits the tympanic artery and veins, the anterior mallear ligament, and the chorda tympani nerve.

The chorda tympani nerve does not follow the entire course through the mallear groove, instead, immediately upon entering the groove, it leaves and extends obliquely, downward and inward, crossing between the downward prolongation of the tegmen tympani and the upper border of the tympanic bone. Thus, the canal containing the chorda tympani nerve is made up of two semi grooves—the petrosal and the tympanic. The posterior orifice of this canal is the anterior *canal of the chorda tympani* or *canal of Huguier*. Running parallel to the inferior margin of the tegmen, it emerges by a small opening on the anterior surface of the tympanic bone. At times, the anterior canal of the chorda tympani extends deep into the inferior prolongation of the tegmen tympani (Bellocq).[11]

Tympanosquamosal Sutures

The tympanic bone is applied against the horizontal part of the squama anteriorly and against the retromeatal portion of the squama posteriorly (see Fig. 15).

Anterior Tympanosquamosal Suture.   This suture is located where the tympanic bone crosses the inferior aspect of the

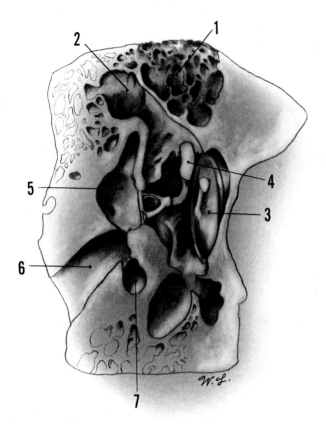

Figure 40.   Vertical section of a freshly cored temporal bone looking posteriorly. 1, The squamosal cells are seen extending anteriorly over the external auditory meatus towards the zygoma. 2, Mastoid antrum. 3, Tympanic membrane. 4, Sectioned incus body. 5, Vestibule. 6, Internal auditory meatus. 7, Basal coil of the cochlea.

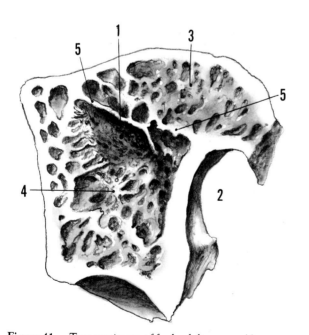
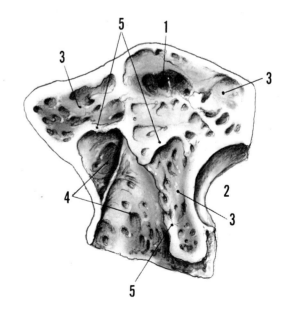

Figure 41.   Two specimens of fresh adult temporal bones cut vertically to illustrate the petrosquamosal lamina. The left one illustrates a high position for the squamosal cells; whereas, the right one shows the cells have extended to a lower level. 1, Mastoid antrum. 2, External auditory canal. 3, Squamomastoid cells. 4, Petromastoid cells. 5, Petrosquamosal lamina.

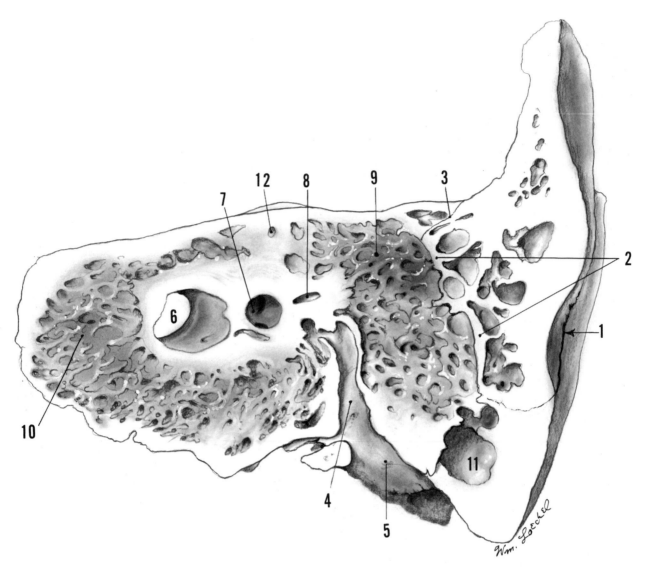

Figure 42. Vertical section of the left adult temporal bone with a squamomastoid, which is very distinct from the petromastoid. The view is directed posteriorly. 1, Posterior external petrosquamosal suture. 2, Petrosquamosal lamina. 3, Internal petroquamosal suture. 4, Facial canal. 5, Digastric groove. 6, Internal auditory meatus. 7, Vestibule. 8, Horizontal semicircular canal. 9, Posterior aspect of mastoid antrum. 10, Apical cells. 11, Petromastoid cell. 12, Superior semicircular canal.

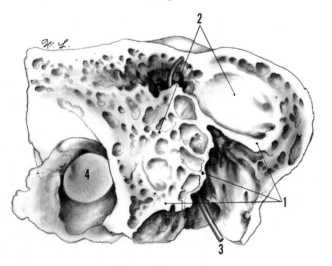

Figure 43. Vertical section through a fresh adult temporal bone, which shows the superficial squamosal cells separated from the deeper petrosal cells by a very distinct petrosquamosal lamina. 1, Petrosquamosal lamina. 2, Squamomastoid cells. 3, Probe in the mastoid antrum. 4, External auditory meatus.

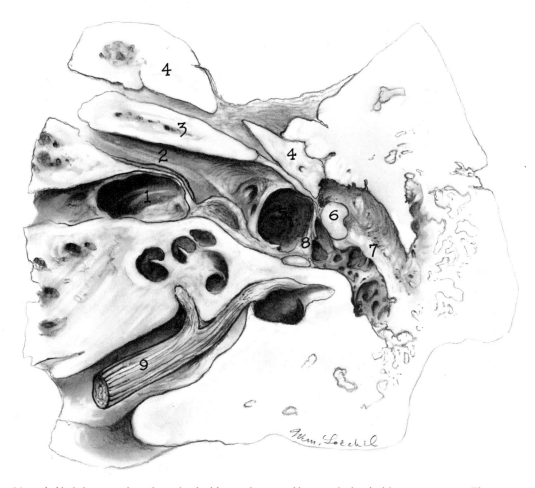

Figure 44. Upper half of a horizontal cut through a freshly cored temporal bone at the level of the protympanum. The intertympanosquamosal crest of the petrosa (3), which is directed posteriorly in the line of the malleus head continues as the petrosquamosal crest. This crest represents the downward thrust of the squamosal tegmen at the internal petrosquamosal suture. 1, Carotid canal. 2, Protympanum. 3, Intertympanosquamosal crest of the petrosa. 4, Squamosa. 5, Supratubal recess. 6, Malleus head. 7, Petrosquamosal crest. 8, Processus cochleariformis. 9, Auditory nerve.

horizontal part of the squama. It lies behind the tympanic crest of the squama and in front of the inward-curving superior border of the anterior surface of the tympanic bone (Fig. 46). The anterior extremity of this suture continues on as the nonbifurcated part of the Glaserian fissure. Another smaller fissure is found at the posterior termination of this suture.

Posterior Tympanosquamosal Suture. It is much longer than the anterior one (see Fig. 14). It corresponds, on the squamosa, to the anteroinferior portion of its retromeatal part, on the tympanic bone, it corresponds to the superior external portion of its posterior surface. At the medial end of this suture lies the sulcus tympanicus, which marks the bottom of the external auditory canal. The suture terminates above the *posterior tympanic spine*. The spine may be pointed or blunt, depending on whether it is formed by the union of the upper border of the tympanic

bone and the sulcus tympanicus, or if it is extended a little further inward at their point of contact (best seen in the newborn).

This spine varies in its relation to the internal border of the squama. It may be external to it (see Fig. 14) or cross it to overlap inside the tympanum.

The posterior tympanosquamosal suture is seen externally as the *external posterior tympanosquamosal suture,* following the external edge of the posterior slope of the tympanic bone. The internal suture (the *internal posterior tympanosquamosal suture*) is less prominent. This inconstant suture is located slightly inside the sulcus tympanicus and continues, below the squama, with the posterior tympanopetrosal fissure. Above, it disappears in the region of the posterior tympanic spine, especially as it approaches the internal lip of the sulcus tympanicus. This relationship is best seen when the spine is flattened and its internal edge is placed inside the sulcus tympanicus.

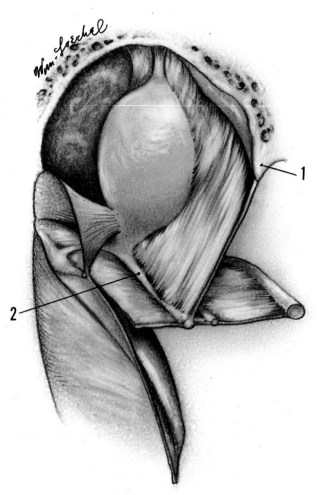

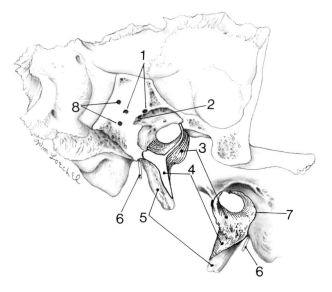

Figure 46. The tympanic bone—its relations. The upper illustration is of a vertical cut through the petrosa looking outward. The lower illustration shows the tympanic bone in the external auditory meatus. 1, Horizontal semicircular canal. 2, Facial canal. 3, Tympanic bone. 4, Vaginal process of tympanic bone. 5, Styloid process. 6, Facial nerve. 7, Tympanomastoid suture. 8, Posterior semicircular canal.

Figure 45. The squamosal tegmen may be deflected downward by the petrosal tegmen to form a petrosquamosal crest seen on the roof of the attic and antrum. This crest may reach low enough to fix the malleus head. A mucosal fold may drop from the crest to the anterior mallear process (S), thus dividing the anterior compartment of the attic into a lateral and medial anterior attic compartment. The crest, when present, may need to be removed when it hinders cleansing of an infected recess, or if it interferes with free movement of the ossicular chain. 1. Petrosquamosal crest. 2. Anterior mallear process.

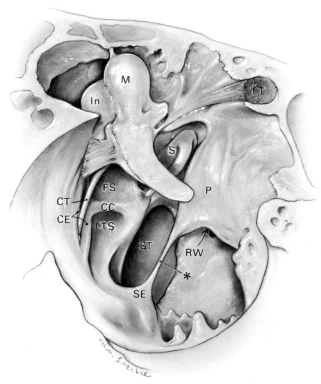

Figure 47. View of the posterior tympanum. Bony bridge from ▶ styloid eminence (SE) to promontory (P). This is vestige indicating that the Reichert's cartilage was once in direct contact with the cartilaginous otic capsule. Separation occurred with development of the middle ear cleft. CE, Chordal eminence. CT, Chorda tympani. CC, Chordal ridge. LTS, Lateral tympanic sinus. ST, Sinus tympani. FS, Facial sinus. RW, Round window. S, Stapes. M, Malleus. IN, Incus.

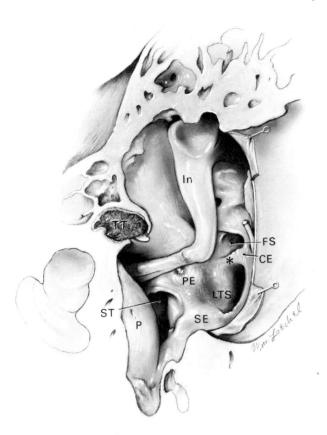

Figure 48. Vertical view of the posterior tympanum. The incus (*IN*) and stapes are in position. The lateral tympanic sinus (*LTS*) is clearly seen between the pyramidal eminence (*PE*), the styloid eminence (*SE*), and the chordal eminence (*CE*). Behind the chordal ridge (*) lies the facial sinus (*FS*). *ST*, Sinus tympani. *TT*, Tensor tympani. *P*, Promontory.

The internal posterior tympanosquamosal fissure is in contact with the styloid complex. At its apex, near the upper end of the internal lip of the sulcus tympanicus, is a small orifice. This is the superior orifice of the *posterior canal of the chorda tympani*. In many cases, it is medial both to the sulcus tympanicus and from the fissure which ends there (Figs. 47-49).

The inferior extremity of the internal posterior tympanosquamosal fissure leads to the point of union of the posterior tympanopetrosal and anterior petrosquamosal sutures. At the point of contact of these fissures in the posterior hypotympanum, we have the point of contact of all four constituents of the temporal bone. The tympanic bone lies external, the petrosa lies internal, and the squama and styloid complex lie in between.

The chorda tympani nerve ascends on the posterolateral aspect of the styloid complex. The orifice of the posterior chordal canal lies on the lateral aspect of the styloid complex. Laterally, it is covered by squamosa or by the tym-

panic bone, especially when the chordal orifice is in contact with the annulus tympanicus, as it always is in the newborn. With growth, the squama may interpose to a variable degree similar to the intrapetrosal situation of the anterior canal of the chorda tympani.

Summary

The sutures we have described are not always found in any one specimen. The four components of the temporal bone are often fused, and suture lines are often obliterated. Their position and course can be predicted by study of the newborn temporal bone—by sectioning the temporal bones with a motor-driven diamond saw, which gives a smooth, clear-cut without variations in the course of the saw, by dissecting and studying decalcified temporal bones, and by studying histologic sections of the temporal bone.

The anterior petrosquamosal fissure is indeed tympanopetrosal, as described by Bellocq.[11] It runs posteriorly along the floor of the hypotympanum. As it approaches the posterior wall of the tympanum, it divides. The external branch is no longer tympanopetrosal; rather, it is tympanosquamosal or stylotympanic. The internal branch, best seen in the newborn, is petrosquamosal or stylopetrosal, depending on the degree of downward growth of the squamosa.

The tympanic bone is in direct contact with the styloid complex posteriorly (second arch origin) so that at the level of the posterior tympanum, we have a stylotympanic suture that extends inferiorly to the point of emergence of the styloid process. Posterolateral to the styloid complex, the tympanic bone is again in contact with the petrosa as the posterior tympanopetrosal suture. On its medial aspect, the styloid complex is in apposition to the petrosa, as the stylopetrosal suture.

In the midportion of the posterior tympanopetrosal suture is a small foramen that permits Arnold's nerve (auricular branch of the vagus) to innervate the skin of the posterior inferior portion of the external auditory meatus and the skin of the posterior part of the auricle. Arnold's nerve spreads from the ganglion of the root of the vagus. It receives a filament of communication from the petrous ganglion of the IX nerve and follows the outer margin of the jugular foramen to an opening between the stylomastoid and jugular foramina. Entering this foramen, it traverses a canal in the temporal bone, which crosses the inner side of the facial canal and terminates between the mastoid process and the external auditory meatus. While traversing the temporal bone, the auricular nerve communicates with the facial nerve and, after reaching its area of distribution, with the posterior auricular nerve.

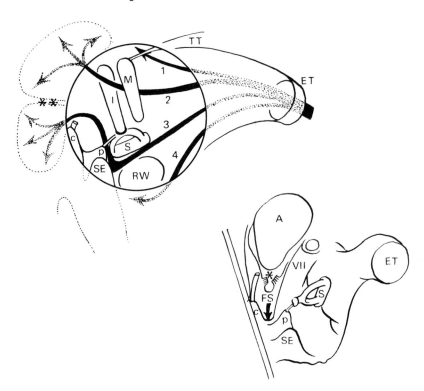

Figure 49. Schema illustrating movement of endothelial pouches of the eustachian tube origin as they develop the middle ear air cell system. 1, Saccus anticus, which may form the supratubal recess. 2, Saccus medius, which leaves the mesotympanum via the anterior tympanic isthmus to form the attic, and goes into the pars petrosal portion of the mastoid. 3, Saccus superior, which ascends over the styloid complex (pyramidal eminence [P], styloid eminence [SE], and chordal eminence [C] and through the posterior tympanic isthmus to form the squamosal portion of the mastoid. 4, Saccus posticus, which forms the hypotympanum, round window niche, sinus tympani, and inferior half of oval window niche. The lower schema shows the styloid complex. The arrow indicates the position of the facial sinus (*FS*) as it descends behind the chordal ridge and drops downward on the lateral aspect of the facial canal. *Posterior incudal ligaments in the fossa incudis. *A*, Antrum.

Variations

The auricular nerve may be absent or may fuse with the main trunk of the facial nerve—its fibers under these circumstances probably reaching their destination through the posterior auricular nerve. Its branch of communication with the facial nerve may be absent (Piersol).[14]

The tympanomeningeal fissure (Hyrtl) and the lateral and medial hypotympanic fissures are of importance in the embryo and are discussed in the section describing the hypotympanum.

3 The Four Parts of the Temporal Bone
Petrosa, Squamosa, Tympanic, and Styloid

Petrosa

The petrosa is in the form of a quadrangular pyramid (see Fig. 7), the summit of which would be anterior and internal; its base would be posterior and external. Its axis is thus oblique anteriorly and medially. Two of its surfaces are intracranial and superior, the two others are extracranial and inferior (Figs. 2, 4, 5, 6, 7).

The intracranial surfaces combine to form the superior rim of the bone, thus one can distinguish an anterior or anterosuperior surface and a posterior or posterosuperior surface.

The extracranial surfaces converge together and form the inferior rim of the temporal bone. This border is less clear than the preceding one. In front is found the anterior or anteroinferior extracranial surface, while behind, we have the posterior or postero inferior extracranial surface.

The extracranial and intracranial surfaces are separated in front by the anterior border of the temporal bone, and behind by the posterior border of this bone.

Anterosuperior (Cerebral) Surface

From the apex laterally (see Fig. 2).

1. Depression for the Gasserian ganglion.
2. Fallopian hiatus.
3. Accessory hiatus.
4. Arcuate eminence.
5. Tegmen tympani anteriorly.

Posterosuperior Surface

The cerebellar aspect of the petrosa:

1. Orifice of the internal auditory meatus.
2. Lateral sinus groove.
3. Orifice of the vestibular aqueduct.
4. Inferiorly, the small groove for the inferior petrosal sinus.

Superior Rim

The superior border, which separates the two preceding surfaces, is indented by the trigeminal nerve and crossed obliquely by the superior petrosal sinus (see Fig. 7). At the level of its midportion lies the vestige of the subarcuate fossa.

Anteroinferior Surface

We can see only the medial part of this surface of the intact temporal bone. It forms the bed for the cartilaginous portion of the eustachian tube (see Figs. 4-5). The rest of this surface is covered by the tympanic bone and by the squama. If we remove these two bones, the anteroinferior surface of the petrosa is seen to be made up of a peripheral zone adherent to the squama (see Figs. 8, 9) and the tympanic bone, and also by a central free zone.

This free zone makes up almost all of the medial wall of the middle ear. It is actually a recess with regard to the adherent zone, which surrounds it (see Figs. 8, 9) so that the anteroinferior surface of the petrosa can be considered as excavated at this level. This free surface corresponds, therefore, in the greater part of its extent to the internal wall of the middle ear. It also forms part of the superior and inferior walls of this same cavity.

Sections through the temporal bone show that the roof of the middle ear is the tegmen tympani, which is of petrosal origin. The anterior portion of the tegmen thickens to articulate with the squama. The posterior portion has less thickening on articulating with the squama. The free edge (laterally) of the anterior tegmen inserts between the squama (see Figs. 14, 16) and the tympanic bone to form a herniation between the two. The medial wall of the tympanum is called the *labyrinthine wall* because of the proximity of the bony labyrinthine capsule.

Posteroinferior Surface

Composed from lateral to medial (see Figs. 8, 9).

1. Mastoid process.
2. Digastric groove.
3. Groove for the occipital artery.
4. Stylomastoid foramen.
5. Styloid process.
6. Jugular fossa.
7. Inferior orifice of Jacobson's canal.
8. Inferior orifice of the carotid canal.
9. One rough surface corresponding to the inferior wall of this canal.

Inferior Rim

It is poorly defined. It is indicated externally by the inferior edge of the tympanic bone, and medially by an indistinct edge, which separated the bed of the cartilaginous eustachian tube from the remainder of the posterior inferior surface.

Anterior Rim

The anterior rim of the petrosa is made up of a free part and an adherent part. The free part articulates with the sphenoid bone. It carries the anterior orifice of the carotid canal medially (see Figs. 4, 7).

The adherent part is represented in the greater part of its length by the anterosuperior rim of the articular surface of the tegmen tympani (see Fig. 22). It is indicated on the intact temporal bone by the internal petrosquamosal suture.

Posterior Rim

This rim contains from medial to lateral:

1. Thick zone of rough bone, which articulates with the occipital bone.
2. Jugular opening (see Figs. 19–21), divided by the jugular spine and bearing the opening of the cochlear aqueduct.
3. Jugular facet opposite the jugular process of the occipital bone.
4. Large, irregular, and strongly convex rim articulating once again with the occipital bone.

Apex

Forms at the junction of the superior, anterior, and posterior rims. It is best seen on the intracranial aspect of an articulated skull.

Base

The petrosal base comes up to the posterior part of the mastoid region (see Figs. 1, 2, 4, 7). It is limited behind by the posterior edge of the petrosa, in front by the external periphery of the anteroinferior surface of the petrosa, and above by the external rim of the petrosa. The base of the petrosa ends freely below, while consituting the greater part of the mastoid process. Its upper limit is also indicated externally by the external petrosquamosal suture (Fig. 1). Its posterior and external borders reunite posteriorly to form the posterior angle of the temporal bone.

The petrosa contains compact bone in its midportion, the interior of which are hollowed-out cavities of the inner ear—the *labyrinthine capsule.* Spongy bone surrounds the capsule to some degree.It is absent anterolaterally at the labyrinthine wall of the middle ear. The spongy bone marrow is constant in the newborn. It is usually replaced to some degree by air cells that invade the petrosa from the middle ear cleft. These petrosal cells are more abundant externally, but they may extend around the labyrinth to pneumatize the apex. Petrosal invasion by air cell tracts may extend:

1. Along the posterior fossa towards the internal auditory meatus (the posteromedial tract of Lindsay).[15]
2. The superior tract—above the superior semicircular canal to the apex.
3. The subarcuate tract—following the subarcuate vessels.
4. Anterior tract—between the cochlea and the carotid canal.
5. The infralabyrinthine tract.

The spongy marrow is enclosed by compact cortical bone, which now forms the surface of the petrosa.

Squama

The squama lies in front of the petrosa and articulates with the greater part of the articulating surface of the anteroinferior surface of this bone (see Fig. 5). The squama is composed of three parts:

1. A superior *vertical* part.
2. An inferoanterior *horizontal* part.
3. A posteroinferior or retromeatal part.

The *zygomatic process,* located on the extracranial surface, contributes to the above division.

Vertical Part

Flat and thin, especially in its midportion, it has a semicircular form. One surface is intracranial and in contact with the brain, the other is extracranial and covered by the powerful temporalis muscle. The free rim articulates with the sphenoid in front and the parietal bone behind. It forms the parietal incisura (see Figs. 1, 7) with the external border of the petrosa. Its inferior margin continues with the other two parts (horizontal and retromeatal) of this bone.

Horizontal Part

The horizontal part of the squama is triangular. Its summit is internal, and its base blends with the vertical part of the squama.

Superior Surface

The superior surface of the horizontal part of the squama continues imperceptibly with the intracranial surface of the vertical portion. It is partially overlapped by the tegmen tympani, which rests on it.

Inferior Surface

The inferior surface is very irregular. It presents from forward backward:

1. Subtemporal plane.
2. Condyle.
3. Mandibular fossa.
4. Tympanic crest.
5. Arch of the external auditory canal.

Anterior Border

The anterior border of the horizontal portion is free. It covers the subtemporal plane and a part of the temporal condyle. It is large and indented. The inferior surface of the horizontal portion does not extend as far forward as its superior surface. It articulates with the great wing of the sphenoid, along with the free edge of the vertical portion of the squama.

Internal Border

The internal border of the horizontal portion articulates with the tegmen tympani, at first by its entire thickness and then only by its superior part. This thick border thickens more in its posterior portion, corresponding to the roof of the external auditory canal. This increase of thickness is accompanied by a change in the orientation of this edge, which is vertical in the greatest part of its extent and oblique below and within—in proportion as it thickens.

Seen from the intracranial surface, this border articulates with tegmen of the petrosa at the level of the internal petrosquamosal fissure. The border is oblique posteriorly and externally and is almost rectilinear in shape. It disappears posteriorly on a vertical portion of the squama.

When examined extracranially, this same border is articular only in its anterior glenoid part. Its posterior part, corresponding to the roof of the external auditory canal, appears free. Its direction has changed. Its anterior glenoid wall remains oblique posteriorly and externally, but its posterior part extends posteriorly and slightly medially. Finally, the inferior part of this internal border (with a free edge at the level of the bottom of the external auditory canal) terminates on the retromeatal portion of the squama.

Thus, while the horizontal portion of the squama disappears posteriorly at the level of the intracranial surface of the temporal bone, it continues below at the level of the extracranial surface of this bone with the retromeatal part of the squama. One can see on a skull that the posterior part of the roof of the external auditory canal is the end point of the two surfaces of this horizontal portion of the squama.

The Summit

The summit of the triangle formed by the horizontal portion of the squama is located at the internal extremity of the submandibular (glenoid) cavity and the temporal condyle. It is determined by the union of the anterior and internal edges of this horizontal portion of the squama. It corresponds to the larger part of this portion of the squama. It coincides with the summit of the angle formed by the free edge of the squama and that of the petrosa.

Retromeatal Part

The retromeatal part of the squama corresponds externally to the posterior wall of the external auditory canal, and to the anterior portion of the mastoid region.

External Surface

The external surface, which includes the spine of Henle or suprameatal spine (see Fig. 1) in the vicinity of the posterosuperior circumference of the auditory meatus, is generally smooth. It is separate behind the base of the petrosa by the external petrosquamosal suture (see Fig. 1). It continues anteriorly to the level of the external auditory canal, with the roof of this conduit formed by the horizontal part of the squama.

Internal Surface

This deep surface is free only in its midportion, where it forms the external wall of the petrous antrum. Everywhere else, it articulates with the petrosa at the level of the external part of the tegmen tympani and with the large inferoexternal surface presented by the anteroinferior surface of this bone. This deep surface of the retromeatal portion of the squama continues imperceptibly, forward and inward, with the internal border of the horizontal portion of the squama.

If we now examine the relations of the whole between the horizontal and retromeatal portions of the squama, we note that when the superior (intracranial) surface of the horizontal portion of the squama disappears, the internal (extracranial) surface and the internal border of the latter continue to the level of the posterosuperior circumference of the external auditory tube—along with the external and internal surfaces of the retromeatal portion of the squama.

The retromeatal part of the squama can be considered as derived from the horizontal part, which would be spread out immediately behind the auditory canal.

Zygomatic Process

The zygomatic process (see Fig. 1) flattens from within outward and originates by a triangular base from the union of the vertical and horizontal parts of the squama.

The superior surface of this base, or root, is gutter-shaped. The inferior surface, concave at the level of its midportion where it forms the external portion of the glenoid cavity, presents anteriorly the anterior zygomatic tubercle and the external extremity of the temporal condyle—and posteriorly the posterior zygomatic tubercle, which terminates externally at the tympanic crest.

The triangular root of the zygomatic process is limited anteriorly by a free rim and extends posteriorly to the supramastoid crest or linea temporalis. This crest marks the level where the vertical and horizontal portions of the squama join. It marks the level of the floor of the middle cranial fossa.

Constitution

The squama is formed (see Figs. 4, 5, 6), by two layers of compact bone (internal and external tables) between which is found a variable amount of spongy tissue or diploe. When the layers of compact bone are separated, the diploe is abundant. When the squama is thinner, the diploe will be missing.

The retromeatal part of the squama, which does not contact the intracranial cavity is made up of a compact layer corresponding to the external surface of the bone and a variable mass of spongy bone. This spongy bone contacts that of the petrosa directly. This spongy mass is fenestrated in its midportion to form the external wall of the petrous antrum. Above, at the level of the internal petrosquamosal fissure, the articulation between the squama and petrosa is established between the inner table of the verticle portion of the squama and the cortex of the anterosuperior surface of the petrosa.

The spongy tissue of the squama is often invaded by pneumatic cells. They are especially frequent in the retromeatal portion of the squama, but are also encountered at the level of the horizontal portion of the squama.

The Tympanic Bone

The tympanic bone is situated behind the petrotympanic fissure. It is below the squama and in front of the petrosa. It articulates with the other constituents of the temporal bone: the petrosa, the squama, and the styloid. It presents in the form of a semicylindrical groove open above (the *tympanic groove*). It forms the anterior inferior, and posterior walls of the bony external auditory canal. Its superior wall is formed by the squama.

The tympanic bone presents two surfaces: one is superficial and the other is deep (Fig.12). It also presents three

borders: anteroposterior, posteroinferior, and external—and an internal extremity.

The Superficial Surface

The *superficial surface* presents two segments:

Anterior Surface

The anterior surface of the tympanic bone is free. It is transversely concave and vertically convex. It is usually smooth, but may be slightly roughened. It represents the tympanic or retroglaserian segment of the mandibular fossa (glenoid cavity). It lodges the deep portion of the parotid gland. The tympanic plate sometimes presents a small deficiency at its center (the *foramen of Huschke*), which is always present until about five years of age.

Posterior Surface

This is the retroauricular segment. It includes the annulus, and is free in its superior part and adherent to the petrosa in its inferior part. It persists externally as a fine groove—a vestige of the tympanomastoid fissure.

The Deep Surface

The deep suface is concave. It corresponds to the bony external auditory canal. In its depth, this surface presents a narrow circular groove—the *tympanic groove* or *sulcus tympanicus*—which houses the tympanic membrane.

Anterosuperior Border

The anterosuperior border is thin. It fuses (1) externally to the squama at the tympanic crest while forming the *anterior tympanosquamosal suture or fissure of Glaser*; and (2) posteriorly to the petrosa.

One can distinguish two segments. One is external, and curvilinear with posterior concavity; at its highest part, this segment is thickened in the form of a rough crest—the *crista spinarum of Henle* (see Figs. 13, 32). The other internal oblique inferiorly, anteriorly, and on the inside. It is in the form of a smooth groove. This is the *sulcus mallearis*, in which proceeds the anterior mallear ligament, the chorda tympani, and the anterior tympanic vessels. The internal extension of this border continues anteriorly to form the anterior wall of the protympanum. Inferiorly, it is adherent to the petrosa.

Posteroinferior Border

The posteroinferior border is large and rough. It is shorter and ascends less than the anterosuperior border. It fuses to the mastoid externally, forming the *tympanomastoid* or *posterior tympanosquamosal suture* (the anterior edge of the mastoid meets the squama). Its medial part fuses with the styloid complex and beyond that to the petrosa.

At the level of the sulcus tympanicus, this border curves inward under a little hooked process called the *the posterior tympanic spine*.

External Border

The external border limits the external orifice of the bony external auditory meatus. Oblique below and externally, it is rough and gradually becomes thinner as it approaches the anterior and posterior borders. It gives insertion for the cartilage of the external auditory canal. Anteriorly, it ends in a spine that extends to the tympanic crest and the posterior zygomatic tubercle. This is the *anterior tympanic spine*. On the anteroinferior side of this spine is attached the tympanic fasciculus of the external pterygoid muscle.

Internal Extremity

The internal extremity is constituted by a triangular process situated at the union of the anteriosuperior border and the the superficial surface (the *tubal process*). This is adherent to the petrosa, except at its superior part, where a groove is formed for passage of the chorda tympani (sulcus mallearis). It delimits with the *inferior extension of the tegmen tympani*—the orifice of the bony portion of the eustachian tube. This orifice is situated in the more external part of the sphenopetrosal suture. Finally, its anterior surface backs up to the spine of the sphenoid.

Vaginal Process

The vaginal process is a bony plate flattened between the entrance of the bony auditory meatus and the tubal process. It prolongs the tympanic bone below (see Fig. 43).

Flattened form behind and outside to within, its anterior surface, which is smooth and slightly concave, continues along the retroglaserian segment of the mandibular fossa. Its posterior surface is adherent to the petrosa and to the styloid process, which forms an imprint on it in the form of a groove—the *styloid groove* (see Fig. 12).

Its inferior edge is irregular, thin, and sharp—at times even jagged. More often, it ends by a small point situated a little in front and inside the styloid process.

The Styloid

We can consider the fourth component of the temporal bone to be the styloid complex. There are two portions to consider: (1) the external or styloid process; and (2) the in-

ternal process, which lies between the tympanic bone and petrosa, forming the posterior wall of the tympanum. The styloid complex is of second-arch origin. It is a part of the hyoid bar.

The styloid process, which is cylindrical and tapering, starts from a point immediately in front of the stylomastoid foramen, and is directed downwards and inwards. The muscular and ligamentous relation of the process are as follows:

1. The stylopharyngeus muscle arising from the inner aspect of the base.
2. The stylohyoid muscle from the posterior and outer aspect of the process near its base.
3. The styloglossus muscle from the front of the process near its tip.
4. The stylomandibular ligament attached just below the styloglossus.
5. The stylohyoid ligament attached exactly to the tip.

The term *styloid* is based on the greek and meaning "peg." Its extratemporal portion is usually thick at its point of origin, and is anterior and slightly medial to the stylomastoid foramen. As it descends, it becomes thinner and finally ends in a point. It varies greatly in length. It descends forward and inward, and continues as the styloid ligament to the lesser horn of the hyoid.

The styloid complex beginning at the stylomastoid foramen continues upward and slightly posteriorly between the tympanic bone and the petrosa as far as the fossa incudis. It forms the posterior wall fo the tympanum. On its posteromedial aspect courses the facial canal (Fallopian aqueduct), housing the facial nerve. The tympanic course of the facial nerve is covered by a thin lamella of bone that is often dehiscent. It enters the styloid portion of the facial canal immediately in front of and below the fossa incudis. The remainder—or descending portion of the facial canal—is covered by a dense bone until the nerve emerges at the stylomastoid foramen, with the exception of the posteromedial wall of the facial sinus, which is usually thin so that it is often possible to see the descending facial canal through it. This makes an excellent guiding landmark while executing the posterior tympanotomy to gain access to the tympanum.

The styloid complex includes:

1. The chordal eminence, which surrounds the iter chordae posticus where the chorda tympani nerve enters the tympanum.
2. The pyramidal eminence housing the stapedius muscle and permitting its tendon to emerge into the tympanum and insert itself on the neck of the stapes.
3. The styloid protuberance of Politzer,[9] which is the blunt projection of the styloid body into the posterior tympanum immediately below the round window niche. It represents the anterolateral bulk of the styloid complex.

The intratemporal portion of the styloid bone is covered anteriorly and laterally by the vaginal process of the tympanic bone. Medially and posteriorly, it articulates with the petrosa.

The styloid process is developed from the proximal part of the cartilage of the second branchial or hyoid arch by two centers—one for the proximal part, the *tympanohyoid*, appears before birth, the other, comprising the rest of the process, is called the *stylohyoid* and does not appear until after birth. The tympanic ring unites with the squama shortly before birth, the petromastoid part and squama join during the first year, and the tympanohyoid portion of the styloid process does so about the same time. The stylohyoid does not unite with the rest of the bone until after puberty—and in some skulls never at all.

4 Cavities of the Temporal Bone

Bony External Canal

The external auditory canal is formed by the squama and tympanic bones. The bony canal varies considerably in shape and size. It is placed horizontally, with the orientation inward and a little forward. This cylindrical canal can be described as having four walls and two orifices.

Anterior Wall

The anterior wall of the external auditory canal is formed entirely by the tympanic bone. Frequent variations of the length of the tympanic bone entail corresponding variations of the anterior wall of the external auditory canal.

This wall is sometimes perforated in its midportion. It is concave in the vertical plane. In the horizontal plane, it can be convex or straight.

Inferior Wall

The inferior wall of the external auditory canal is represented by the bottom of the tympanic gutter (see Fig. 11). It is concave from front to back. In the horizontal plane, it can be slightly convex or smooth and straight in this same direction.

Posterior Wall

The external auditory canal is formed behind by a tympanosquamosal wall (see Fig. 1). It is tympanic in its inferomedial part, where it corresponds to the posterior slope of the tympanic gutter, and is squamosal in its superior and external part, which corresponds to the anterior zone of the retromeatal part of the squama. The tympanosquamosal fissure marks the superior and external extremity of the posterior tympanosquamosal suture. This wall, concave from above downward, is straight or slightly convex in the transverse direction.

Superior Wall

The superior wall of the external auditory meatus is concave in the horizontal and anteroposterior directions. It is completely squamosal, corresponding to the posterior part of the horizontal portion of the squama.

This wall is completely absent in the newborn, except for its more internal part. The horizontal portion of the squama is a structure peculiar to adults. It does not exist at birth, and appears progressively in the infant as the growth of the brain causes a transverse growth of the base of the cranium.

External Orifice

The external orifice of the external auditory canal is well marked out anteriorly and inferiorly by the external rim of the tympanic gutter (see Fig. 11). On the squamosal portion of the external meatus, the superior and posterior walls continue gradually onto the neighboring part of the squama.

Internal Orifice

The bottom of the external auditory canal is clearly indicated by a groove—*tympanic groove* or *sulcus tympanicus*—belonging to the tympanic bone (see Fig. 13). The sulcus tympanicus does not describe a complete circle. Posteriorly, it stops at the summit of the posterior slope of the tympanic gutter. Anteriorly, it continues up to the point where the superior border of the tympanic bone crosses the inner rim of the squama.

This groove, which is generally distinct, is less marked at its two extremities. Posteriorly, it may be concealed by the posterior tympanic spine and inward-curving portion of the tympanic bone placed immediately lateral.

The deep orifice of the external meatus is indicated in the greater portion of its circumference by the sulcus tympanicus of the tympanic bone. Only the superior segment

39

of this orifice is formed by the squama, which is represented at this level by the inferior free part of its internal edge (internal border of its horizontal portion).

The internal orifice has a complex orientation. It is directed down, out and forward. Vertical cuts through the bone show it very oblique below and inward. The angles determined by the plane of this orifice and the two superior and inferior walls are very different. Above, the angle is large and strongly obtuse; below, it is narrow, very acute, and reduced further by the convexity of the inferior wall. The obliquity of the internal orifice is of the same direction as that of the external orifice of this canal, but it is much more accentuated.

Horizontal cuts also demonstrate the obliquity of the internal orifice. The angle is obtuse posteriorly and very acute anteriorly. Thus, the length of the canal walls is unequal. The anterior becomes the larger wall and the posterior is the smaller wall. The posterosuperior quadrant of the drumhead is the most accessible one; the anteroinferior quadrant is least accessible.

Middle Ear

The middle ear is formed by the union of the four constituents of the temporal bone. A longitudinal cut along the anterior border of the petrosa and parallel to the plane of the drumhead gives a good view of the entire middle ear cleft. Three main divisions are recognized: the eustachian tube, the tympanum, and the petrous antrum.

The Tympanic Cavity

External Wall

The external or tympanic wall of the tympanum is made up, in large part, by the deep orifice of the external auditory canal. The wall is much smaller in front of the canal orifice, as well as below. Superiorly, however, this wall angulates laterally and is relatively large. The wall is formed in front and below by the tympanic bone, above and in front by this bone and the petrosa, and above by the squama.

1. The squama is represented by its inner border.
2. The petrosa is represented by the inferior prolongation of the tegmen tympani (anterior).
3. The tympanic bone is represented in front and below by its posterior surface, adjoining the sulcus tympanicus, and above by a portion of its superior border, indicated by the crest of the mallear gutter.

The inferior prolongation of the tegmen tympani, projecting above the superior border of the tympanic bone, transforms the mallear gutter into an important canal for the passage of:

1. The chorda tympani nerve for a short part of its course.
2. The anterior tympanic artery and veins.
3. The anterior mallear ligament.

This canal, whose posterior or tympanic orifice (see Fig. 32) is bordered externally by the posterior tympanic spine (which is always clearly visible), opens anteriorly at the level of the posterior branch of the Glaserian fissure (see Fig.14).

Internal Wall

The internal or labyrinthine wall of the tympanum (see Figs. 24, 47, 48) is more extensive behind than in front. The oval window divides this wall into two parts. The inferior part is opposite the deep orifice of the external auditory canal, and is directly explorable through this canal. The superior, less extensive part is opposite the external wall of the tympanum, which is above the level of the deep orifice of the external auditory canal. Thus, it is not directly visible through this canal.

The *oval window* has three concave borders—superior, external and internal. The inferior window is straight or convex, thus giving the oval window a kidney shape. It is directly down, forward, and outward. Its great axis is more often oblique downwards and outwards.

The inferior part of the internal wall, in its midportion, is raised to form the *promontory*. Grooves are often seen on the promontory for the branches of Jacobson's nerve. These grooves converge below, towards the upper opening of the canal of Jacobson. On occasion, instead of grooves, one may find shallow tunnels of bone ascending the promontory to transmit these nerves.

The promontory, limited above and behind by the oval window, is confined below and behind by the orifice of entrance into a niche—the *round window niche*, which quickly leads to the round window. A ridge of bone runs from the posterior lip of the round window niche to the styloid eminence (subiculum). Another ridge of bone extends from the pyramidal eminence to the inferior margin of the oval window niche (ponticulus). Between the two ridges lies the sinus tympani (infrapyramidal fossette), which varies greatly in size. It may extend as far posteriorly as the bony posterior vertical semicircular canal. Above the ponticulus and, at times, as far superior as the horizontal semicircular canal is the posterior tympanic sinus. At times, there is no ponticulus present. There results a large cavity made up of the combined sinus tympani and the posterior tympanic sinus. These recesses are important to recognize at surgery. Should they be involved with cholesteatoma, they may not be removed completely enough to control progression of the disease.

The inferior part of the internal wall of the tympanum contains a canal superiorly and anteriorly that is often incompletely closed on its outer side—the *canal for the tensor tympani muscle* (see Fig. 24). It runs obliquely medial and inferior. It is placed immediately below the tegmen tympani, but separates from it on approaching the oval window. As soon as it reaches the anterior edge of the oval window, it curves externally and forms the *processus cochleariformis* (Greek for spoon-shaped). Internally, this canal ends at the level of the angle formed by the squama and the petrosa.

The superior part of the internal wall of the tympanum is marked by two superimposed projections. The inferior prominence runs obliquely below and behind as the *second portion of the facial canal*. It follows the superior edge of the oval window, often overlapping it. This fact, plus the promontory below, creates an oval window niche. The bone covering the second portion of the facial canal may be dehiscent, so that the facial nerve itself may reach the stapedial crura. Above the facial canal, we can often see a groove separating it from the prominence directly above.

Above the facial canal, we find the smooth prominence of the external or horizontal semicircular canal. Compact, thick, and strong, this wall is very different from that of the facial canal, which is thin, fragile, and at times dehiscent.

Superior Wall

The superior or cranial wall, oblique below and in front and also medially (see Fig. 25) is formed by the tegmen tympani, which projects laterally and anteriorly from the petrosa to articulate with the squama. Posteriorly, where the tegmen tympani does not articulate with the superior portion of the inner edge of the horiztonal part of the squama, the junction of the superior and lateral walls of the tympanum forms the petrosquamosal suture. Anteriorly, however, this junction is formed by the inferior prolongation of the tegmen tympani and of the tegmen itself. The superior wall is thin and sometimes dehiscent, so that cerebral tissue is in contact with the tympanm.

Inferior Wall

The inferior or jugular wall is very variable and runs obliquely forward and slightly inferior. It is entirely petrous, and separates the tympanum from the jugular dome below. The wall may be very thick, or it may be very thin and convex. In the newborn, this wall is very thin and, at times, dehiscent. The floor thickens with growth, with the degree of thickening depending on the development of the jugular bulb. It would be very thin and even dehiscent if the jugular bulb bulges into the interior of the tympanum, or it becomes very thick if the bulb remains distant from the tympanum. The inferior wall is usually covered over with bony trabeculations running from medial to lateral (Figs. 49-53), which makes it irregular and can obscure its convexity.

Posterior Wall

The posterior or mastoid wall of the tympanum can be considered completely closed by irregularly but systematically shaped bone up to the level of the pyramidal eminence. Above this level and anteriorly lies the attic, and directly above the pyramidal eminence lies the aditus ad antrum. The wall lies between the annulus tympanicus and the medially places labyrinthine capsule.

Embryology.   The posterior bony wall of the tympanum is derived from the second branchial arch, which contains

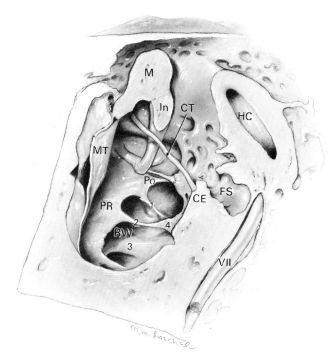

Figure 50.   A posterolateral view of the posterior tympanum in an adult showing a bony bridge (2), which indicates that the styloid eminence (4) was once in direct contact with the bony labyrinth. A ridge (3) across the floor of the round window niche (*RW*) is also indicative of the former close relationship. Note the position of the facial sinus (*FS*). *CE,* Chordal eminence. *PO,* Ponticulus extending from promontory (*PR*) to the pyramidal eminence. *CT,* Chorda tympani nerve. *HC,* Horizontal semicircular canal. *MT,* tympanic membrane. *M,* malleus. *IN,* Incus and VII descending facial nerve. The sinus tympani lies between the ponticulus (PO) and the subiculum (1).

Reichert's cartilage as its skeletal support. Coursing on its posteromedial surface is the nerve of the second arch (facial nerve).

Examination and dissection of the fetuses shows Reichert's cartilage extending up to the posterior aspect of the oval window. It is easily separated from both the cartilaginous labyrinth, and the cartilaginous annulus tympanicus (Fig. 54). The tympanic membrane in a six- to nine month-old fetus is nearly the size of an adult tympanic membrane,[16] and it is nearly in a horizontal plane (15° to 25°) (Fig. 55). It lies under the relatively large cartilaginous labyrinth, and is separated from it by a narrow band of gelatinous material containing the primitive endothelium, that is to line the future tympanum and its viscera.

Subsequently during childhood, the neck grows at a more rapid pace compared to the skull, so that the inferior portion of the drum rotates outward, enlarging the hypotympanum, while the mastoid is pulled down and out by the growth of th sternomastoid muscle. This growth pattern facilitates the expansion into the middle ear cleft of the endothelial-lined pouch originating from the primitive eustachian tube. Evidences in the adult of this middle ear

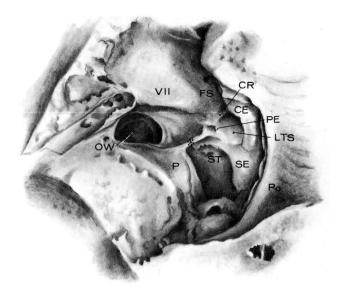

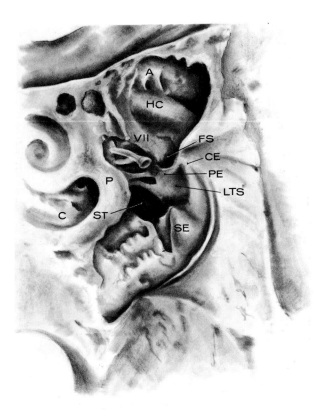

Figure 51.   View of the posterior tympanum with a ponticulus (*) separating a large posterior tympanic sinus above from the sinus tympani (*ST*) below. The pyramidal eminence (*PE*) is short. The stapedial tendon would be very long, and the facial canal is descending at a point more posterior than normal. The lateral tympanic sinus (*LTS*) is shallow and lies between the three eminences (pyramidal [*PE*], styloid [*SE*], and chordal [*CE*]). The facial sinus (*FS*) lies between the facial canal and the chordal ridge (*CR*). *OW*, Oval window. *P*, Promontory, with prominent sulcus promontori for Jacobson's nerve.

Figure 52.   The posterior tympanum viewed from in front and slightly lateral. Note the area concamerata lying between the styloid eminence and the round window niche. Its ridges are directed sagittally. The styloid complex (pyramidal eminence [*PE*], styloid eminence [*SE*], and chordal eminence [*CE*], with its lateral tympanic sinus (*LTS*), is quite distinct. The sinus tympani (*ST*) is large, and extends upward beneath the two bony bridges between the pyramidal eminence and promontory (*P*) to reach the facial canal. *FS*, Facial sinus. *VII*, Facial canal. *HC*, Horizontal canal. *A*, Antrum. *C*, Cochlea.

cleft-widening process are seen in Figures 47, 50 and (1) the various bony ridges, which always cross the floor of the hypotympanum from a medial to a lateral position; (2) the subiculum, which persists from the styloid eminence to the posterior lip of the round window niche; (3) the ponticulus, which extends as a ridge or bridge from the pyramidal eminence to the promontory immediately below the oval window niche; and (4) bony bridges from the styloid complex to the promontory.

The outward rotation of the bony inferior portion of the annulus tympanicus plus the expanding endothelial pouches are accompanied by changes in the contour of Reichert's cartilage and its eventual conversion to form the ossified posterior tympanic wall (Fig. 56). Reichert's cartilage is the skeletal portion of the second branchial arch. The entire second arch structure, composed of cartilage plus other arch mesodermal structures, can be referred to as the *styloid complex*.[5] The antrum and mastoid air cell system develop by passage of the saccus superior of the primitive eustachian tube up and over the styloid complex to form that portion of the mastoid derived from the pars squamosa.[4] The saccus medius extends posteriorly above the saccus superior to eventually pneumatize that portion of the mastoid derived from the pars petrosa. It is extremely rare for pneumatization of the mastoid to occur at a lower level by way of the sinus tympani.

The Adult Morphology.   The upper portion of the second branchial arch or styloid complex eventually ossifies to form three permanent projections that can be seen in all adult temporal bones: (1) the pyramidal eminence; (2) the styloid eminence; and (3) the chordal eminence.

Sinuses of the Posterior Tympanic Wall.   Sinuses of the posterior tympanum are related to the remnants of this second branchial arch (styloid complex). They are formed by the abutting of the primitive pouches against solid cartilaginous or bony walls. They are: (1) sinus tympani; (2) lateral tympanic sinus; (3) posterior tympanic sinus; and (4) facial sinus.

The sinus tympani lies in the posterior tympanum between the labyrinthine capsule and the styloid complex (Fig. 56). It is limited above by bone around the facial canal and by the dense bony capsule around the lateral semicircular canal. Posteriorly, it is contained by the dense capsule around the posterior vertical canal (Fig. 57). Inferiorly,

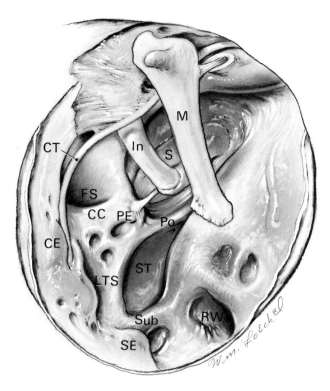

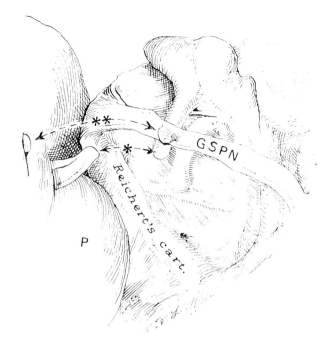

Figure 53. A view into the posterior tympanum laterally and slightly anteriorly. The round window niche (*RW*) has, at its margins, a thick tegmen and thick postis posterior to which are attached a heavy subiculum (*SUB*). The lateral tympanic sinus (*LTS*) contains three large bony pits. The ponticulus extends from the inferior aspect of the pyramidal eminence (*PE*) to the promontory edge below the oval window. *SE,* Styloid eminence. *CE,* Chordal eminence. *CC,* Chordal crest or ridge. *FS,* Facial sinus. *CT,* Chorda tympani nerve. *IN,* Incus. *M,* Malleus. *S,* Stapes.

Figure 54. Fetus at approximately 10 weeks gestation. The tympanum is forcibly opened anteriorly. The annulus tympanicus and ossicles were rotated outward. The facial nerve was cut at the genu (**) and the incus separated from the stapes (*). Reichert's cartilage is closely wedged between the cartilaginous annulus tympanicus and the cartilaginous labyrinth. *GSPN,* Greater superficial petrosal nerve. *P,* Promontory.

the sinus is limited by the bony ridge between the styloid eminence and bony labyrinth (subiculum) (Fig. 58) and, to a variable degree, by the jugular wall.

In many specimens, there is a bony or membranous ridge or bridge (ponticulus) from pyramid to promontory, which would divide this space into a larger inferior sinus (sinus tympani) and a somewhat smaller sinus superiorly known as the posterior tympanic sinus (Fig. 51).

In the interval between the three eminences of the styloid complex lies a shallow, superficially placed sinus that has been known for some time as the lateral tympanic sinus (see Figs. 48, 51, 52).

Behind the styloid complex—and between it and the descending facial canal—lies the facial sinus (Figs. 48-51). The facial sinus appears to develop as a result of the method by which membrane bone has divided the primordial facial canal (of the 21-week-old fetus) into the definitive canal and a cul de sac situated between the membrane bone and Reichert's cartilage. This process may be facilitated by the widening of the middle ear cleft.

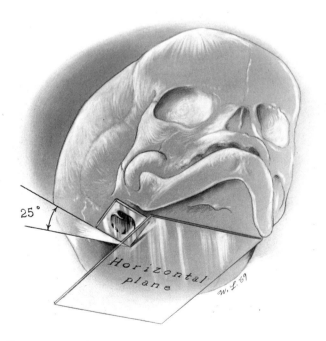

Figure 55. At the time of birth, the tympanic membrane and annulus fibrosus are a 25° angle from the horizontal plane. With development of the middle ear cleft and sternomastoid and splenicus capitus muscles attached to the temporal bone, there is an outward rotation of the drumhead from 25° to approximately 80° with the horizontal plane.

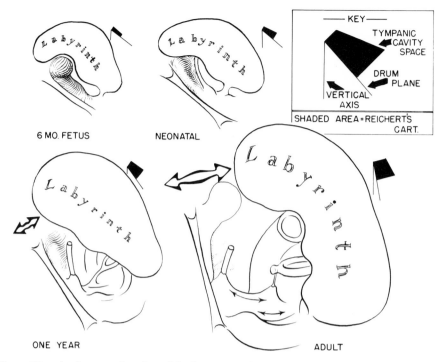

Figure 56. A schema to show lateral displacement and rotation of the tympanic ring away from the labyrinth with growth of the neck. The second arch structure (Reichert's cartilage) forms the posterior tympanic wall. Evidence of this movement with growth can be seen in the configuration of the posterior tympanic wall. As the second branchial arch is stretched laterally in the process, the three eminences (styloid, pyramidal, and chordal) develop.

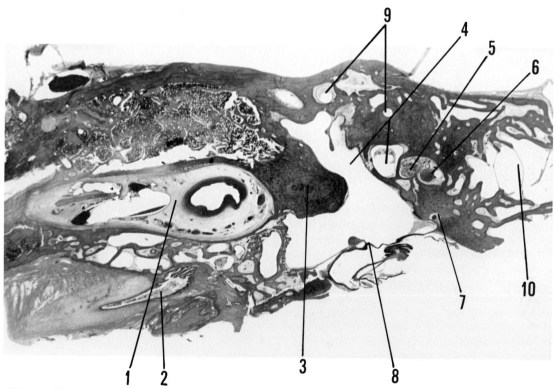

Figure 57. Horizontal histologic section of a temporal bone showing relationships of the third part of the facial canal just below its second turn. 1, Carotid canal. 2, Eustachian tube. 3, Base of cochlea. 4, Sinus tympani. 5, Stapedius muscle. 6, Facial nerve. 7, Chorda tympani nerve. 8, Umbo. 9, Posterior semicircular canal. 10, Mastoid antrum. Note the dense bone of the styloid complex lateral to the facial nerve and the dense bony labyrinth medial to it.

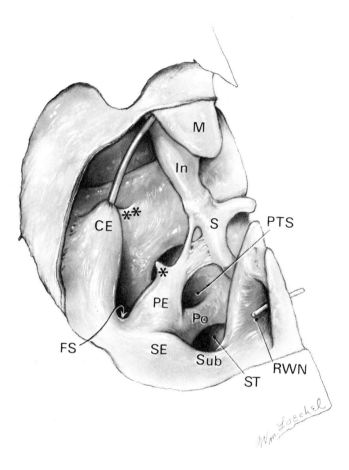

Figure 58. View into the posterior tympanum looking upward and medially. The chordal eminence (*CE*) is very prominent. A ridge extends from it to the facial canal (**). The chordal ridge can hardly be distinguished. A stump of a chordal bridge (*) can be seen on the pyramidal eminence. The facial sinus (*FS*) extends downward along the course of the descending facial canal. A thick ponticulus (*PO*) is present, which separates the posterior tympanic sinus (*PTS*) from the sinus tympani (*ST*). The subiculum (*SUB*) is seen extending from the styloid eminence (*SE*) to the posterior lip of the round window niche. Bristles pass through the round window membrane (*RWN*).

Bony Ridges of the Styloid Complex.   Between the three eminences of the styloid complex, one can distinguish three ridges. These are best seen when the lateral tympanic sinus is well formed (see Figs. 48, 51, 52). The most prominent ridge and occasional bridge extends from the chordal eminence to the facial canal (see Fig. 52). This structure will be referred to as the chordal ridge: Posterior to it lies the facial sinus. A slight bony ridge extends from the chordal eminence to the styloid eminence (styloid ridge), and a third from the styloid eminence to the pyramid (pyramidal ridge).

Other bony ridges extend from the styloid complex to the bony labyrinth. A prominent ridge extends from the styloid eminence to the posterior lip of the round window niche and is called the subiculum. It limits the sinus tympani inferiorly. There may be several bony ridges from the

styloid eminence to the floor of the round window niche, and even bridges to the lip of the promontory directly above (see Figs. 47, 51).

Finally, a ridge is often seen extending from the pyramidal eminence to the promontory. It is often a bony bridge, so that this structure has been termed the *ponticulus* (see Figs. 48, 50).

Practical Considerations.   If the posterior bony canal wall is preserved in surgery for chronic middle ear disease, one must always be sure that the mastoid cells can easily obtain air from the tympanum. This air flow can occur through the anterior or posterior tympanic isthmuses.[4] If these are obliterated, it may be possible to establish air flow by one of several means: (1) by removal of the tensor fold when the attic is large or when the malleus head is missing or has been removed; (2) by removal of the incus body and short crus, leaving the long crus attached to the stapes (enlarging the posterior tympanic isthmus)[4]; or (3) by creating a facial recess from the mastoid through the interval between the descending facial canal and the chorda tympani nerve into the posterior tympanum.

When the temporal bone is small and not well pneumatized, all three means of improving aeration may be undertaken. In the small temporal bones, the bony annulus tympanicus may lie closer to the labyrinthine capsule, so that the surgically created facial recess can be very narrow, which makes for a difficult dissection.

In chronic middle ear disorders, the facial sinus is always found to contain pathologic tissues. Failure to clear the disease from the facial sinus in a radical or modified radical mastoidectomy will result in continued discharge and crusting of the facial ridge in the posterior tympanum; in tympanoplasty procedures, it is a frequent cause of failure. Numerous dissections have failed to show any communication between the facial sinus and the mastoid cells. It was noted that the facial sinus often extends down to the level of emergence of the chorda tympani nerve from the facial nerve. When approached from behind, this sinus is found directly lateral to the descending facial canal (Figs. 58-60). It is an important landmark for guidance to the facial nerve in this area. Confidence in the knowledge of this anatomy makes it possible to open the facial canal, where it lies immediately medial to the facial sinus. The course of the facial canal across the tympanum is an excellent guide for the position of the facial canal at the beginning of this descending segment. This is a faster and safer exposure than the digastric exposure of the facial nerve. It is often possible to remove the bony cover over the facial nerve up to the geniculate ganglion without displacing the incus, once the facial recess is opened. Further exposure can be obtained, when necessary, by cutting the posterior incudal ligament and elevating the short process, taking care not to injure or displace the stapes.

If the sinus tympani must be explored, the anterior approach via the meatus must be used. Both the pyramidal eminence and the components of the styloid complex may require extensive removal. In some temporal bones, removal of bone anterior to the descending facial canal

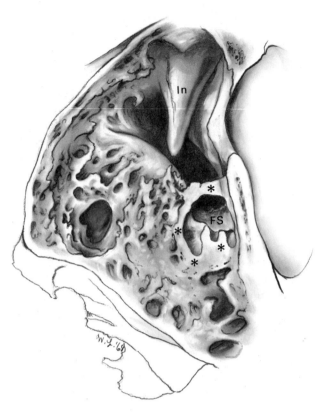

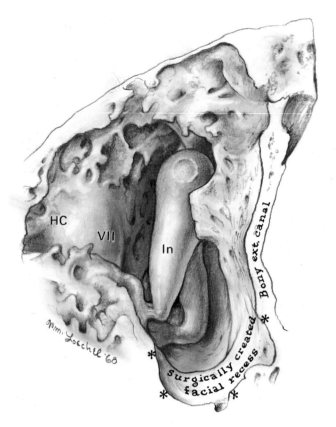

Figure 59.   Creation of the facial recess for improved ventilation between tympanum and mastoid. The facial sinus does not communicate with the mastoid cells. A bony portion must be removed (****) to gain access to the facial sinus from behind. The incus has not been disturbed.

Figure 60.   The facial recess between the descending facial canal and the bony annulus has been created to give wider access directly into the tympanum, thus bypassing ventilation through the attic and the anterior and posterior tympanic isthmi.

may fail to expose the full limits of this sinus; and in such an event, additional retrofacial dissection may be effective in removal of diseased tissue, particularly cholesteatoma. Care must be taken to avoid opening the posterior vertical canal or injuring the facial nerve.

The Anterior Wall

The anterior (tubocarotid) wall contains an orifice in its superior part—the posterior orifice of the eustachian tube. Below, the anterior wall is often bulging due to the presence of the carotid canal. The internal carotid artery is separated from the tympanum by a wall that is usually thin and sometimes dehiscent. This wall is usually perforated with several minute openings for passage of the carotico–tympanic vessels into the tympanic plexus. Beside the arteries and veins, sympathetic fibers pass through these openings to the tympanic plexus from the superior cervical ganglion. The anterior wall may be thick and covered by bony trabeculae or pneumatic cells. The latter may be confined to the interval between the carotid canal and tubal lumen (peritubal cells), or they may develop between the cochlear capsule and the carotid canal in its

horizontal portion to reach into the petrous apex. This anterior wall is formed entirely from the petrosa.

The Attic

The attic (*recessus epitympanicus*) is limited medially by the superior portion of the internal wall of the tympanum (overlying the oval window), externally by the free portion of the internal border of the squama, and above by the tegmen tympani. It contains the greater part of two ossicles of hearing—the *malleus* and *incus*—and presents three important relationships aside from the facial nerve: posteriorly with the petrous antrum, above with the brain, and externally with the external auditory canal.

The tegmen tympani is a thin wall that is transparent at times and even dehiscent. It often presents bony trabeculae, which may be developed enough to present actual air cells. These cells communicate not only with the tympanum, but even with neighboring cells: (1) periantral cells posteriorly; (2) perilabyrinthine cells medially; and (3) cells of the superior wall of the external meatus externally.

The external wall of the attic is oblique below and inwards. It forms a very acute angle with the superior wall of

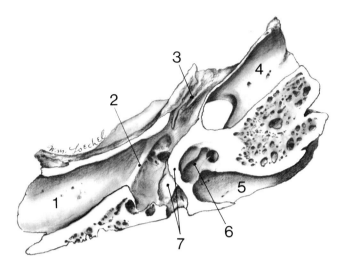

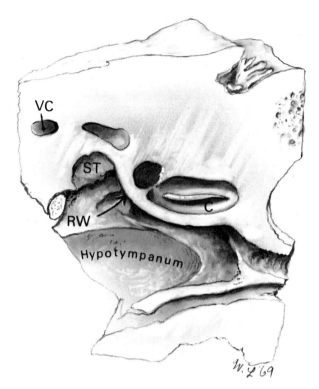

Figure 61. Horizontal cut—inferior segment. 1, External auditory canal. 2, Sulcus tympanicus. 3, Eustachian tube. 4, Carotid canal. 5, Internal auditory meatus. 6, Cochlea. 7, Promontary (posterior segment—tegmen of round window niche.)

Figure 62. Horizontal section. A view into the basal coil of the cochlea (C) and the hypotympanum. Note the position of the sinus tympani (ST) between the round window niche (RW) and the descending facial nerve. The sinus tympani is limited posteriorly by the dense bony capsule surrounding the inferior curvature of the posterior vertical semicircular canal (VC).

the external auditory canal, which has been termed the *scutum* by the anatomist Leidy of the University of Pennsylvania. The scutum may be very thin if it is well pneumatized, and may erode with extended disease processes to open directly into the meatus.

The Hypotympanic Sinus

The hypotympanic sinus occurs where the external (tympanic) wall and the inferior (petrosal) wall of the tympanum meet (Figs. 61–63). It is closed in front and behind by the anterior and posterior walls of this cavity. It is absent when the tympanic bone and petrosa meet at the level of the tympanic sulcus. The further away from the sulcus tympanicus that this suture occurs, the greater the size of the hypotympanic sinus. In many cases, the hypotympanic sinus appears as a hollow diverticulum in the petrosa that is directed downward toward the jugular bulb, or down and out under the inferior wall of the external meatus.

This sinus is the lowest point in the tympanum. Numerous trabeculae or cells may make this region very irregular. Necrosis of bony walls will endanger the jugular bulb below and the internal carotid artery in front.

The walls of this sinus may be very thin and, at times, dehiscent. The jugular bulb may be uncovered in the floor of the tympanum and likely to be injured in the course of a myringotomy.

Petrous Antrum

The petrous antrum constitutes the posterior part of the middle ear. Situated behind and outside the tympanum, it

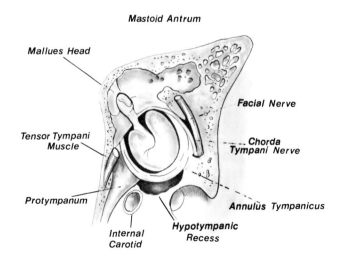

Figure 63. Lateral schema of tympanum showing the position of the hypotympanic recess or sinus.

is variable in its form and dimensions. It is limited externally by the squama, which represents its surgical wall. Elsewhere, it is hollowed out at the expense of the petrosa.

Above, it is separated from the cranial cavity by the tegmen antri, which may be thin or contain cells. Medially and anteriorly, we find the prominence of the horizontal semicircular canal. The bone surrounding the antrum may be diploic (spongy tissue), pneumatic (air cells), or pneumodiploic.

The antrum is related below to the cerebellar wall of the petrosa (posterosuperior wall), posteriorly to the lateral sinus, externally to the squamosal surface of the mastoid region, and superiorly to the cerebrum. The antrum varies considerably in size. In the small sclerotic mastoid with little or no pneumatization, it can be quite small. When pneumatization is extensive, it can be voluminous. The spine of Henle and the position of the linea temporalis above help to mark the position of the antrum on the surface. In pneumatization, the growth of the mastoid air cells is directed posteroinferiorly from the antrum.

Aditus ad Antrum

The petrous antrum opens anteriorly at the level of the superior part of the tympanum (attic) by a narrow passage— the *aditus ad antrum*.[17] The superior wall of the aditus blends imperceptibly with the tegmen tympani in front and the tegmen antri behind. The external wall of the aditus is formed by the squama. On its internal wall can be seen the prominence of the horizontal semicircular canal. The inferior wall varies in width, but it is the top of the styloid complex, with its small articular facet for the reception of the short process of the incus. The inferior wall is relative with the terminal part of the second portion of the facial canal, which lies on the posteromedial aspect of the styloid complex. The facial nerve is injured at surgery most often in the region immediately below the floor of the aditus ad antrum.

The Attic (recessus epitympanicus)

The attic is bounded superiorly by the roof-like tegmen tympani, medially by the prominence of the lateral semicircular canal and the prominence of the facial canal, laterally by the scutum (the free portion of the internal border of the squama), posteriorly by the fossa of the incus and the irregular bony surface just behind it, and inferiorly by the tympanic diaphragm. It contains the greater part of the two ossicles (malleus and incus), and presents three important relations besides the facial canal:

1. Posteriorly with the petrous antrum.
2. Above with the brain;
3. Externally with the external auditory canal.

The *tegmen tympani* is a thin wall that is sometimes transparent and even perforated. Very often, it presents bony trabeculi developed enough, in certain cases, to form

actual air cells. The latter are not only in communication with the tympanum, but even with the neighboring cells:

1. Periantral cells behind.
2. Perilabyrinthine cells medially.
3. Cells of the superior wall of the external auditory canal externally.

The *internal or medial wall* of the attic is more extensive posteriorly. The canal for the tensor tympani muscle and the processus cochleariformis form the lower limit of the attic. The tensor canal detaches from the tegmen posteriorly, while directing itself toward the oval window to form the processus cochleariformis.

The internal wall of the attic has two superimposed projections:

1. The more inferior projection is an oblique prominence below and behind that is the second part of the facial canal. It follows the superior circumference of the oval window, while often overlapping it toward the base.
2. Above, it is separated by a groove from the lateral semicircular canal that is compact, thick, and strong in contrast with the thin, fragile, and often dehiscent bone of the facial canal.

The attic may be divided into a lateral and medial compartment along its entire length when the petrosquamosal suture is deformed by overgrowth of the petrosal tegmen over the squamosal tegmen, forcing the latter downward into the tympanum (see Figs. 31, 44, 45).

The *anterior wall* of the attic quickly narrows as the tegmen tympani drops at an acute angle down to the level of the tympanic diaphragm,[17] which is attached to the tensor canal. Often, the tensor fold does not develop fully due to extension of the saccus anticus in the fetal stage past the tensor canal up to the tegmen. This forms a supratubal recess in direct contact with the mesotympanum. In such cases, an anterior attic compartment is not present.

A partial or complete bony septum occurs in a plane transverse to the long axis of the epitympanum (mallear plate). A bony niche lying in the medial wall of the anterior attic was described by Wigand and Trillsch[13] in 1973, who called it the *epitympanic sinus*. I termed this the *geniculate sinus*. It may be dehiscent over the geniculate ganglion— hazard of injury to the facial nerve with surgery in this sinus. Nonlamellar new bone formation in the anterior attic recess was reported by Hawke et al.[18] in 1975. They felt that this was a normal feature of this portion of the epitympanum. They speculated that inflammatory diseases could provoke the development of a bony bar enclosing the ossicles or bridging the attic.

Attention has been called to the transverse *mallear plate* by Gacek.[19] It is an excellent landmark for locating the geniculate ganglion, which lies medial to this plate and forms a part of the facial canal at this point.

Posterior atticotomy is designed to improve aeration of the mastoid from the eustachian tube across the length of the attic. Diseased mucosa and cholesteatoma must be removed. The transverse mallear plate is removed to open into the supratubal recess. Pathology must be removed from the geniculate sinus. If a tensor is present, it is removed.

Aeration of the mastoid region through the mesotympanum to the eustachian tube is obtained by removing bone between the tympanic ring and the descending facial canal (Figs. 64-67)—a *posterior mesotympanotomy*—which improves exposure of the sinus tympani, round window niche, and hypotympanum. Preservation of this route in the post surgical period requires judicious use of a plastic (silastic) sheeting to prevent stenosis and the development of retracting pockets, adhesive otitis media, and recurrent cholesteatoma.

Anteriorly on the lateral wall, the petrosal tegmen passes beneath the horizontal squama to form the petrosal hernia in the Glaserian fissure. Beneath the hernia, we find the tympanic bone, which at this level forms the spine of Henle (the mallear crest), and the anterior and posterior tympanic spines (see Fig. 32). Here, we also see the sulcus mallearis for the anterior mallear ligament, tympanic artery and veins, and chorda tympani.

Laterally, the attic extends over the horizontal part of the squama to form the scutum of Leidy over the bony external auditory meatus. Thus, it projects itself entirely on the superior wall of the bony external auditory meatus so that an attic abscess can open directly into the meatus.

Posteriorly on the lateral wall, the tegmen of the retromeatal part of the squama contacts the petrosal tegmen

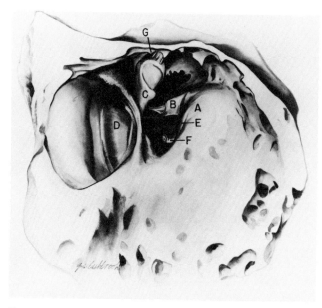

Figure 65 Posterior atticotomy. Bone is removed down to the floor of the fossa incudis. The incus has been removed. C, Malleus. F, Stapes, A, Horizontal semicircular canal. E, Facial canal. B, Processus cochleariformis. D, Tympanic membrane. G, Superior mallear ligament. Note the transverse attic septum in its position anterior to the malleus head.

at the internal petrosquamosal fissure, and it extends further posteriorly up to near the level of the aditus.

Petrosal Antrum

A posterolateral extension of the attic constitutes the posterior part of the middle ear. Located behind and outside the tympanum, it is variable in form and size. It is limited externally by the squama, which represents its surgical wall. It is hollowed out elsewhere at the expense of the petrosa. Superiorly, it is very close to the brain—from which it is separated by the tegmen antri, which is thin or else covered with cells like those found at the tympanic level. Medially and anteriorly, we see the prominence of the lateral semicircular canal. Elsewhere, it is surrounded by bone tissue of the mastoid (diploic, pneumatic, or pneumatic-diploic).

The antrum with adjacent diploic or pneumatic bone corresponds below to the cerebellar wall of the petrosa (posterosuperior wall), posteriorly to the lateral sinus, and externally to the squamosal surface of the mastoid region.

The spine of Henle marks its position well on the external surface of the temporal bone. The mastoid region corresponds to the antrum in only a small part of its extent. The latter is placed at its anterosuperior part.

Aditus ad Antrum

The petrous antrum opens anteriorly at the level of the superior part of the tympanum (attic) by a narrow part—the *aditus ad antrum*.[17]

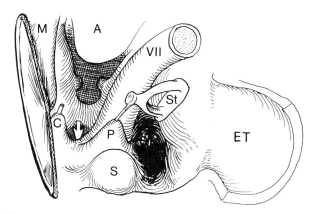

Figure 64. A schema of the posterior or mastoid wall of the tympanum. It lies between the tympanic bone and the labyrinth, and is of second-arch origin (styloid). The facial nerve, also being of second-arch origin, is in intimate association with the styloid portion of the temporal bone. The styloid eminence (S) projects into the posterior tympanum. Two other eminences of bone surround second arch structures: the chordal eminence (C) and the pyramidal eminence (P). A bony ridge passes between the chordal and pyramidal eminences (chordal ridge), and behind it (arrow) lies the facial sinus, which follows the facial nerve to the point of emergence of the chorda tympani nerve. Above and posterior is the fossa incudis with the bifid posterior incudal ligament. A, Antrum. M, Malleus handle. S, Stapes. ST, Sinus tympani. ET, Eustachian tube orifice.

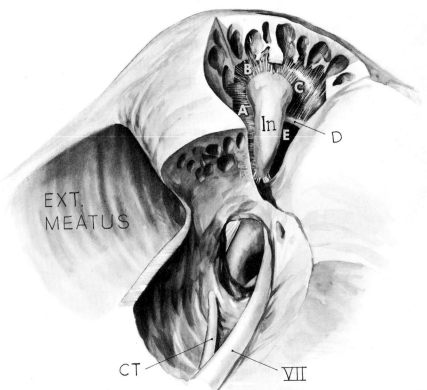

Figure 66. The lower control window of Wullstein for exploration of the posterior tympanum. The creation of this window can result in much improved ventilation of the mastoid air cell system. The window also makes possible a more direct view into the round window niche to ascertain mobility of the round window membrane. This is usually done by seeking light reflex movements of fluid in the niche itself when the stapes is moved. The window is made in the interval between the chorda tympani nerve (*CT*) and the descending portion of the facial nerve (*VII*). Note that the lateral incudal fold (*A*), lateral mallear fold (*B*), and superior mallear fold (*C*) limit access to the mesotympanum via the anterior tympanic isthmus (*E*) above. This lies between the stapes head and the tendon of the tensor tympani (*D*).

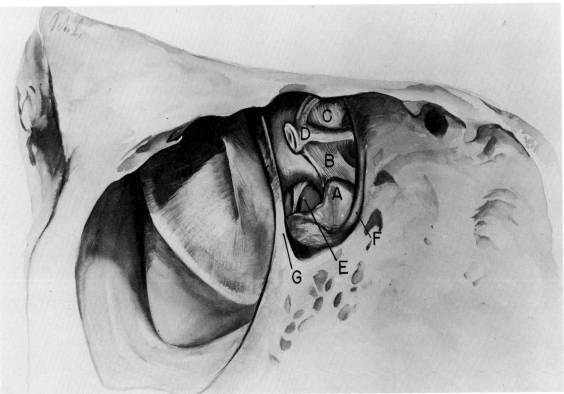

Figure 67. Posterior atticotomy. Dissection showing stapes at the floor of the fossa incudis. This allows good control of the attic (posterior atticotomy). If the heavy bone is dissected downward between the bony external meatal wall and the descending (third part) facial canal, we begin exposure of the mesotympanum below the tympanic diaphragm (posterior tympanotomy). In this view, the dissecting microscope is tilted inferiorly. A, Pyramidal eminence. B, Plica stapedis and stapedial tendon. C, Membrane obtoraturia. D, Stapes head. E, Sinus tympani. F, Facial canal. G, Annulus tympanicus.

The superior wall of the aditus corresponds to the tegmen tympani in such a way that they pass imperceptibly, following the inferior surface of this tegmen from the superior wall of the petrous antrum to that of the tympanum.

Externally, the external wall of the aditus is like that at the level of the antrum and the attic formed by the squama. Internally, on the internal wall, one again finds the prominence of the external semicircular canal, which extends from the highest part of the tympanum to the level of the petrous antrum. Finally, the inferior wall below, varying in cases, occasionally presents a small articular facet for the incus. This interior wall is in relation (and more often at a distance) with the terminal part of the second portion of the *facial canal* (more internal than the aditus).

Of the three parts of the middle ear, the tympanum is the only one formed by all four components of the temporal bone. It is petrosquamostylotympanic, whereas the antrum is petrosquamosal and the eustachian tube is petrotympanic.

The Hypotympanum

Summary

Recent advances of surgery into the skull base will often involve the hypotympanum. For this reason, the complicated anatomy of the region is carefully reviewed and updated. The jugular bulb and carotid canal have a larger role to play in the anatomy of the area (see Fig. 23), and are to be carefully evaluated surgically both by the clinical examination of the patient and by the several radiologic techniques now available for their scrutiny.

The hypotympanum is that part of the tympanum lying below the level of the floor of the external auditory canal (Fig. 62). Its floor is somewhat dome-shaped, with its concavity facing inferiorly (see Fig. 24). Anteriorly, it extends to the carotid wall and posteriorly to the styloid complex (Fig. 68). These borders, however, may be quite variable, depending on the specific anatomy of a temporal bone.

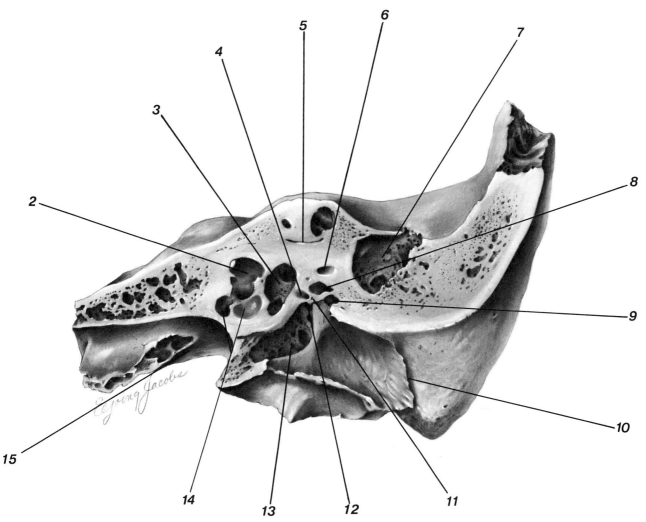

Figure 68.   Oblique horizontal cut through a temporal bone showing hypotympanum and its relations—carotid canal (15), internal auditory meatus (2), vestibule (3), posterior tympanic sinus (4), subarcuate tract (5), lateral semicircular canal (6), mastoid antrum (7), facial canal (8), facial sinus (9), tympanomastoid suture (10), pyramidal eminence (11), sinus tympani (12), hypotympanum (13) and basal coil cochlea (14), carotid canal (15).

The inferior or jugular wall (paries jugularis) is narrow and runs oliquely forward and scantily inferior. It is entirely petrous, and separates the tympanum (fundus tympani) from the jugular dome below (see Fig. 25). The wall may be very thick, or it may be very thin and convex. In the newborn, this wall is very thin and occasionally dehiscent. The floor thickens with growth—the degree of thickening depending on the development of the jugular bulb. It would be very thin and even dehiscent if the jugular bulb bulges into the interior of the tympanum, or it becomes very thick if the bulb remains distant from the tympanum. The inferior wall is usually covered over with bony trabeculation running from medial to lateral, which makes it irregular and can obscure its convexity.

The Hypotympanic Sinus

This occurs where the external (tympanic) wall and the inferior (petrosal) wall of the tympanum meet (see Figs. 62, 63). It is limited posteriorly by the styloid complex and anteriorly by the tubocarotid wall. It is absent when the tympanic bone and petrosa meet at the level of the tympanic sulcus. The further away from the sulcus tympanicus that this suture occurs, the greater the size of the hypotympanic recess. In many cases, the hypotympanic recess appears as a hollow diverticulum in the petrosa that is directed downward toward the jugular bulb, or down and out under the inferior wall of the external meatus. This recess is in the lowest part of the tympanum. Numerous trabeculae or cells make this region very irregular. If cells are infected, they should be removed to avoid jugular inflammations.

Sublabyrinthine Cell Tracts

Pneumatic cells may originate from the hypotympanum and extend medially toward the petrous apex (Fig. 69). These tracts are posterior to the carotid canal. Their size depends on the structure of the petrosa and the height of the jugular dome. If the jugular dome rises to a high level, the sublabyrinthine cell tracts may only reach the otic capsule; but if the jugular dome is absent, a larger sublabyrinthine cell tract will be present.

In about 70% of the temporal bones, the jugular dome rises to a high level and occupies the whole of the posterior region of the sublabyrinthine space, barring the route to the apex for cells lying behind the mastoid portion of the facial canal and more deeply in the occipitojugular region. It is possible in this group to find a few cells under the cochlea, but they rarely extend into the apex (see Figs. 24, 25). If they do, a long narrow subcochlear cell tract leaves from the hypotympanum, engages below the subvestibular part of the cochlea (between the carotid canal in front and the jugular dome behind), and finally opens into the petrous apex below the internal auditory canal (see Fig. 69).

The jugular dome is absent or slightly indicated in 30% of the temporal bones. Here the route to the apex is largely open, with cells arising from the hypotympanum, retrofacial, and occiptojugular regions (see Fig. 69). These cell

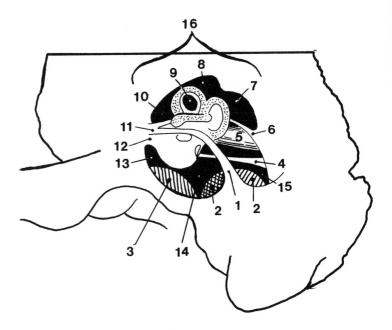

Figure 69.   Schema of perilabyrinthine tracts originating from the tympanum, antrum, and mastoid region.[36] 1, Stylomastoid foramen. 2, Jugular dome. 3, Carotid canal. 4, Cochlear aqueduct. 5, Internal auditory canal. 6, Vestibular aqueduct. 7, Superior retrolabyrinthine cell tract. 8, Petrosal crest cell tract. 9, Subarcuate tract. 10, Superior prelabyrinthine cell tract. 11, Geniculum. 13, Precochlear cell tract. 14, Anterior sublabyrinthine cell tract. 15, Inferior retrolabyrithine cell tract. 16, Superior perilabyrinthine cell tracts. 12, Adherent zone of cochlea to petrosa cortex.

groups fuse under the labyrinth, and continue from there to extend toward the petrous apex gliding on the cortex of the inferior wall, passing under the cochlear aqueduct—then under the internal auditory canal, skirting in front of the basal region of the cochlea and the upper region of the carotid canal to finally open into the apex. In large petrosas, an inferior retrolabyrinthine cell tract is sometimes seen behind the posterior semicircular canal and below the vestibular aqueduct.

The sublabyrinthine cell tract exists in about one third of petrosas with an absence of the jugular fossa (about 10% of cases). If we add to this figure of 10 the percentage of 6%, concerning the petrosas with well-marked jugular fossae, we verify a total of 16% where this cell tract exists.

Inferior View of the Temporal Bone

The inferior aspect of the petrosa, upon scrutiny, will help in the orientation of the hypotympanum (see Figs. 4, 14). Externally, the petrosa contacts the mastoid tip and includes the variable-shaped digastric groove. A much smaller vascular groove for the occipital artery parallels the median border of the digastric groove. The stylomastoid foramen lies at the anterior end of the digastric groove. Sometimes a smaller foramen is seen in front of and external to the stylomastoid foramen, through which passes the chorda tympani nerve (the posterior canal of the chorda tympani). Usually, this orifice does not present on the surface, but rather may be found on the anterior wall of the descending facial canal at a variable distance.

Medially and slightly anterior is the styloid process, directly in front of which is the vaginal process of the tympanic bone. Behind the styloid process is the *jugular facette* (jugum petrosum), which is a ridge joining the petrosa and squamosa that continues posteriorly and externally (see Fig. 4). It can be of considerable size when the mastoid cells extend medial to the digastric groove.

In the medial portion of the jugular facette lies the jugular fossa of variable size. The posterior border of this fossa is in relation to the posterior part of the jugular foramen (Figs. 19-21). In the interior of the jugular fossa are on its external or anteroexternal wall is a small orifice for the auricular branch of the vagus nerve (Arnold's nerve) (see Fig. 4).

The jugular fossa is a venous depression for the jugular bulb, which raises the floor of the hypotympanum in its posterior portion. Anteriorly and medially is found the inferior orifice of the carotid canal. This orifice and the initial portion of the canal are immediately posterior and medial to the tympanic bone (see Fig.14). The turn of the carotid canal raises the anterior floor of the hypotympanum. On the anteroexternal wall of the initial portion of this carotid canal are seen several tiny foramina (carotico-tympanic foramina) for transmission of sympathetic fibers to the tympanic plexus, as well as for passage of the caroticotympanic vessels. Instead, large foramen may occasionally be found so that the tympanic wall may be dehiscent, permitting the carotid artery to present in the protympanum. Posterior to the inferior orifice of the carotid canal, we see the pyramidal fossette, which is the anterior nerve-containing (IX to XI cranial nerves) portion or compartment of the jugular foramen (see Figs. 4, 14, 19-21).

The inferior orifice of Jacobsen's canal (for transmission of Jacobson's nerve—a branch of the IX cranial nerve is found on the bony septum between the jugular fossa and the carotid canal—either on its crest or jugular slope, or on its carotid slope (see Figs. 4, 19–21). The inferior aspect of the petrosa is rough (see Figs. 4, 14) especially in its posterior portion, anteriorly, it is smoother to accommodate the cartilaginous eustachian tube (sulcus tubaris). The tympanic bone (internal portion) forms the anterior wall of the bony portion of the eustachian tube; at its termination, it constitutes the anterior periphery of the bony tubal orifice (see Fig. 22). The remaining circumference of the bony tubal orifice is completed (posteriorly and superiorly) by the petrosa, which continues laterally and posteriorly as a lamina to form the bony roof of the protympanum, and to continue to divide the squamosa from the tympanic bone as the petrosal hernia—thus creating two parallel sutures, one of which is internal and small to permit passage for the chorda tympanic nerve into the infratemporal fossa and the other is lateral and larger (Glaserian fissure) both for exit of the spenomandibular ligament (Meckel's cartilage remnant) and anterior tympanic veins

and for the entrance of the anterior tympanic artery (see Figs. 14, 22). On the endocranial surface, we see this as the petrosquamosal suture.

When looking into the tubal orifice, we see a transverse bony septum. The upper smaller compartment is the canal for the tensor tympani muscle (see Fig. 22). Below the tubal orifice and on the external wall of the carotid canal lies a roughened area of bone on the petrosal, which serves as the site of origin of much of the fibers of the levator palati muscle (see Fig. 22).

The inferior aspect of the petrosa in its posterior third presents a rough surface for its articulation with the occipital bone. Behind this very rough articular surface lies the groove for the inferior petrosal sinus, which ends externally in the jugular fossa and internally at the apex of the petrosa on its endocranial surface (see Figs. 19, 21).

Relations of the Labyrinth With the Inferior Petrosal Wall

The labyrinth view from below presents:

1. The inferior aspect of the cochlear cone.
2. The posterior third of the floor of the vestibule.
3. The ampullary arm of the posterior semicircular canal.

The underlying sublabyrinthine portion of the petrosa is very uneven. It is always occupied anteriorly by the carotid canal and immediately posterior by the jugular dome. Between these structures, the bone varies in thickness, and may be either compact, spongy, or cellular.

Relations With the Carotid Canal.   The carotid canal is cylindrical with a diameter of 6 to 7 mm. The canal consists of a vertical portion rising from the base of the petrosa, an elbow that contacts the inferior aspect of the capsule of the cochlea, and a horizontal portion that extends toward the petrous apex. In a very large petrosa, the carotid canal contacts only the lowest edge of the larger basal turn of the cochlea. In a small petrosa, the carotid canal contacts the inferior edge of all three spiral turns of the cochlear capsule.

The height of the vertical portion of the carotid canal varies. It may rise to the level of the promontory (small petrosa), or it may be as much as 5 mm below the cochlea, with a recess between canal and cochlea. Thus, the cochlea is separated from the inferior aspect of the petrosa by the height of the vertical area of the carotid canal, which is about 5 mm. The presence of the internal carotid artery at the bottom of the tympanum is a constant danger when a surgeon opens the cochlea. The best landmark is the oval window. The carotid canal lies 4 to 9 mm (average, 7 mm) below and slightly anterior to the anterior wall of the oval window niche.

Relations With the Jugular Dome.   In about 30% of temporal bones, the jugular dome is small and creates only a slight depression on the inferior surface of the petrosa. It may be separated from the labyrinth by a distance of 8 to 10 mm. This creates a large space under the posterior labyrinthine capsule extending from the carotid canal in front to the cerebellar fossa behind. This space is usually well pneumatized from the hypotympanum as the sublabyrinthine tract, which may extend to the petrous apex (see Fig. 69). The hypotympanum is large and low, and may extend under the external auditory meatus (hypotympanic sinus) (see Figs. 62, 63) more often, the jugular fossa is large enough to admit the tip of the index finger (see Fig. 25). It would narrow the sublabyrinthine space. At surgery, the jugular dome may be seen medial and anterior to the descending facial canal.

The inferior aspects of the cochlea capsule, the carotid canal, and the jugular dome form the sides of a triangular space with the summit below and whose base is the cochlear capsule above. This triangle is the subcochlear space, which is made up of sublabyrinthine cell tracts.

The jugular dome may be large and fill the posterior sublabyrinthine spaces as far as the round window, up to the floor of the vestibule, and up to the ampullary arm of the posterior semicircular canal, which sometimes indents the dome and forms a ridge under the vault. If the opposite internal jugular vein is absent or rudimentary, the sole-functioning jugular bulb may be massive and insinuate between the posterior semicircular canal and the cerebellar wall of the petrosa.

The vestibular aqueduct may be in intimate contact with such a large jugular bulb. The course of the vestibular aqueduct may be distorted, and may be elevated toward the petrosal crest to occupy the interval between the lateral sinus externally and the internal auditory meatus internally. Large jugular bulbs may be a hazard in surgery to the ear. An X-ray study of the skull base will both indicate a large jugular dome and alert the surgeon as to its size. Vascular anomalies have important surgical implications. Presurgical radiographic examination—with particular attention to the size and position of the jugular dome, lateral sinus, carotid canal, and eustachian tube, the pneumatization of the temporal bone and the overall size of the temporal bone—are mandatory if one is to be prepared to handle every eventuality at surgery.

The cochlear aqueduct connects the labyrinthine perilymphatic spaces with the fluid system in the cerebellar fossa. It arises on the posterior wall of the tympanic scala by a small orifice located in front of the crest that stands out from the inferior external edge of the round window. It passes under the spiral lamina and is directed backwards, outwards, and inferiorly under the ampullary arm of the posterior semicircular canal. It proceeds almost parallel to the internal auditory canal to empty into the cerebellar fossa at the level of the inferior surface of the petrosa by a wide orifice called the *pyramidal fossette* (also contains the IX to XI cranial nerves), which is found 4 to 5 mm below the internal auditory meatus (see Figs. 21, 69). The aqueduct is 10 to 12 mm long. The aqueduct is surrounded by a thick layer of compact bone that may block extension of a cellular sublabyrinthine air cell tract into the petrous apex.

Embryology[20]

Growth of the petrosa from the canalicular otic capsule region towards the tympanic bone separates the hypotympanum from the posterior cranial fossa. At that time, two fissures are formed in the region of osseous fusion with the otic capsule and the tympanic bone. These are the medial and lateral hypotympanic fissures. The medial fissure transmits the tympanic branch of the glossopharyngeal nerve (Jacobson's nerve) and an artery and vein originating from the posterior cranial fossa. These vessels provide circulation to the medial hypotympanum and round window niche. They accompany Jacobson's nerve to the cochlear promontory. In addition, these vessels anastomose with the vessels that enter the hypotympanum via the lateral hypotympanic fissure.

The lateral hypotympanic fissure lies in the fusion plane between the petrosal ledge of bone and the tympanic bone. It is the passageway for an artery and vein from the external carotid circulation. These supply the lateral hypotympanum and the medial surface of the tympanic membrane.

Medial to the round window niche in a 16 to 18-week-old fetus is the primitive cochlear aqueduct, which contains three structures:

1. The tympanomeningeal fissure (Hyrtl's fissure).
2. Periotic duct.
3. Inferior cochlear vein.

This area is continuous with the posterior fossa dura-connective tissue surrounding the inferior petrosal sinus and the superior ganglion (jugular ganglion) of the IX cranial nerve (Fig. 21).

Hyrtl's fissure closes by fusion of the medial ossification center of the canalicular otic capsule to the cartilaginous bar, which forms the medial lip of the round window rim (24-week-old fetus). The two hypotympanic fissures remain patent until one month postpartum. The process of fusion formation and narrowing occurs during the lag phase of hypotympanic growth, and is primarily a function of periosteal petrosal bone growth. During this time, the hypotympanum is sequestered into the middle ear and separated from the jugular bulb and posterior cranial fossa.[20]

Embryology and Anatomy of the Eustachian Tube

The auditory tube was described in some detail by Eustachius in 1563. The structure was mentioned again by Valsalva in 1717. In 1818, Carus published his observations on amphibian embryos. He found structures suggestive of the gill structures in fish, and concluded that the development of the eustachian tube was related to the respiratory tract. In 1825, Rathke published similar conclusions from his work with pig embryos. By the end of the 19th century, the theory that the middle ear complex developed from the pharynx was universally accepted. The exact mechanism of development, however, is contested to this day.

Hammar[21] of Upsala, using wax reconstruction, studied fetuses from three weeks to birth. He described three stages of development: (1) the anlage period; (2) the demarcation period; and (3) the transformation period.

In the first period (three to seven weeks), a slit-like pouch develops from the visceral groove of the pharyngeal wall and extends through undifferentiated mysenchyme to establish temporary contact with the ectoderm of the first branchial cleft.

In the second period (seven to nine weeks), the second branchial arch grows rapidly and constricts the midportion of the tubotympanic recess. The lateral part was considered by Hammar[21] as the primary tympanic cavity, and the medial part was the anlage of the auditory tube.

In the early portion of the third period (ninth week until birth), the dense mesoderm surrounding the primitive tympanum is replaced by loose connective tissue. Later, the cavity radically increases in size due to absorption of the gelatinous tissue. During the fourth fetal month, the eustachian tube lengthens and its lumen becomes slit-like.

Frazer[22] susequently contested Hammar's concept of the origin of the tympanic cavity. He believed that the primitive tympanic cavity was formed by forward growth of the third branchial arch, which contacts the first arch in the anterior wall of the recess, thus forming the anterior and medial walls of the tympanic cavity, while the floor would originate from the second branchial arch and second visceral groove.

This double layer of entodermal cells from the third arch disappears quickly, but it may persist as a vestigial remnant, as Frazer[22] suggested. It would lie below the eustachian tube, behind the tensor palati muscle, and in front of the carotid and stylopharyngeus muscle (Figs. 70-73).

During the fourth month, the cartilaginous portion of the tube develops by a process of chondrification in four centers of the adjacent mesoderm. In the fifth month, junction between the tube and middle ear becomes apparent. In the sixth month, the cartilaginous tube is relatively long and reaches the posterior border of the promontory. During the seventh month, the tympanic cavity is shaped by ossification and growth of the petrosquamous and tympanic portion of the temporal bone.

Of interest is the rare hamartoma (Fig. 74) which may be found in relation to the eustachian tube. Such a growth was recently reported by Eichel and Hallberg.[23] In their case, the growth originated in the eustachian tube and filled the middle ear. According to Jacobson,[24] these growths represent a disturbance in cell differentiation, which is brought about by embryonic induction. Embryonic induction is an interaction between one tissue (the inductor) and another responding tissue, resulting in the responding tissue taking a course of differentiation it would otherwise not have followed. Thus, most organs form as a result of gradual

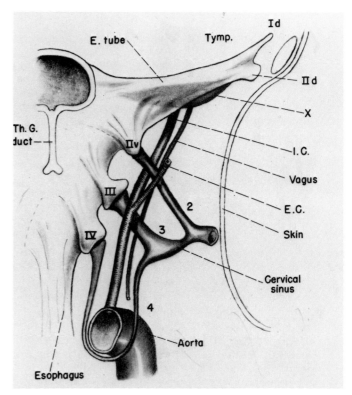

Figure 70. Potential branchial fistulous tracts between the entodermal pouches and ectodermal clefts. At X is a double layer of entodermal cells from the third arch, which may persist and form a branchial cyst in the lateral wall of the nasopharynx (see Figs. 72 and 73). *Id* is the first branchial pouch, dorsal end. *IIv*, Second branchial pouch, ventral end. *Ic*, Internal carotid artery. *Ec*, External carotid artery. 2, 3, 4, Second, third, and fourth branchial clefts. *Th G-duct*, Thyroglossal duct. *E*, Eustachian tube. *Tymp*, tympanum.

cumulative effects of interactions among embryonic tissues.

It is well to review the anatomy of the eustachian tube on occasion and to relate it to new concepts of its function, pathology, and methods of treating abnormal and diseased states.

The protympanum or bony portion of the eustachian tube is the site of some tubal occlusions, and we are concerned with normal structures so that we can deal better with abnormal and diseased structures.

The structure of the mobile cartilaginous tube makes an interesting study, particularly with the play of adjacent muscles and supporting structures. A basic knowledge of anatomy helps to understand function, and both are necessary to interpret and treat diseases of the eustachian tube.

Anatomy

From its pharyngeal orifice, the auditory tube extends posteriorly, laterally, and superiorly to its tympanic orifice. The

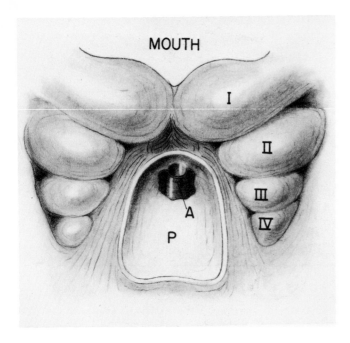

Figure 71. Inferior aspect of the branchial arches in the embryo illustrating how arch III can pass arch II to contract arch I. A double layer of entodermal cells may persist as a vestigial remnant and form a branchial cyst in the lateral nasopharyngeal wall. Mesodermal tissue from the occipital myotomes posterior to arch IV moves forward under the arches to arch I, carrying the hypoglossal nerve, and ultimately forming the tongue musculature. *A,* Aorta. *P,* Pericardium.

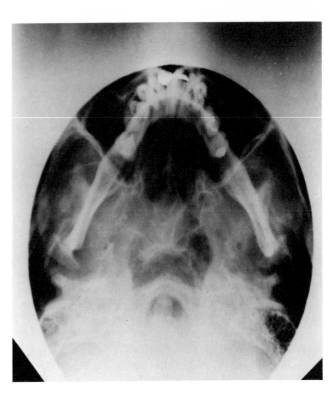

Figure 72. Axial view of a branchial cyst of arch III origin in the left lateral nasopharyngeal wall.

tube consists of an anteromedial cartilaginous two thirds and a posterolateral bony tube (protympanum).

The length of the entire tube varies from 31 to 38 mm[6]; the bony tube, 11 to 12 mm; and the fibrocartilaginous tube, 24 to 25 mm. In the infant, the bony tube is relatively longer.

The vertical diameter of the orifice varies from 3 to 11 mm, and its horiztonal diameter varies from 2 to 5 mm. The lumen is shaped like two cones meeting at their apex, which in this case is the isthmus.

The direction of the tube in the adult inclines superiorly at an angle of 30° to 40° with the horizontal plane. Thus, the pharyngeal orifice is about 15 mm lower than the tympanic orifice. In the child, the direction is more horizontal with perhaps a 10° superior angle. From a sagittal plane through the pharyngeal orifice, the tube passes laterally at an angle of 45°. The tube lies obliquely laterally and posteriorly and forms an angle of 130° to 140° with the sagittal axis of the nasal fossa. The eustachian catheter is shaped to this angle. It is inserted in a sagittal plane, and its inferiorly directed tip should be rotated clockwise 120° to 130° in order to engage the tubal orifice. The bony and cartilaginous tubes meet at an obtuse angle of 160°.

Morphologically, three types have been described[11]: (1) type 1 (48%), which is a primitive infantile form without a

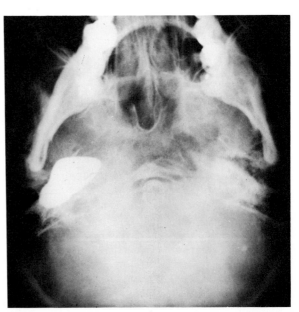

Figure 73. Axial view of a branchial cyst of arch III origin filled with lipoidal (right lateral nasopharyngeal wall). When large, these cysts bulge through the sinus of Morgagni, stretching the fascia pharyngobasilaris ahead of it. These cysts can usually be peeled out by blunt dissection via the oral route to the nasopharynx.

distinct isthmus and with a strait lumen seen in brady-cephalics, susceptible to ear infections; (2) type 2 (30%), which is the average type and is slightly spiral; and (3) type 3 (22%), which has a marked angulation at the isthmus level, with narrowing and torsion, an easily obstructed lumen, and is seen in dolicocephalics.

The isthmus is 1 mm wide and 2 mm high. In the infant, the height is 3 mm according to Tröltsch. The protympanum is 5 mm high and 2 mm wide. The pharyngeal orifice is 9 mm high and 5 mm wide.

The eustachian tube is one of the most complicated structures in the human body. Its anatomy is certainly very complicated, its physiology is still incompletley understood, and its pathologic states are infrequently examined and difficult to interpret.

The eustachian tube consists of an anteromedial cartilaginous two thirds and a posterolateral bony third (protympanum). When considering the cartilaginous tube, one must always include its adnexae (levator veli palatini, tensor veli palatini, and salpingopharyngeal muscles, its fascial and suspensory system, and the submucosal structures of the tubal lumen), since they are so vitally concerned with this function.

Bony Portion

The bony portion of the eustachian tube lies within the temporal bone, and is a prolongation of the anterior portion of the tympanic cavity directed inward, forward, and downward toward the nasopharynx. The boundary between the tympanic cavity and the bony eustachian tube or protympanum is most distinct on its floor, where the obliquely rising anterior wall of the tympanic cavity curves toward the inferior wall of the osseous tube. Above lies the tympanic osteum of the eustachian tube. Its height is 4.5 mm and its width 3.3 mm.[1] The lumen of the bony canal is usually only about 2 mm and narrows only slightly at its junction with the cartilaginous portion of the eustachian tube (isthmus) Figs. 75, 76.

The roof of the protympanum is composed of both the bony semicanal for the tensor tympani muscle (Figs. 76, 77) and the smooth concave roof of the protympanum itself. Lateral to the roof of the protympanum lies the canal of

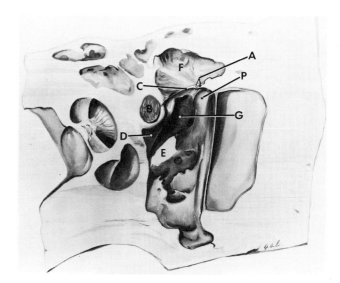

Figure 75. Frontal view through the right temporal bone to expose the anterior tympanum. Laterally lies the anterior mallear ligament (A), which will pass forward through the Glaserian fissure. Medially lies the chorda tympani nerve, which will pass forward through the canal of Huguier. Immediately below lies a slight bony ridge separating the semicanal for the eustachian tube (G) from the pretympanic recess, which extends laterally to the sulcus tympanicus. B, Tensor tympani muscle. D, Semicanal for the tensor tympani. E, Tubal isthmus. C, Mucosal fold of the tensor tympani. F, Anterior compartment or recess of the attic.[2]

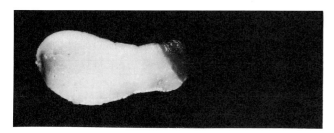

Figure 74. Hamartoma of the nasopharynx from a six-month- old female infant. It appeared to originate from the eustachian tube orifice.

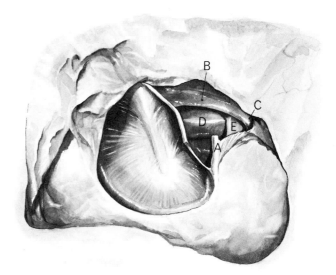

Figure 76. Lateral view of pretympanic recess. The anterior edge of the drum is reflected posteriorly. The anterior tympanic spine has been removed. The annulus fibrosus (A) is left in its normal position, with the mucosa of the lateral wall of the pretympanic recess (E) attached to it. Above, on the roof, can be seen the anterior mallear ligament (B). The semicanal for the tensor tympani (D) is seen on the medial tympanic wall.

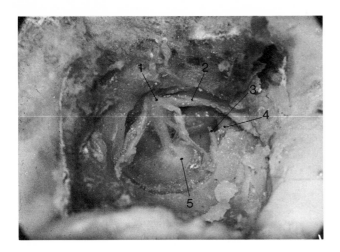

Figure 77. Dissection into the anterior tympanum. 1, Short process of malleus. 2, Anterior mallear process and tendon. 3, Annulus fibrosus. 4, Pretympanic space. 5, Tympanic membrane.

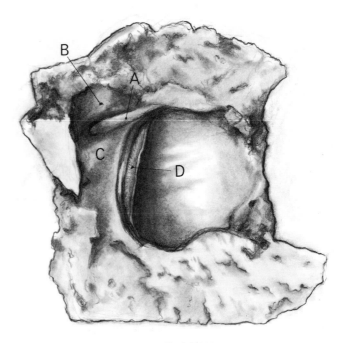

Figure 78. Anterolateral view of the pretympanic sinus. The lateral wall of this sinus (C) is smooth. The anterior compartment of the attic may extend forward (B), or this space may be a supratubal recess. The chorda tympani nerve lies on the medial side of the anterior mallear ligament as they go forward (A). A portion of the drum (D) with the external auditory meatus is shown on the right.

Huguier through which passes the chorda tympani nerve, the narrow intertympanosquamosal crest of the petrosa, the petrotympanic or Glaserian fissure, and a shallow pretympanic recess[2] (Figs. 78-82).

The lateral wall of the protympanum is the thin tympanic plate of the tympanic bone. The medial wall is the thin bony carotid wall (see Fig. 82) which usually has several perforations for passage of the carotico-tympanic vessels. Sometimes only one large vessel passes through a large foramen; occasionally, the carotid wall may be dehiscent, so that the carotid artery may actually project into the protympanum. At birth, the protympanum is short and wide; but with growth of the carotid canal, the carotid wall bulges into the protympanum narrowing it.

The floor of the protympanum is narrow and irregularly ridged by the junction of the petrosal and tympanic portions of the temporal bone at this point.

The superior wall of the protympanum terminates where it meets the anterior-most extent of the anterior compartment of the attic. The attic, however, may extend forward only as far as the superior mallear ligament and fold.[4] The space anterior to the ligament would then be a direct continuation of the superior tubal wall, and would represent a supratubal recess (see Fig. 82).

Fibrocartilaginous Tube

The cartilaginous portion of the eustachian tube is about 25 mm in length, and is firmly attached to the rough oblique margin of the anterior end of the bony protympanum. Its posterior wall is formed by a plate of cartilage, the upper margin of which is curled outward upon itself to form a gutter that presents as a hook on a transverse section. The interval between the margins of this cartilaginous groove presents outward and forward, and is closed by a strong fibrous membrane, thus completing the canal (Fig. 83).

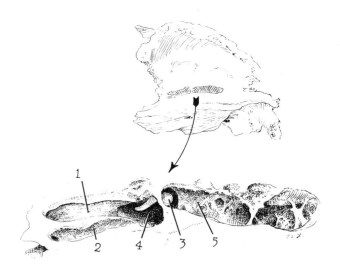

Figure 79. The middle ear cleft has been opened from the cranial cavity. 1, The Protympanum is 1 cm long and about 2 mm wide. It does not narrow down to an isthmus itself. 2, Semicanal for the tensor tympani. 3, Malleus head. 4, Tympanic cavity. Note how the tympanic cavity drops below the level of the tympanic orifice of the protympanum and below the level of the antrum (5).

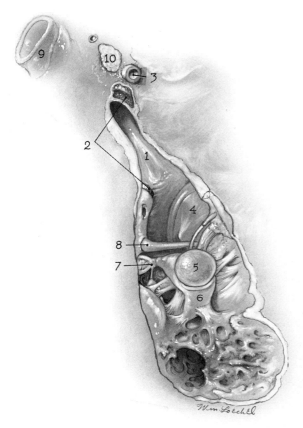

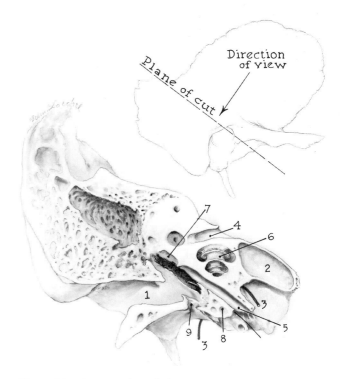

Figure 80.   Middle ear cleft opened from above in a wet specimen. 1, Protympanum. 2, Cut ends of tensor tympani muscle (muscle and its canal removed in part). 3, Middle meningeal artery. 4, Tympanic membrane. 5, Malleus head. 6, Incus. 7, Stapes. 8, Tendon of the tensor tympani muscle. 9, Internal carotid artery. 10, Trigeminal nerve (mandibular branch). Insertion of the cartilaginous tube is just beyond the anterior end of the dissected protympanum. A surgical approach to the bony eustachian tube from the middle cranial fossa would be most difficult.

Figure 81.   A section through the temporal bone in the axis of the canal for the tensor tympani muscle (5). The Canal measures 15 mm in lenth. 1, External auditory meatus. 2, Large apical cell in the petrosa. 3, Carotid canal. 4, Internal auditory meatus. 6, Cochlea. 7, Facial canal in its tympanic segment. 8, Intertympanosquamosal crest of the petrosa. 9, The same for the Glaserian fissure. The protympanum lies below the intertympanosquamosal crest and the semicanal for the tensor tympani.

Figure 82.   Horizontal cut through a temporal bone at the level of the protympanum (2). The upper half of the cut shows a supratubal recess (5), since there is no anterior compartment to the attic. 1, Carotid canal, with a tiny, bony carotid wall separating it from the protympanum. 3, Intertympanosquamosal crest of the petrosa. Note how this edge of the petrosa is directed posteriorly in the line of the malleus head (6), continuing as the petrosquamosal crest (7). Overriding of the squamosa here can be a cause of malleus fixation and conductive deafness. 4, Squamosa. 8, Processus cochleariformis. 9, Auditory nerve.

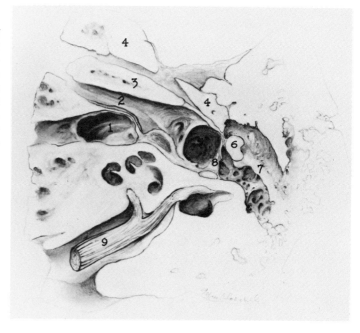

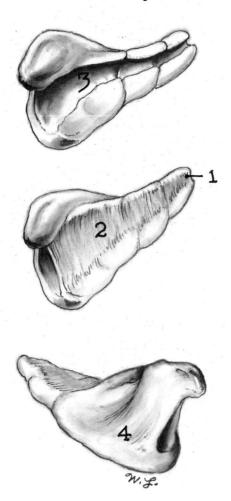

Figure 83. Cartilages of the left eustachian tube. The cartilages arise from two or three centers of condrification. A sliding joint persists throughout life, permitting free movement of the pharyngeal end of the tube, while the tympanic end remains fixed at the isthmus. 1, Tympanic end. 2, Fibrous tissue of the anterolateral wall. 3, Cavity of the tube. 4, Posteromedial wall, modified from E.B. Jamieson, *Illustrations of Regional Anatomy* (Livingson, 1942).

Superiorly, the cartilaginous tube is in contact with the base of the skull, occupying a groove (sulcus tubaris) from which it is suspended by the superior tubal ligament (Fig. 84). The cartilaginous tube is composed of three or four segments that originate from three or four centers of condrification (see Fig. 83). Thus, there are two or three sliding joints that permit the pharyngeal end of the eustachian tube to whip around with swallowing. The narrower end of the cartilage at the isthmus is always fixed. Diseases or injuries to the cartilaginous tube and its suspensory ligaments could interfer with normal tubal function.

Musculature of the Eustachian Tube and Soft Palate

The muscles concerned with function of the eustachian tube, in the order of their greatest influence are: (1) tensor veli palatini; (2) levator veli palatini; (3) superior pharyngeal constrictor; (4) salpingopharyngeal; and (5) tensor tympani. Other muscles to be considered because of their actions on the soft palate are: (1) palatopharyngeus; (2) palatoglossus; and (3) musculus uvulae.

The two tensor muscles are extrapharyngeal, and are supplied by the V cranial nerve. The remaining muscles are intrapharyngeal and are innervated from the pharyngeal plexus (IX to XI cranial nerves).

The tensor veli palatini and the levator veli palatini originate from the base of the skull—the former in front of the eustachian tube and the latter behind. The eustachian tube fits snugly in the interval between these two muscles. The anterior muscle (tensor) descends almost vertically between the two pterygoid wings and almost perpendicular to the tube, whereas the posterior muscle (levator) takes a parallel direction.

The buccopharyngeal fascia, which supports the pharynx, continues upward above the level of the superior constrictor muscle of the pharynx as the pharyngobasilaris fascia to insert into the base of the skull. The interval between the upper border of the superior constrictor muscle and the base of the skull is called the *sinus of Morgagni*. The eustachian tube and levator palatini pass through this sinus to become intrapharyngeal and mobile. The buccopharyngeal fascia attaches to the inferior aspect of the cartilaginous tube and covers the inner or pharyngeal aspect of the extrapharyngeally placed tensor veli palatine (*salpingopharyngeal fascia of Tröltsch*). Thus, the tensor veli palanti is lateropharyngeal, whereas the levator veli palatini is intrapharyngeal and proceeds directly under the palatal mucosa. The anterolateral surface of the tensor veli palatini is covered by the fascia of Weber-Liel, which is an offshoot from the buccopharyngeal fascia and attaches to the pterygoid crest and the sphenoid spine (Fig. 85).

Tensor Veli Palatini Muscle (dilator tubae)

This muscle originates from the scaphoid fossa at the root of the medial pterygoid plate, the spine of the sphenoid, and the lateral membranous part of the eustachian tube; it becomes tendinous and bends at right angles around the bursa of the hamulus, and is continued inward to be inserted partly into the posterior border of the palate bone and chiefly into the aponeurosis of the soft palate above the other palatal muscles (Figs. 85–89). It is fan-shaped, with its superior base attached to the entire length of the anteroexternal wall of the cartilaginous tube. The axis of the muscle and the axis of the tube form an acute angle open below and in front. Zollner[25] quoting Terracol et al.,[26] have called attention to the division of this muscle into two distinct anatomic and functional planes; one is external or superficial and the other is internal or deep.

The superficial layer originates from several points.

1. Posteriorly, fibers originated: (a) on the internal aspect of the sphenoid spine (intermingling with fibers of the tensor tympani muscle); (b) from the scaphoid fossa; and (c) from a crest that unites the external lip of the

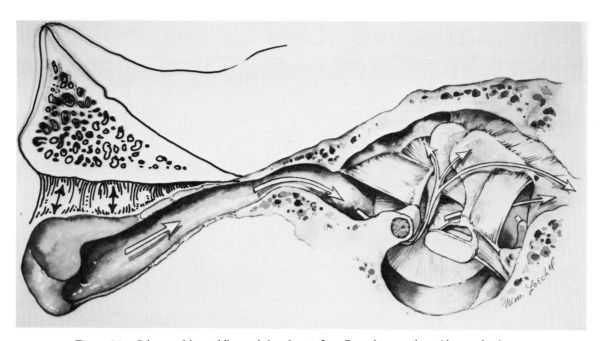

Figure 84. Schema of the middle ear cleft and its air flow. Eustachian cartilages (three or four) are suspended from the base of the skull by the superior tubal ligament. The segmented cartilaginous tube has two or three sliding joints that permit the pharyngeal end of the tube to whip around with swallowing, while the tympanic end of the cartilaginous tube is firmly fixed at the isthmus. White arrows indicate the movement of air through the tympanic isthmi to reach the attic and antrum. Black arrows indicate movements of the cartilaginous tube to and from the base of the skull.

Figure 85. Relations of the pterygoid muscles and the interpteryoid fascia seen on a transverse cut passing behind the pterygomaxillary fossa—right side, inferior segment of the cut. 1, Maxillary sinus. 2, Medial pterygoid plate. 3, Lateral pterygoid plate. 4, Tensor veli palatini. 5, Internal pterygoid. 6, Levator. 7, Superior constrictor of the pharynx. 8, Fascia of Weber-Leil. 9, External pterygoid. 10, Sphenomaxillary ligament. 11, Condyle. 12, Sphenopalatine artery. 13, Salpinogopharyngeal fascia of Troeltsch. 14, Buccopharyngeal fascia. 15, Ligament of Civinini. 16, Interpteryoid fascia. 17, Lingual nerve. 18, Inferior dental nerve. 19, Middle meningeal artery. 20, Internal maxillary artery. 21, Superficial temporal artery.

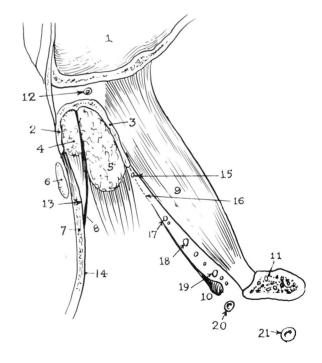

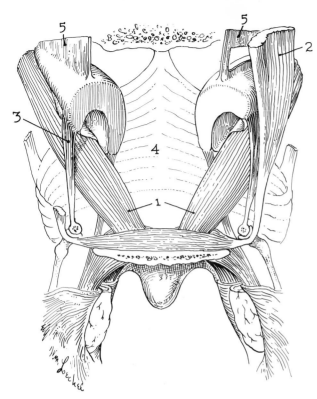

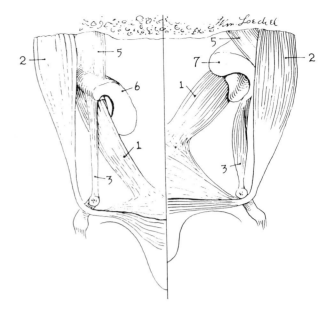

Figure 86. Schema showing the position of the levator muscle (1) with respect to the eustachian tube, superior tubal ligament (5), and two components of the tensor veli palatini muscle—one which tenses the palate (2) and the other which pulls the hook of the eustachian cartilage downward (3). 4, Superior pharyngeal constrictor muscle.

Figure 87. Schema to illustrate the action of the tubal muscles. On the left, the tube is at rest. On the right, the position of the tube is illustrated during swallowing. The levator (1) pulls the soft palate up, back, and lateral to help close the nasopharynx, and to elevate and help rotate the tubal cartilage. Forward rotation is checked by the superior tubal ligament (5). Medial fibers of the tensor (3) pull the hook of the cartilage downward and dilate the tubal lumen, thus opening it. Lateral fibers of the tensor (2) tense and elevate the soft palate.

scaphoid fossa to the sphenoid spine (the pterygospinal crest). Weber[27] called the latter the apophysis of the tensor veli palatini muscle. It frequently exists in the adult, but is always very distinct in the fetus.

This superficial bed slopes laterally and does not have direct relations with the tube. Its purpose is to tense the palate. The superficial portion of the tensor veli palatini muscle passes as a tendon around the hamulus at right angles, and then fans out to insert into the palate. The tendon is separated from the hamulus by a little serous bursa.

2. Anteriorly, the muscle, corresponding to its ventral portion originates from the fascia of Weber-Liel. It possesses some very short fibers that insert on the posterior part of the hard palate.

The deep layer of the tensor muscle is less complicated. On an external view (after removal of the superficial layer), it is muscular in its superior half and tendinous in its inferior half. On an internal view, the reverse is true. It is tendinous superiorly and muscular below. The inner aspect of the deep muscular layer originates from the fibrous sheath, which is attached along the tip of the cartilaginous hook and may actually coil under the hook. Towards the

pharyngeal orifice of the tube, this sheath continues on as the salpingopharyngeal fascia of Tröltsch. Some fibers also originate from the anterior aspect of the lateral cartilaginous lamina. The deep fibers converge into a slender tendon, that inserts on the hamulus. The fibrous sheath is distinct from the fibroelastic membrane, which forms the anterior wall of the fibrocartilaginous tube. Zollner,[25] however, on histologic sections, demonstrated connective tissue bands passing from the submucosal bed of the tube above the lateral fat body of Ostmann and between the fibroelastic tube and the fibrous sheath of the deep muscular bed.

Levator Veli Palatini Muscle

The levator muscle has a double origin: (1) from the cranium; and (2) from the cartilaginous tube (see Figs. 85–89). It originates: (1) from that portion of the temporal bone directly in front of the carotid orifice; and (2) from the tubal apophysis of the tympanic bone; and (3) from the petrosa (anterior fibers). They are separated from the adjacent protympanum by pneumatic cells.

The muscle is fixed in its posterior third onto the medial cartilaginous lamina, which adheres to the sphenoid in this region. Some fibers may be attached to the tubal floor in the isthmus region.

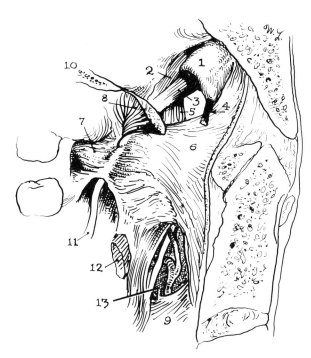

Figure 88. Lateral view of the nasopharynx and oropharynx, showing superior constrictor of the pharynx (6), which is shown attaching to the hamulus and pterygomandibular raphe, continuing as the buccinator (7). The levator (3) and the tubal cartilage (1) are shown descending and passing around the hamulus (8). 4, Salpingopharyngeal. 5, Medial pterygoid. 9, Middle constrictor. 10, Hard palate. 11, Lingual nerve. 12, Palatoglossus. 13, Facial artery.

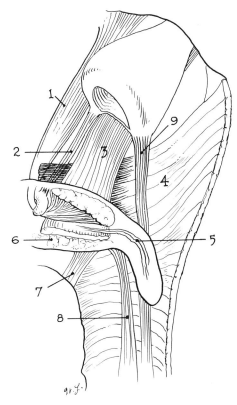

Figure 89. Lateral view of the nasopharynx, showing the position of tubal and palatal muscles, and their mode of action on the eustachian tube. 1, Anterolateral portion of the tensor veli palatini; its primary function is to tense the palate. 2, The posteromedial portion of the tensor veli palatini; its function is to pull the eustachian hook downward and forward to open the tube. 3, Levator veli palatini, which elevates the tube and helps with its rotation, while elevating the palate to close the nasopharynx, during swallowing. 4, Superior constrictor of the pharynx, which assists tubal elevation with swallowing. 5, Musculus uvulae. 6, Palatal glands. 7, Palatoglossus. 8, Palatopharyngeus. 9, Salpingopharyngeus.

In its anterior two thirds, the muscle has no direct relation with the tube. It is separated from the elastic tubal wall by connective tissue in the middle third, and in the anterior third by fatty tissue. The rounded belly of the muscle descends parallel to the tube, is closely applied to the membranous portion that forms the floor of the tube, and is inserted in a radiating fashion into the dorsal surface of the soft palate below its pharyngeal orifice.

Some of the anterior fibers from the tubal origin insert on the posterior edge of the hard palate, constituting the salpingopalatinus muscle, while others descend in the lateral wall of the pharynx, covered by mucous membrane, beneath the salpingopharyngeal fold. They make up the salpingopharyngeus muscle.[26] Most of the fibers of the levator cross the midline in the front part of the soft palate. Some of the fibers form loops with an upward concavity with fibers from the opposite side. Near the hard palate, this decussation completely divides the glandular layer.

The action of this muscle is not confined to the soft palate alone. It also raises the floor of the eustachian tube through shortening and swelling of its fibers. This causes the pharyngeal orifice to become smaller and the resistance of the tube to lessen due to widening of its lumen (see Fig. 87).

Superior Pharyngeal Constrictor Muscle

The superior constrictor muscle of the pharynx is attached to the pharyngeal tubercle and to the median raphe posteriorly. It extends forward between the pretubal (tensor) and retrotubal (levator) muscles to insert on the inferior third of the posterior margin of the inner wing of the pterygoid (see Figs. 85, 88, 89) and its hamulus, to the pterygomandibular raphe (see Fig. 88), to the alveolar process of the mandible above the posterior end of the mylohyoid line, and by a few fibers to the side of the tongue. The superior fibers curve below the levator veli palatini and the eustachian tube, so that contraction of the superior constrictor muscle also assists in the elevation of the eustachian tube with swallowing (see Figs. 88, 89).

Salpingopharyngeal Muscle

The muscle originates in the inferior aspect of the torus tubarius and occasionally from the floor of the tube. It averages 3.8 cm in length. Its inferior portion is divided into two heads, one of which inserts on the superior horn of the thyroid cartilage and the other into the posterior wall of the pharynx. The muscle may intermingle with the pharyngopalatinus muscle, or it can descend independently. In the latter event, the intermuscular space contains the elastic fibers of the pharyngotubal ligament of Zuckerkandl.[28] During swallowing, the muscle assists in opening the eustachian tube. In the resting stage, the salpingopharyngeal fold is only a ridge on the lateral wall of the nasopharynx; but during contraction of the muscle, the fold stands out and narrows the nasopharynx.

Tensor Tympani Muscle

The tensor tympani muscle arises from: (1) the top of the cartilaginous part of the eustachian tube (posterior fibers); (2) the adjacent portions of the great wing of the sphenoid adjacent to the carotid canal; and (3) the wall of the osseous canal through which the muscle passes. It is about 2 cm long. The fibers converge in a feather-like manner to the tendon, which begins within the muscle about the middle of the canal. The muscle is contained in the bony canal above the protympanum from which it is separated by the septum canalis musculotubaris.

The rounded tendon of this bipenniform muscle leaves the canal at the rostrum cochleare (processus cochleariformis), extends in a direction almost at right angles to the belly of the muscle across the tympanic cavity, and is inserted on the inner margin of the handle of the malleus just below the short process. The tendon of the tensor tympani, which can be followed some distance into the canal, lies in its free course in a sheath (Toynbee's tensor ligament). Occasionally, but not constantly, the anterior portion of the tensor tympani is connected with the tensor veli palatini, either immediately or by tendinous tissue.

Palatopharyngeus Muscle

The muscle originates in layers from the border of the hard palate, the hamulus, the lower surface of the palatal aponeurosis, and fibers of the levator veli palatini. Some fibers originate in the midline and pass down and lateral over the musculus uvulae, whereas others pass beneath the glandular layer. The muscle passes down near the posterior edge of the soft palate and then into the pharyngopalatine arch, where it mingles with the stylopharyngeus and the salpingopharyngeus. A part inserts into the posterior border of the thryoid cartilage and superior horn. It also expands into a thin layer just superficial to the mucous membrane of the back of the pharynx, meeting its opposite fellow in the midline, and inserting into the pharyngeal aponeurosis behind the larynx.

Pataloglossus Muscle

The palatoglossus muscle is a small muscle bundle that is narrower in the middle than at either end. It arises from the anterior surface of the soft palate, where it is continuous with its fellow from the opposite side and passing downward, anterior to the palatine tonsil, to insert into the side of the tongue spreading over the dorsum and also passing deep to intermingle with the transversus linguae.

Musculus Uvulae

The musculus uvulae arises from the tendinous fibers of the tensor veli palatini just behind the posterior nasal spine. Its course is down into the uvula, but on reaching the base, it is already broken up into separate bundles that pass about and through the glandular core of the uvula. The belly of the muscle lies near the dorsal surface between the fibrous expansion of the tensor veli palatini and levator veli palatini, which decussates on its oral surface (see Fig. 89).

Function of the Tubal and Palatal Muscles

With every swallow, the tensor veli palatini muscle certainly (the levator muscle probably) opens the tubal lumen. This is the brief moment when the middle ear is aerated. At the same instant, the tensor tympani muscle regulates the degree of tension of the tympanic membrane. This synergism of action is made possible by a common innervation via the otic ganglion. At the same time, the chorda tympani is stimulated to secrete submaxillary and sublingual saliva.

The levator opens the pharyngeal orifice while lifting the cartilage upward by pulling outward on the fibrous wall of the cartilaginous tube. This action opens the inferior or pharyngeal third of the fibrocartilaginous tubal lumen.

The posterior portion of the tensor, which attaches to the entire length of the hook of the eustachian cartilage, pulls the hook downward toward the hamulus as far as the superior tubal ligament will permit (see Fig. 87). At the same time, the cartilaginous hook is pulled away slightly from the posterior lamina of the eustachian cartilage so that the tubal lumen is opened momentarily. This action is more effective in the upper two thirds of the cartilaginous tube. Thus, the levator opens the lumen in the lower third of the tube, and the tensor opens the lumen in the upper two thirds of the tube. The entire tube opens with synergistic action of the two palatal muscles.

The superior constrictor muscle assists in elevating the tube, particularly the torus tubarius during swallowing. The salpingopharyngeus appears to help elevate the larynx during swallowing, since it contracts when the eustachian tube is elevated to the roof of the nasopharynx by the stronger levator and superior constrictor muscles.

Peritubal Aponeuroses. The pharyngeal aponeurosis is formed by two fibrous sheaths: one is intrapharyngeal and the other is peripharyngeal. Between these two fibrous sheaths are placed the various muscles. The intrapharyngeal fascia is modified to form the pharyngotubal ligament. The peripharyngeal fascia superiorly supports the various constituent elements of the eustachian tube.

These structures play an important role in the movements of this region. Contractions of the tubal muscles follow axes different from those of the pharyngeal muscles. The palatal muscles form the muscular support of the lateral nasopharyngeal wall above the upper border of the superior constrictor muscle.

The lateral aponeurosis of the nasopharynx is separated from the muscles of the region by variable thicknesses of cellular and adipose tissue. Posteriorly, it is fixed to the stylopharyngeal membrane in its superior portion. It is not attached to the prevertebral fascia. Anteriorly, it is attached just external to the tube to a portion of the great wing of the sphenoid adjacent to the tubal cartilage and below to the posterior edge of the internal lamina of the pterygoid bone.

The pharyngobasilaris fascia passes internally to the tensor veli palatini muscle, at which level it is the fascia of Tröltsch. On the external surface of the tensor palatini muscle lies the fascia of Weber-Liel. The fascia of Tröltsch is attached to the inferior and external edge of the tube.

Bony Tube and Pneumatization

Cells frequently develop about the bony tube. In the very pneumatic mastoid, they may completely encircle the canal (paratubal cells). They may penetrate the lumen of the bony canal (intratubal cells). They may extend in front of the labyrinth and behind the carotid towards the petrosa, as Lindsay[15] has so elegantly demonstrated.

Blood Supply of the Eustachian Tube

The eustachian tube receives its blood supply from three vessel systems: (1) the internal maxillary; (2) the ascending pharyngeal; and (3) the ascending palatine arteries.

From the internal maxillary system, blood in the descending palatine artery travels chiefly to the palate. The middle meningeal artery gives of a small branch to the exterior of the cranium, and the vidian artery gives off a branch to the pharyngeal orifice of the tube.

The ascending pharyngeal artery gives branches to the fossa of Rosenmueller, along with branches from the ascending palatine artery. It arrives at the base of the cranium between the carotid foramen and the superior insertion of the levator veli palatini muscle. It descends forward and medially following the posteroinferior border of the levator veli palatini muscle. As it crosses the roof the nasopharynx, it gives off the posterior meningeal and the inferior tubal artery. From its descending portion, it gives off branches to the palatal muscles. The inferior tubal artery passes under the superior origin of the levator muscle (to which it fur-

nishes twigs) and terminates in the inferior part of the eustachian tube.

The ascending palatine artery originates, in most cases, from the facial artery. It may originate from the external carotid artery, or from a common trunk with the ascending pharyngeal artery. It can be absent. It passes up between the styloglossus and stylopharyngeus muscles to which it sends branches; then it comes to lie upon the outer surface of the superior constrictor of the pharynx. It terminates by sending branches to the soft palate, tonsil, and auditory tube. The latter is the superior tubal artery, which supplies the superior segment of the pharyngeal portion of the tube.

Levator Veli Palatini Muscle. This muscle receives, on its superficial surface, one or two branches of the ascending palatine artery; on its deep surface, it receives branches originating from the descending pharyngeal artery or from the inferior tubal artery.

Tensor Veli Palatini Muscle. This muscle receives arterial branches only in its extrapalatal course. On its superficial aspect, it receives: (1) two or three branches from the inferior palatine artery; (2) a branch from the internal maxillary artery; and (3) a branch from the middle meningeal artery to join the nerve of the tensor palatine muscle. On the deep aspect, branches are received from the anteroexternal branch of the ascending palatine artery.

Tubal Lumen. The pharyngeal orifice is supplied by the ascending pharyngeal and ascending palatine arteries, while the tube itself receives branches from the middle meningeal artery.

Veins. A venous plexus is located in the submucosa of the tube. It is drained almost entirely by the pterygoid plexus and by the carotico-tympanic veins to the paracarotid venous plexus. The tubal venous plexus extends along the entire tube and communicates with the tympanic veins. They may give rise to tubal varices. This plexus communicates with the plexus of the middle meningeal foramen, the anterior lacerated foramen, and the foramen ovale, thus assuring the liaison of the venous circulation of the tube and of the intracranial circulation.

Lymphatics

A lymphatic plexus exists in the region of the pharyngeal orifice. In the interior of the tube, this plexus decreases in density, depending upon the thickness of the mucosa and the abundance of lymphoid elements.

The collecting trunks reach the cervical nodes by four routes. The retropharyngeal trunk passes along the lateral pharyngeal walls and ends in the retropharyngeal nodes. The retrostyloid trunk ends in the jugular nodes. The trunks pass through the parapharyngeal space, where the lymphatic ducts from the nasal fossa also gather. Paresis of palatal muscles, in the course of rhinosinusitis, can be explained by infection in this space. The prestyloid trunk also ends in the internal jugular nodes. The accessory transtympanic route goes via the bony tube, tympanic membrane, and external auditory canal to the parotid nodes.

In 1874, Gerlach,[26] described a lymphoid mass in the cartilaginous tube of a six-month-old infant. Wolff,[30] in 250 subjects of all ages, did not encounter such a lymphoid mass. Farrior[3] also did not find lymphoid tissue in or around the lumen of the tube.

Innervation

Motor Innervation-Levator Veli Palatini.   This muscle is innervated from the vagus through the pharyngeal plexus by fibers that probably have their origin in the anterior part of the nucleus of the spinal accessory nerve.

Tensor Veli Palatini.   This muscle is supplied by the motor or masticator part of the trigeminal nerve, by way of the mandibular division, through the tensor veli palatini branch that passes through the otic ganglion.

Sensory Innervation-Pharyngeal Orifice and Fossa of Rosenmueller.   This anterior wall of tubal orifice is innervated by a branch from the nerve to the tensor veli palatini muscle (from otic ganglion). The posterior wall of tubal orifice and fossa of Rosenmueller is innervated via the plexus located in the prestyloid space. It is also richly supplied from the pharyngeal plexus. The superior wall is innervated by the pharyngeal nerve of Bock—a branch from the sphenopalatine nerve.

Eustachian Tube and Protympanum.   The tubal branch of Arnold is innervated from the tympanic plexus and ramifies in the anterolateral wall of the cartilage and mucosa. The protympanum also receives branches from Jacobson's nerve.

The midportion of the eustachian tube is innervated by four or five filaments from the pharyngeal plexus (plexus of Haller), and also by filaments originating from the greater superficial petrosal nerve.

The eustachian tube derives its innervation from three sources: (1) The anteroinferior portion of the pharyngeal orifice and the fibrous tube are innervated by the tubal branch of the nerve to the tensor veli palatini muscle. The anterosuperior portion receives its innervation from the pharyngeal nerve of Bock. (2) The posterior portion of the tubal orifice and the posteromedial cartilaginous lamina receive their innervation by numerous twigs from the pharyngeal plexus. (3) The bony tube (protympanum), the anterolateral cartilaginous lamina, and the tubal mucosa are innervated by the tubal branch of Jacobson's nerve and the tympanic plexus.

The glossopharyngeal nerve plays the predominant role in tubal innervation. Complete anesthesia of the tubal mucosa has followed the intracranial section of the nerve. Innervation of the fossa of Rosenmueller is derived from the pharyngeal plexus. Inflammations produce otalgia, vertigo, and nausea.

Sympathetic Innervation.   The tensor veli palatini is dependent on the otic ganglion. The levator veli palatini is dependent on the sphenopalatine ganglion and vidian nerve. The tube derives this innervation from the otic ganglion. The palate obtains the sympathetic innervation from the sphenopalatine ganglion and facial nerve. The innervation of the tubal mucosa is more complex. It is dependent on the sphenopalatine ganglion (pharyngeal nerve of Bock), the otic ganglion (submucosal branch of the tensor veli palatini nerve), the petrosal nerves (greater superficial petrosal and paired facial), Jacobson's nerve (paired glossopharyngeal), and the carotico-tympanic nerve.

The Development Of The Middle Ear Spaces And Their Surgical Significance

The recent advances in techniques for surgery of the middle ear cleft have revived interest in microanatomy of the middle ear. In the present study,[4] the previous works of anatomists and otologists working in this field were intensively reviewed. Fresh temporal bones were then procured at autopsy and preserved by deep freezing. Later, microdissections were made, photographed, and then sketched by a competent medical illustrator.

Our attention will be directed to the contents of the middle ear, to the embryologic origin, and to the surgical significance of these structures.

The middle ear contains the ossicular chain with its ligaments and the tendons of the tensor tympani and the stapedius muscles. Along with the chorda tympani nerve, these structures may be considered as the "viscera" of the tympani cavity.[4]

Attached to the ossicular chain are various mucosal folds, which are are of considerable clinical importance because they carry blood vessels to the ossicles and divide the middle ear into several definite compartments. They may be considered the "mesenteries" of the tympanic cavity. These mucosal folds are easily seen in living and frest temporal bones. They disappear or disintegrate rapidly if the temporal bones are permitted to dry or are immersed in fixative solutions. They may also disintegrate in disease processes involving the middle ear. Mucosal folds and their remnants are often considered as residues of inflammation or as adhesions. It must be emphasized, therefore, that they occur in fairly constant anatomic positions that can be explained by the embryologic development of the middle ear.

Compartments and Folds of the Middle Ear

The attic or epitympanum is almost completely separated from the mesotympanum by the ossicles and their folds except for two small but constant openings, which we propose to call the isthmus tympani anticus and the isthmus tympani posticus (Fig. 90). The anterior opening lies pos-

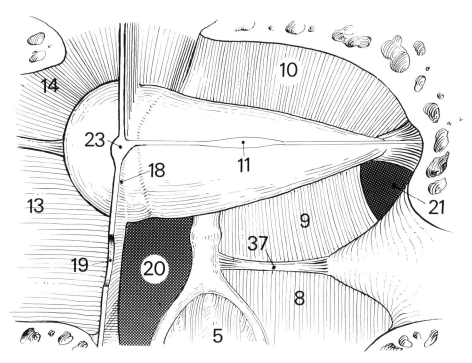

Figure 90. Floor of attic viewed from above. The mesotympanum is almost completely separated from the attic by the ossicular chain and mucosal folds. The only constant communication are the isthmus tympani anticus and the isthmus tympani posticus. 5, Obturatoria stapedis. 8, Plica stapedis. 9, Media incudal fold. 10, Lateral incudal fold. 11, Superior incudal fold. 13, Tensor tympani fold. 14, Anterior mallear (anterior fold of van Troeltsch) fold. 18, Superior mallear fold. 19, Incisura tensoris. 20, Isthmus tympani anticus. 21, Isthmus tympani posticus. 23, Superior mallear ligament. 37, Stapedius tendon.

terior to the tensor tympani tendon and anterior to the stapes, and medial incudal fold. The posterior opening is bounded posteriorly by the pyramidal process and posterior tympanic wall, laterally by the short process of the incus and posterior incudal ligament, and anteriorly by the medial incudal fold, which extends from the short to the long process of the incus. Its medial boundary is the stapes and the stapedial tendon.

The attic usually extends forward through the incisura tensoris and anteriorly to the tensor tendon as the anterior mallear space or anterior compartment of the attic. This space lies above the tensor fold, which extends laterally from the semicanal for the tensor tympani muscle to the anterior mallear ligament.

The attic, however, may extend anteriorly only to the level of the tensor tendon, where it is limited by a medial extension of the superior mallear fold instead of by the tensor fold, which in such an instance does not form. The space anteriorly would be in communication with the mesotympanum and eustachian tube. This space, when present, is called the supratubal space.

Posterior to the transversely placed superior mallear fold lies the larger posterior compartment of the attic. That portion of this compartment lateral to the superior incudal fold may be considered the superior incudal space, and that portion medial to the superior incudal fold may be the

medial incudal space. Laterally, the floor of the superior incudal space is formed by the lateral mallear fold and by the lateral incudal fold, which extends posteriorly to the posterior incudal ligament.

The entrance into Prussak's space is usually located between the lateral mallear fold and the lateral incudal fold.

Medially, the posterior compartment of the attic is separated from the mesotympanum by the dihedral-shaped medial incudal fold, which extends from both crura of the incus to the pyramidal eminence and stapes (Figs. 91, 92).

Beneath the floor of the attic and in the upper mesotympanum, there are three compartments. They are the inferior incudal space and the anterior and posterior pouches of von Troeltsch (Fig. 93).

The inferior incudal space extends from the inferior surface of the incus laterally to the posterior mallear fold (Fig. 94). It is limited medially by the median incudal fold and anteriorly by the interossicular fold, which lies between the long crus of the incus and the upper two thirds of the malleus handle.

Between the posterior mallear fold and the tympanic membrane lies the posterior pouch of von Troeltsch (Figs. 93, 95). The chorda tympani nerve lies in the free margin of the posterior mallear fold, although it may cross

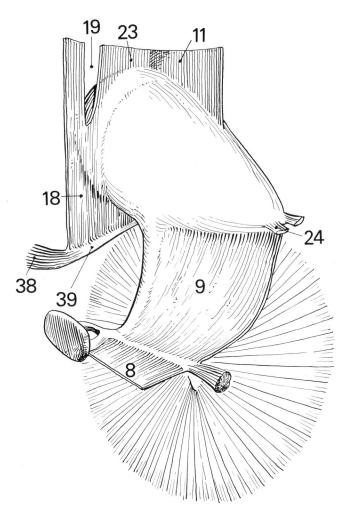

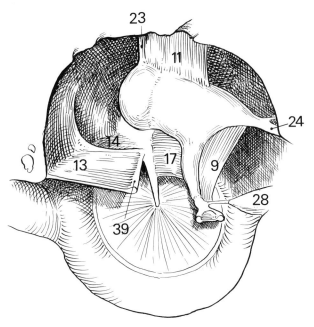

Figure 92.   Lateral view of tympanum. Note the anterior compartment of the attic with the tensor fold as the floor, the interossicular fold between malleus and incus and the medial incudal fold with the isthmus tympani posticus behind. 9, Medial incudal (incudal-stapedial) fold. 11, Superior incudal fold. 13, Tensor tympani fold. 14, Anterior mallear (anterior fold of von Tröltsch) fold. 17, Interossicular fold. 23, Superior mallear ligament. 24, Posterior incudal ligament. 28, Pyramidal eminence. 39, Tensor tympani tendon.

Figure 91.   The ossicles viewed from posterior, superior and medial. The medial incudal fold extends medially and postero-inferiorly from the incus crura to the stapedial tendon. 8, Plica stapedis. 9, Medial incudal fold (incudo- stapedial). 11, Superior incudal fold. 18, Superior mallear fold. 19, Incisura tensoris. 23, Superior mallear ligament. 24, Posterior incudal ligament. 38, Tensor tympani muscle. 39, Tensor tympani tendon.

the posterior tympanum independent of this fold.

The shallow anterior pouch of von Troeltsch lies between that portion of the drumhead anterior to the malleus handle and the anterior mallear fold, which is draped on the anterior mallear ligament (Figs. 93, 95).

Between the malleus handle and the drumhead and superior to the umbo lies the shallow manubrial fold. (Fig. 95)

Five folds may be recognized as stapedial folds (Fig. 96). They are: (1) the obturatoria stapedis between the crura; (2) the anterior stapedial fold between the promontory and anterior crus; (3) the posterior stapedial between the promontory and posterior crus; (4) the plica stapedis between the pyramidal eminence and the posterior crus; and (5) the superior stapedial folds, which extend from the long crus of the incus to either crus of the stapes or from the facial canal to the crura.

Prussak's Space

The annulus fibrosus—the dense fibrocartilaginous ring to which the radial fibers of the drum attach—leaves the sulcus tympanicus posteriorly (Fig. 97). Its outer fibers insert on the posterior tympanic spine or extend in the stria membrana tympani posticus to the short process of the malleus. Its inner fibers insert on the medially placed pretympanic spine[4] or radiate out, forming the supporting structure for the poseterior mallear fold and attaching on the posteromedial aspect of the upper third of the malleus handle. Between the posterior mallear fold and the drum lies the posterior pouch of von Tröltsch.

Anteriorly, the annulus fibrosus leaves the sulcus tympanicus to attach in part to the anterior tympanic spine and then continues on: (1) as the stria membrana tympani anticus to the short process; (2) to radiate out to help form the floor of Prussak's space; (3) to interdigitate with fibers of the lateral mallear fold; and (4) to attach to the bony rim of the notch of Rivinus.

The lateral mallear fold arises from the junction of the malleus head and neck and radiates out to insert on the entire bony rim of the notch of Rivinus, thus forming a firm roof for Prussak's space (Figs. 98, 100).

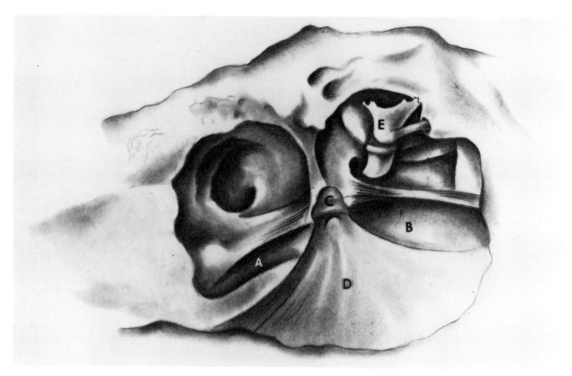

Figure 93. A view of the anterior and posterior pouches of von Tröltsch looking up into the tympanum after removal of the floor of the tympanum. A- anterior pouch of von Tröltsch B- posterior pouch of von Tröltsch. C- umbo. D- tympanic membrane. E- stapes head with attached stapedial tendon.

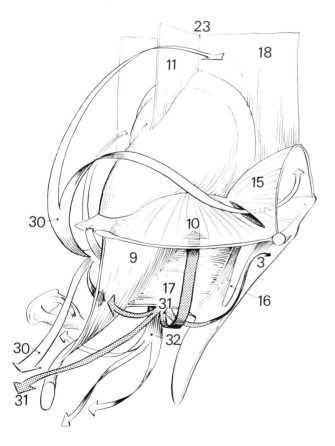

Figure 94. Postero-superior and lateral view of middle- ear contents showing embryological origin. Saccus medius forms the superior incudal space, Prussak's space and extending posteriorly into the mastoid (pars petrosa).Saccus superior forms the inferior incudal space, posterior pouch of von Tröltsch and extending into that portion of the mastoid developed from pars squamosa. Saccus posticus forms the round window niche, sinus tympani and lower half of oval window niche. 3, Posterior pouch of von Tröltsch. 9, Medial incudal fold. 10, Lateral incudal fold. 11, Superior incudal fold. 15, Lateral mallear fold. 16, Posterior mallear fold. 17, Interossicular fold. 18, Superior mallear fold. 23, Superior mallear ligament. 30, Saccus medius. 31, Saccus superior. 32, Saccus posticus.

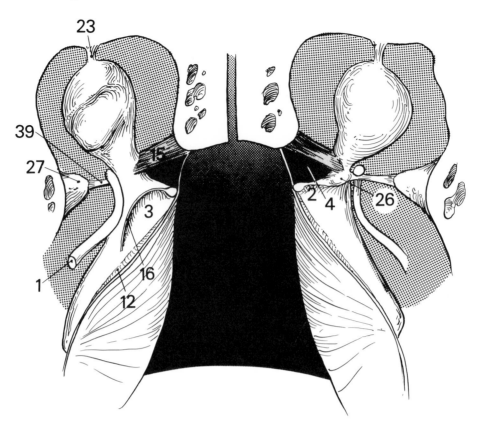

Figure 95.   Section of malleus. Anterior aspect (right) and posterior aspect (left). Note anterior and posterior pouches of von Tröltsch. 1, Chorda tympani nerve. 2, Anterior pouch of von Tröltsch. 3, Posterior pouch of von Tröltsch. 4, Prussaks space. 12, Manubrial fold. 15, Lateral mallear fold. 16, Posterior mallear fold. 23, Superior mallear ligament. 26, Anterior mallear process. 27, Processus cochleariformis. 39, Tensor tympani tendon.

Embryology

Between the third and seventh fetal month, the gelatinous tissue of the middle ear cleft is gradually absorbed. At the same time, the primitive tympanic cavity develops by a growth into the cleft of an endothelial-lined fluid pouch extending from the eustachian tube (Fig. 99). Four primary sacs or pouches then bud out. They are the saccus anticus, saccus medius, saccus superior, and saccus posticus.[4] Where these pouches contact each other, mucosal folds are formed. Between the mucosal layers of the folds are remnants of the mesoderm, including blood vessels supplying the "viscera" of the tympanic cavity.

The saccus anticus is the smallest of the pouches. It extends upward anteriorly to the tensor tendon to form the anterior pouch of von Tröltsch. Its upward extent may be limited at the level of the semicanal for the tensor tympani by contact with the anteriormost saccule derived from the faster-developing saccus medius (Fig. 100). The fold formed is the tensor fold, and above it is the anterior compartment of the attic. The saccus anticus may, however, extend upward to the tegmen and as far posterior as the superior mallear fold. In this instance, a supratubal space is

developed instead of an anterior attic compartment (Fig. 101).

The saccus medius forms the attic. It extends upward through the isthmus tympani anticus and usually breaks into three saccules. The anterior saccule may form the anterior compartment of the attic; the medial saccule forms the superior incudal space by growth over the malleoincudal body to the lateral incudal fold and posterior incudal ligament. Occasionally, the medial saccule extends only to the level of a superior incudal fold, in which case the lateral incudal fold is absent. The superior incudal space would, in such an instance, be developed from the saccus superior. The posterior saccule of the saccus medius extends posteriorly to the anterior crus of the stapes, passes medial to the long crus of the incus, and eventually pneumatizes that portion of the mastoid air cell system derived from the pars petrosa of the temporal bone.

The saccus superior extends posteriorly and laterally in the interval between the malleus handle and the tip of the long crus of the incus. It forms the posterior pouch of von Tröltsch and the inferior incudal space. Its upper limit is the lateral incudal fold, although it may extend to the level of a complete superior incudal fold and also extend into

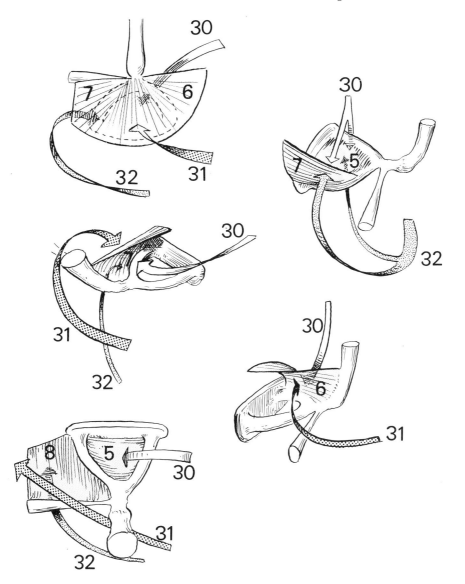

Figure 96.   Five combinations of the various stapes folds showing their embryological origin. 5, Obturatoria stapedis. 6, Anterior stapedial fold. 7, Posterior stapedial fold. 8, Plica stapedis. 30, Saccus medius. 31, Saccus superior. 32, Saccus posticus.

Prussak's space. Posteriorly, the saccus superior extends medially to pass over the pyramidal eminence into the antrum. Eventually, it pneumatizes that portion of the mastoid derived from the pars squamosa. Persistence and further development of the mucosal fold between the saccus superior and saccus medius in the antrum and mastoid of the adult will result in a bony partition known as Körner's septum.

The saccus posticus extends along the hypotympanum to form the round window niches, sinus tympani, and greater portion of the oval window niche. When the plica stapedis and membrana obturatoria are present, they indicate the furthest advance of the saccus posticus. The saccus

posticus, however, often extends under the stapedial tendon to pneumatize the posterior tympanic sinus.

In the region of the oval window niche, three pouches play an intimate part in the development. The saccus posticus extends upward from the hypotympanum, hugging the bony medial wall of the tympanum and forming the lower half of the niche itself. The saccus superior passes lateral to the long crus of the incus over the saccus posticus and stapedial tendon on its way to the antrum. The saccus medius extends medial to the long crus of the incus between the stapes crura and facial canal and superior to the saccus superior to enter the antrum.

Figure 97. Detail of Prussak's space. Terminal fibers of annulus fibrosus spread out to help form the boundries of Prussak's space. The roof is formed by the lateral mallear fold which fans out to attach along the rim of the notch of Rivinus. 16, Posterior mallear fold. 25, Short process of malleus. 26, Long process of malleus. 33, Spina pretympanicus (tuberculum tympanicum posticus). 34, Posterior tympanic spine. 35, Anterior tympanic spine. 41, Stria membrana tympani anticus. 42, Stria membrana tympani posticus.

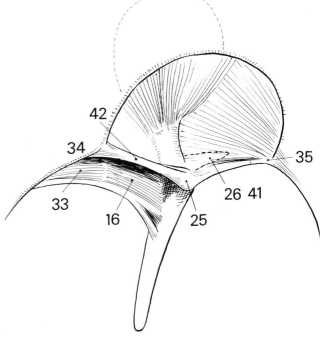

Figure 98. Prussak's space. Frontal section showing the posterior two-thirds of this space. Note the anterior mallear fold extending from the anterior process of the malleus to the stria membrana tympani anticus. 1, Chorda tympani nerve. 13, Tensor tympani fold. 14, Anterior mallear fold. 15, Lateral mallear fold. 18, Superior mallear fold. 26, Long process of malleus. 38, Tensor tympani muscle. 40, Pars flaccida. 41, Stria membrana tympani anticus.

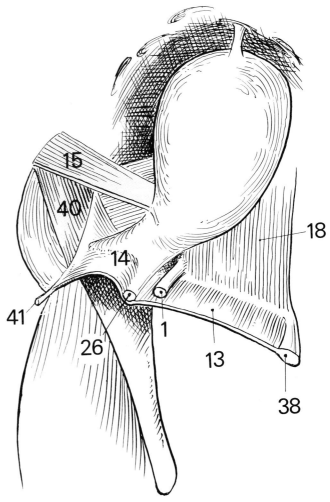

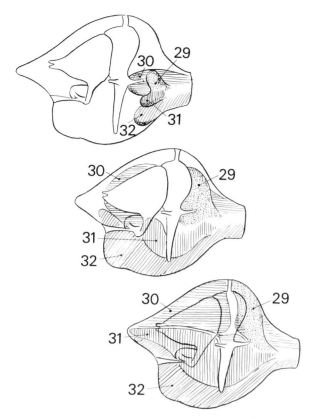

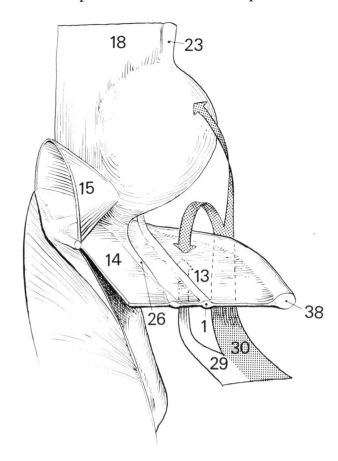

Figure 99.   Illustrates growth of pouches into the middle ear of 3 to 7 month-old embryos. 29, Saccus anticus. 30, Saccus medius. 31, Saccus superior. 32, Saccus posticus.

Figure 100.   Development of anterior compartment of the attic by saccus medius with the saccus anticus stopping at the level of the semicanal and tensor tympani tendon resulting in formation of the tensor fold. 1, Chorda tympani nerve. 13, Tensor tympani fold. 14, Anterior mallear fold. 15, Lateral mallear fold. 18, Superior mallear fold. 23, Superior mallear ligament. 26, LONG process of malleus. 29, Saccus anticus. 30, Saccus medius. 38, Tensor tympani muscle.

Surgical Significance

It is of considerable benefit to the otologic surgeon to recognize the mucosal folds in both normal and diseased conditions. It is a challenge to recognize them when they are edematous and distorted. These folds carry an important share of the blood supply to the ossicles.[32] By compartmenting the middle ear, these various folds may limit disease for a considerable time to one or more compartments. Cholesteatomas have been followed in various sequences of compartments. Examples are from Prussak's space into the superior incudal space, then into the medial incudal space, and finally into the anterior compartment or into the antrum. From Prussak's space, they may extend downward into the inferior incudal space. Cholesteatomas of posterior marginal origin extend into the inferior incudal space, and then via the isthmus tympani posticus into the antrum (occasionally eroding the short process of the incus), the sinus tympani, or inferior aspect of the oval window. If the cholesteatoma is contained in its sac, it may be possible to remove the sac in its entirety, preserve the underlying mucosal folds and the "viscera," and exteriorize the involved compartments to prevent recurrence. This is essentially the older concept of a modified radical mastoidectomy. The surgeon should preserve the

functioning structures of the middle ear as much as possible. Reconstruction is better performed from the point where the disease process can be controlled.

We can now consider briefly the problem of chronic middle ear cleft effusion (Fig.102). Blue drums, cholesterol granulomas, and tympanosclerosis may be included in this group. Whenever the aero- and hydrodynamics of the middle ear cleft are interfered with, the exudates and transudates from the mucosal lining of the air cell system are trapped. We usually think in terms of eustachian tube obstruction. However, attention is called to the significance of the isthmi tympani anticus and posticus. If these small openings from the attic into the mesotympanum are occluded by swollen mucosa, cholesteatoma, or tympanosclerotic deposits, these exudates will accumulate above the level of obstruction. If the obstruction is correctable at surgery or if it is reversible, then surgery can be planned so that the mastoid air cell system can communicate normally again with the mesotympanum. New communications can

Figure 101. Development of the anterior compartment of the attic by extension of saccus anticus to superior mallear fold. 1, Chorda tympani nerve. 15, Lateral mallear fold. 18, Superior mallear fold. 23, Superior mallear ligament. 26, Anterior mallear process. 29, Saccus anticus. 30, Saccus medius. 31, Saccus superior. 32, Saccus posticus. 38, Tensor tympani muscle. 39, Tensor tympani tendon. 41, Stria membrana tympani anticus.

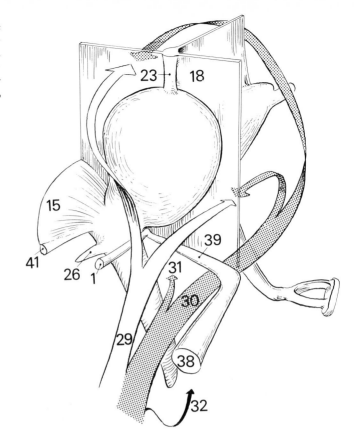

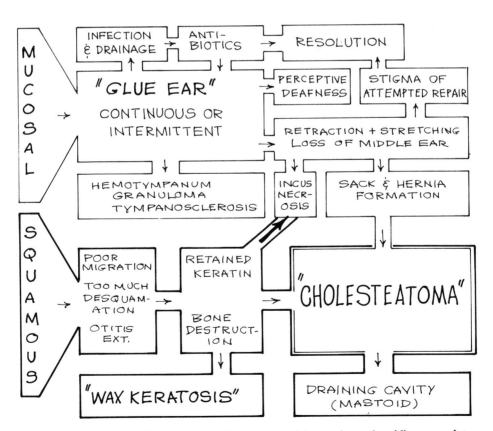

Figure 102. Schema to illustrate means of progression of various diseased middle ear conditions. (Courtesy of R. Thomas, York, England).

be created in several ways. The tensor fold may be removed, and often with it the tensor tendon to establish a passage directly from the attic into the anterior portion of the mesotympanum. On several occasions, persistent effusion, despite a normally functioning eustachian tube, the incus body was removed after cutting the long crus free and leaving it attached to the stapes. The drumhead can easily be shifted the short distance to the preserved long crus. By removal of the incus body, the fluids normally formed in the mastoid can once again pass into the mesotympanum. If communication is thus reestablished, there will not be the need to remove the mastoid cells in these nonsuppurating ears.

It is hoped that this presentation will stimulate interest in anatomy of the middle ear. This interest will put the surgeon in a better position to interpret the extent of the pathologic process, to plan a more exacting control of the disease, and finally to help obtain the best possible hearing result.

The Tympanic Diaphragm and Aeration of the Middle Ear Cleft

The middle ear cleft is an air-filled space that begins in the nasopharynx at the pharyngeal end of the eustachian tube, extends up the tubal lumen to the tympanum, up through the tympanic diaphragm into the epitympanum or attic, through the aditus into the antrum, and finally dissipating out into the remotest mastoid and petrosal air cells. (Figs. 103–116).

Normally, air flow up through this system is precisely controlled by a complex mechanism of muscles and ligaments that open the tubal lumen under certain normal physiologic conditions. Conversely, we have a reverse flow of secretions down this system to the nasopharynx.

We usually think of malaeration in this middle ear cleft in terms of tubal mucosal swellings, tubal fibrosis, or bony stenosis, or paratubal lesions in the nasopharynx or infratemporal fossa. We must also learn to consider obstruction at the level of the tympanic diaphragm as a cause of impaired aeration (Figs. 117–120).

The tympanic attic (Leidy) or epitympanic recess (Schwalbe) is usually defined as the upper portion of the tympanic cavity above the tympanic membrane. The attic contains the head of the malleus and the body of the incus. Politzer[9] stated that it was bounded above by the tegmen tympani and below by the horizontal portion of the facial canal and the tendon of the tensor tympani muscle.

Careful dissection of fresh temporal bones with preservation of mucosal folds reveals that the attic is separated from the mesotympanum by a diaphragm (the tympanic diaphragm) made up of the malleus head and neck, the incus body and short crus, the anterior mallear ligament, the posterior incudal ligament, the lateral mallear ligament, the lateral and medial incudal folds, the tensor fold, and even the plica stapedis and membrana obturatoria when present (Figs. 91–96). The folds commonly seen are:

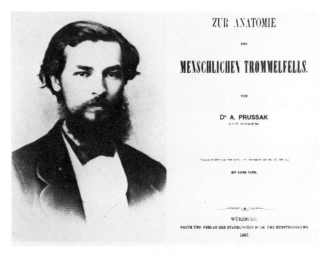

Figure 103.   In 1867 Prussak[108, 109] published his studies on the anatomy of the human tympanic membrane wherein he describes the space for which he is noted. He became the first Professor of Otology at the Medico-Surgical Academy of St. Petersburg in 1870 and occupied this chair for 25 years.

1. *Tensor fold*—between the semicanal for the tensor tympani muscle and the chorda tympani nerve and anterior mallear process.
2. *Lateral incudal fold*—between the incus body and lateral bony attic wall (scutum of Leidy).
3. *Medial incudal fold*—between the crura of the incus.
4. *Lateral mallear fold*—between the malleus neck and bony rim of the notch of Rivinus.
5. *Stapedial fold*—between the posterior crus of the stapes and posterior tympanic wall following the stapedial tendon and pyramidal eminence (Fig. 96).
6. *Obturator fold*—between the stapedial crura.

The tympanic diaphragm is best seen by removal of the tegmen tympani in fresh temporal bone specimens. Cadaver dissections will not demonstrate them because mucosal folds are poorly preserved. The mucosal folds are normally very thin and carry small blood vessels to the ossicles,[32] so that they may be considered as mesenteries. Because of their delicate structure, they rapidly dry out and disappear when exposed to hot dry air.

The tympanic diaphragm always has two small openings that permit aeration between the attic above and the mesotympanum below. They are the anterior tympanic isthmus between the tensor tympani tendon and the stapes, and the posterior tympanic isthmus between the medial incudal fold and the bony posterior tympani wall (styloid complex) (Figs. 91, 104).

The malleus head and neck and the incus occupy a large share of the attic space (Figs. 104, 111, 121). The aditus ad antrum is the only communication from the middle ear into the mastoid antrum and air cell system. Inflammatory swelling of the mucosa covering the attic and aditus walls, and the mucosa covering the ossicles as well as the

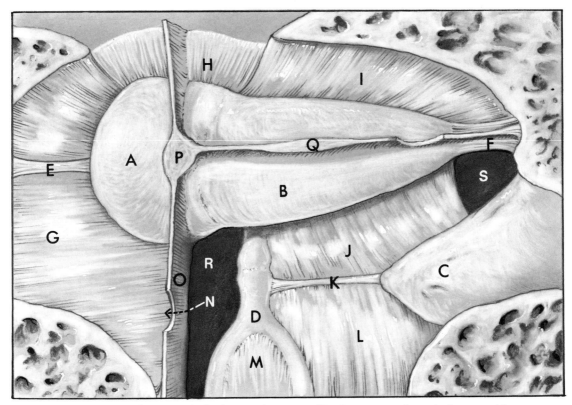

Figure 104. The Tympanic diaphragm. The attic roof has been removed in a fresh temporal bone specimen. The attic floor is surprisingly complete with the exception of the anterior tympanic isthmus (R) and the posterior tympanic isthmus (S). A, Malleus head. B, Body of incus. C, Pyramidal eminence. D, Stapes. E, Anterior mallear ligament. F, Posterior incudal ligament. G, Tensor fold. H, Lateral mallear fold. I, Lateral incudal fold. J, Medial incudal fold. K, Stapedial tendon. L, Plica stapedis. M, Membrana obturatoria stapedis. N, Incisura tensoris. O, Superior mallear fold. P, Superior mallear ligament.

Figure 105. Prussak's space can develop from saccus superior (B) via the inferior incudal space. It would then commuicate with the mesotympanum instead of with the attic. Cholesteatomas originating in Prussak's space would first extend into the inferior incudal space before extending into the attic. A, Saccus medius. B, Saccus superior. 1, Lateral incudal fold. 2, Lateral mallear fold. 3, Interossicular fold. 4, Medial incudal fold. 5, Stapedial fold. 6, Superior mallear fold.

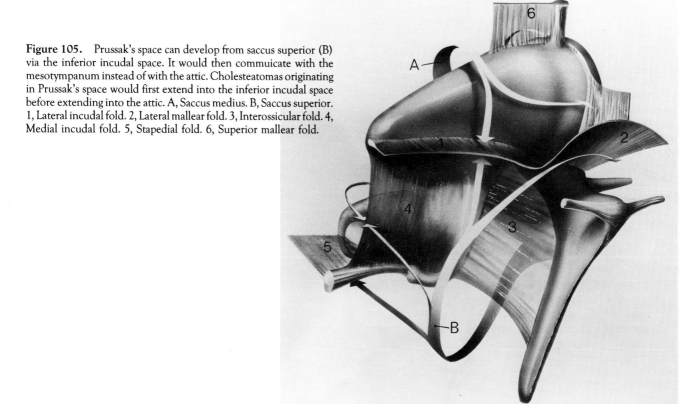

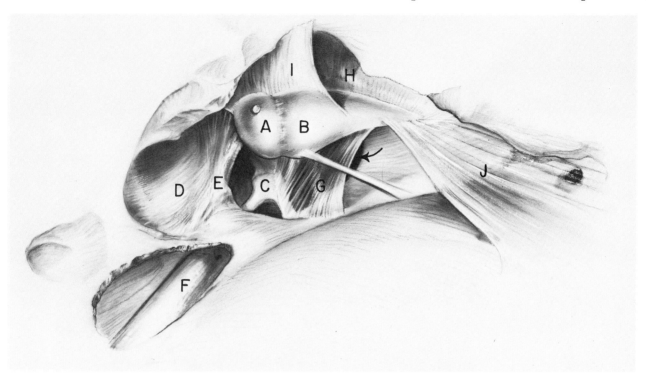

Figure 106.   The roof of the tympanum has been removed in a fresh temporal bone specimen to reveal the mucosal folds. A, Malleus head. B, Incus. C, Stapes. D, Tensor fold and floor of anterior compartment of the attic. E, Tendon of tensor tympani muscle. F, Exposed tensor tympani muscle in tensor canal. G, Medial incudal fold. H, Lateral incudal fold. I, Lateral mallear fold fused with an oblique superior incudal fold. J, Fold passing into the mastoid antrum, which is a persistence of the contact between the pars media and pars superior in the development of the mastoid. The arrow points to the posterior tympanic isthmus. The anterior tympanic isthmus lies between the tensor tympani tendon (E) and the stapes (C).

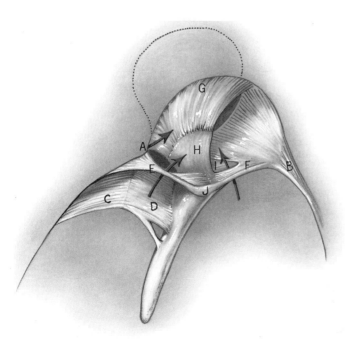

Figure 107.   Prussak's space and anterior and posterior pouches of von Troeltsch, with arrows indicating the three possible routes for pneumatization of Prussak's space. Reversal of the arrows would indicate routes that cholesteatomas may follow as they expand out of Prussak's space. A, Posterior tympanic spine. B, Anterior tympanic spine. C, Pretympanic spine. D, Posterior mallear fold (the space between it and the removed drumhead is the posterior pouch of von Troeltsch). E, Stria membrana tympani posticus. F, Stria membrana tympani anticus. G, Lateral mallear ligament inserting along rim of notch of Rivinus. H, Malleus neck. I, Anterior mallear process. J, Short process of malleus. The anterior pouch of von Troeltsch is very shallow and lies between anterior mallear process and the tympanic membrane.

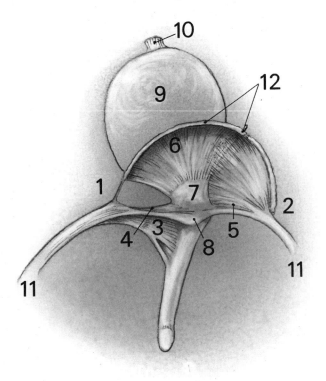

Figure 108. Prussak's space lies between the notch of Rivinus, the anterior and posterior tympanic spines, and the short process of the malleus. It is limited above by the lateral mallear fold, and anteriorly and inferiorly by the terminal flaring out of the annulus fibrosus as it leaves the anterior tympanic spine. On leaving the posterior tympanic spine, fibers of the annulus fibrosus end at the malleus neck, forming the posterior floor of the annulus fibrosus floor of Prussak's space. They also spread to attach to the malleus handle, forming the posterior mallear fold. 1, Posterior tympanic spine. 2, Anterior tympanic spine. 3, Posterior mallear fold with the posterior pouch of von Tröltsch between it and the tympanic membrane laterally. 4, Lower edge of communication between Prussak's space and the attic. 5, Anterior mallear fold with the anterior pouch of von Tröltsch beneath it. 6, Lateral mallear fold. 7, Neck of the malleus. 8, Short process of the malleus. 9, Head of the malleus. 10, Superior mallear ligament. 11, Annulus fibrosus. 12, Attachment of the lateral mallear fold to the notch of Rivinus.

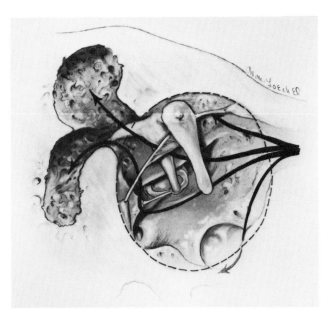

Figure 109. Lateral schema of aeration of the middle ear cleft. The anterior pouch forms the anterior pouch of von Troeltsch. The medial pouch extends into the attic and pars petrosa of the mastoid via the anterior tympanic isthmus. The superior pouch passes lateral to the pyramidal eminence, and the stapedial tendon (through the posterior tympanic isthmus) passes low in the fossa incudis and into the pars squamosa of the mastoid. The petrosquamosal lamina (Körner's septum) divides the pars petrosa and pars squamosa portions of the mastoid.

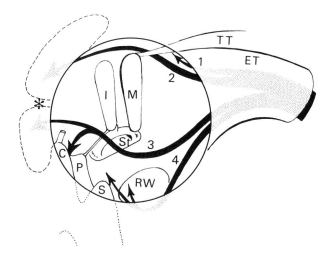

Figure 110. Schema showing movement of the embryonic pouches through the tympanum and into the mastoid. 1, Saccus anticus. 2, Saccus medius. 3, Saccus superior. 4, Saccus posticus. *TT,* Tensor tympani. *ET,* Eustachian tube. *M,* Malleus handle. *I,* Long crus of incus. *ST,* Stapes. *RW,* Round window. *Petrosquamosal lamina (Körner's septum). The styloid complex is represented by: *C,* Chordal eminence; *P,* Pyramidal eminence; and *S,* Styloid eminence. The lower arrow of the saccus superior is directed down into the facial sinus.

mucosal folds, can easily close the tympanic isthmuses and the aditus to aeration—and prevent the normal flow of exudates into the mesotympanum and eustachian tube (see Figs. 117–1120).

Anatomic Origin

The structure and development of the tympanic diaphragm was clearly described by Hammar[21] of Uppsala in 1902 in his wax constructions of the developing ear in fetuses.

In the three-to-seven-week-old embryo, and endothelial-lined pouch progresses as a lateral endodermal pouch of the first and second branchial arches up through the

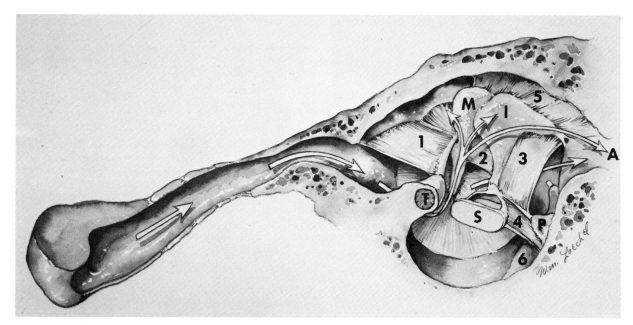

Figure 111. Medial wall of the middle ear removed to show air flow (arrows) from the eustachian tubal orifice to the antrum (A). The cartilaginous tube consists of four overlapping cartilages. Air reaches the attic by passing through the anterior isthmus located between the tensor tympani tendon and the long crus of the incus (1). Air also passes lateral to the long crus of the incus and the medial incudal fold (3), and through the posterior tympanic isthmus to enter the mastoid antrum. T, Tensor tympani muscle. S, Stapes. M, Malleus. 1, Tensor fold. 2, Interossicular fold. 3, Medial incudal fold. 4, Stapedial fold. 5, Lateral incudal fold. 6, Styloid eminence. The chordal eminence with the emerging chorda tympani nerve is seen directly above the pyramidal eminence (P).

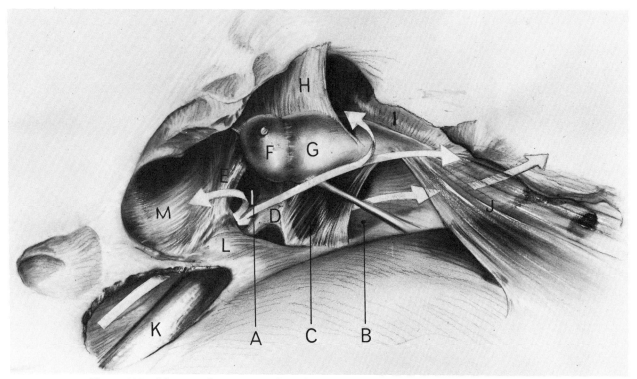

Figure 112. View into the tympanum from above. Arrows indicate the route of advance of primitive pouches into the middle ear cleft. These routes persist throughout life for aeration of the cleft. A, Anterior tympanic isthmus for passage of the medial pouch. B, Posterior tympanic isthmus for passage of the superior pouch. C, Medial incudal fold. D, Stapes. E, Tendon of the tensor tympani muscle. F, Malleus head with superior mallear ligament. G, Incus. H, Superior incudal fold. I, Lateral incudal fold. J, Mucosal (petrosquamosal) fold extending into the antrum (residual of contact between medial and superior pouches of the fetus). K, Tensor tympani muscle exposed in its semicanal. L, Rostrum of processes cochleariformis.

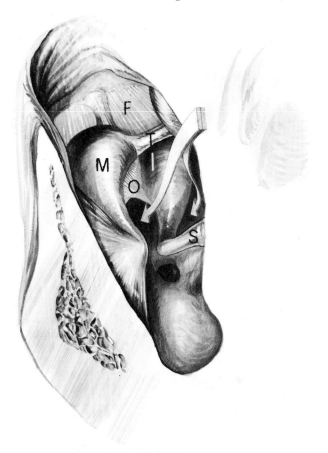

Figure 113. View from the anterior tympanum directed posteriorly. The anterior tympanic isthmus is indicated by the arrow to the right. The left arrow indicates the route to the posterior tympanic isthmus. M, Malleus. I, Incus. S, Stapes. O, Interossicular fold. T, Tensor tympani tendon. F, Superior mallear ligament and fold. In this specimen, the tensor fold is absent, and there is a supratubal recess (anterior compartment of the attic is nonexistent).

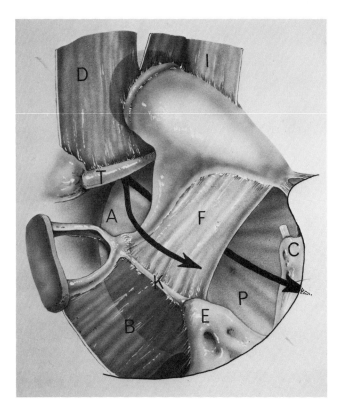

Figure 114. The ossicles viewed posteriorly, superiorly, and medially. The medial incudal fold (F) extends medially and posteroinferiorly from the incus crura to the stapedial tendon (K). The medial pouch enters the attic through the anterior tympanic isthmus (A) and passes posteriorly on the medial aspect of the medial incudal fold; whereas the superior pouch (S) passes posteriorly on its lateral aspect to emerge in the posterior tympanic isthmus (P), and then into the mastoid. The arrows indicate the direction of air flow. B, Plica stapedis. E, Pyramidal eminence. C, Chordal eminence. T, Tensor tendon. I, Superior incudal fold. D, Superior mallear fold with incisura.

loose mesenchyme between the tympanic ring and the cartilaginous labyrinthine capsule (Fig.99). This pouch, which is slowly propelled by the swallowing act of the fetus, encounters the firm structure of the ossicular chain and its ligaments. It divides around the ossicles into four smaller pouches (anterior, medial, superior, and posterior pouches). The anterior pouch forms the anterior pouch of von Tröeltsch (see Fig. 93) and the roof of the protympanum (Figs. 95, 99–101). The medial pouch forms the attic (Figs. 94, 99–101) by passing upward between the tensor tympani tendon and the stapes (anterior tympanic isthmus). It continues on to form the part of the mastoid air cell system located in the petrosa (see Figs. 94, 109). The superior pouch extends posteriorly in the interval between the malleus handle and the long crus of the incus to form the inferior incudal space (Figs. 94, 105, 110) and posterior pouch of von Tröeltsch before it enters the antrum to even-

tually form the part of the mastoid air cell system originating from the squamosa. The posterior pouch (see Figs. 94, 110) extends along the hypotympanum to form the round window niche, sinus tympani, and lower half of the oval window niche.

Where these pouches contact each other, there is formed a double layer of epithelial cells lying back to back, and carrying blood and lymph vessels very much like the abdominal mesenteries. This has recently been demonstrated by Hamberger et al.[32]

Practical Considerations

During the years when a complete mastoidectomy for acute suppurative mastoiditis was common, and attempt was always made to enlarge the aditus opening from

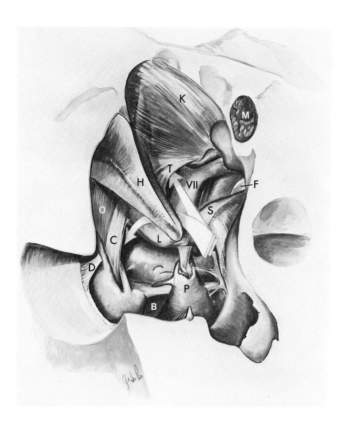

Figure 115. A view of the posterior tympanum and attic floor viewed inferiorly and anteriorly. The arrow on the left is passing posteriorly in the interval between the malleus handle (*H*) and long crus of the incus (*L*), and medial to the chorda tympani nerve (*C*) in the posterior mallear fold (*O*) to pass through the posterior tympanic isthmus. The arrow on the right passes through the anterior tympanic isthmus between the stapes (*S*) and tensor tendon (*T*) to enter the attic. *F*, Stapes foot plate. *VII*, Facial nerve. *D*, Cut edge of the tympanic membrane. *P*, Pyramidal eminence. *B*, Facial sinus. *K*, Tensor fold. *M*, Tensor tympani muscle.

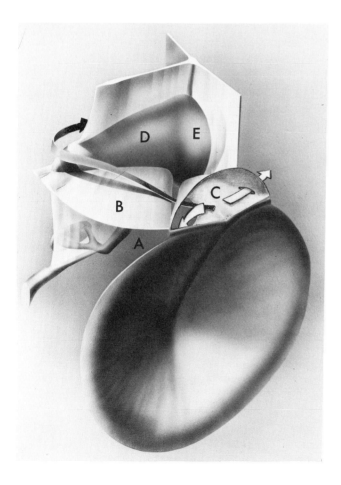

Figure 116. Aeration of Prussak's space. The arrows indicate the three routes that cholesteatomas may follow when they extend beyond Prussak's space. They follow the route for which the space was created during fetal life. The black arrow indicates the medial pouch route, which is most common. The posterior white arrow dips into the inferior incudal space (superior pouch route). The anterior white arrow extends into a supratubal recess (anterior pouch route). The latter is a rare occurrence. A, Inferior incudal space. B, Lateral incudal fold. C, Prussak's space. D, Incus body. E, Malleus head.

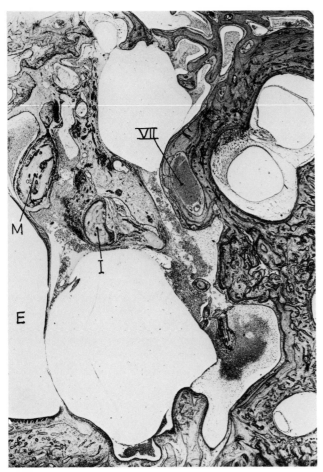

Figure 117. Vertical section showing inflammation of the mucosa at the level of the attic floor. M, Malleus. *I*, Incus. *VII*, Tympanic course of the facial nerve. These structures with their swollen mucosa could easily block the tympanic isthmi and obstruct ventilation of the attic and mastoid air cell system. Note how little swelling there is of the mucosa in the mesotympanum. *E*, External meatus.

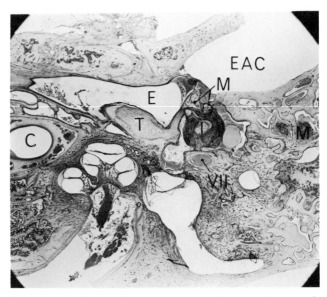

Figure 118. Horizontal histologic section of a temporal bone with marked swelling of the mucosa around the incus (I). Note the absence of diseased mucosa in the protympanum (*E*). The sluggish ventilation through the attic resulted in retained exudates in the mastoid cells (M). Tensor tympani at the processus cochleariformis (*T*), malleus neck (*M*), and carotid artery (*C*).

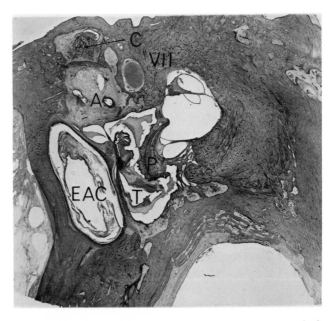

Figure 119. Vertical histologic section of a temporal bone, which shows firm fibrous occlusion of the attic air passages. Exudates, as well as air, are absent in the mastoid air cells. Clefts of cholesterol crystals (C) are seen in the upper portion of the attic. The reaction in the tympanum (*T*) is mildly inflammatory with a purulent exudate. *P*, Promontory. *EAC*, External auditory canal. *A*, Attic. *VII*, Facial nerve.

behind to promote adequate drainage and ventilation into the attic and the mesotympanum. In trying to accomplish this, the incus was sometimes dislodged, causing disruption of the ossicular chain. We may see the end result of this mishap many years later when the ear is explored to determine the cause of a conductive-type of hearing loss.

Throughout life, air is circulated up into the middle ear cleft in exactly the original passageway that forms in the fetus. Exudates and transudates constantly flow in a reverse direction aided by ciliary action, gravity, and suction of the swallowing act.

When we examine histologic sections of the temporal bone in cases of middle ear cleft inflammations, we find marked swelling of the mucosa in the acute stages at the level of the tympanic diaphragm (see Figs. 114–117). Exudates are dammed up in the mastoid, while the protympanum and mesotympanum have relatively little swelling

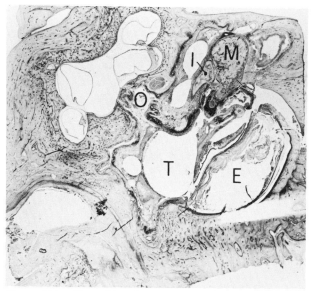

Figure 120.   Vertical histologic section of a temporal bone, which shows swelling of ossicular mucosa that would impair ventilation of the attic and mastoid air cell system. *M,* Malleus. *I,* Incus. *O,* Oval window niche. *T,* Mesotympanum. *E,* External auditory meatus.

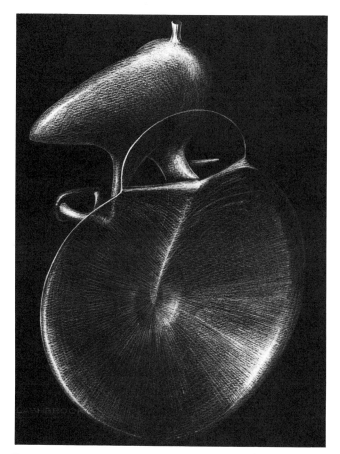

Figure 121.   The relative position of the tympanic membrane and the ossicular chain. The malleus head and incus body are in the epitympanum or attic.

of the mucosa and exudates are quickly emptied down the eustachian tube and into the nasopharynx.

When middle ear inflammations reach the chronic state (see Figs. 117–120), we see on histologic examination that there is organization and thickening of the mucosa at the tympanic diaphragm level. Partial aeration may occur in the attic (see Fig. 117). Such cases would present some degree of conductive hearing impairment. When the attic is completely occluded (see Fig. 118) and aeration above the tympanic diaphragm is impossible, we see evidence of long-standing accumulation of exudates with organization and retention of cholesterol crystals. In some cases, the healing process stimulates new bone formation that may completey occlude the aditus.

Clinical application of the principles of aeration to otologic surgery is seen in the poseterior atticotomy and posterior tympanotomy techniques (see Figs. 59, 60). It is clearly evident that preservation of the posterior bony canal wall is highly desirable when performing surgery upon chronic ear suppurations and cholesteatomas, provided that the disease can be controlled and progression arrested. However, if the posterior bony canal wall is preserved, the mastoid must be assured of aeration.

Improved aeration is accomplished in one of two ways. First, we widen the aditus in all directions until the attic is well opened from behind (posterior atticotomy) (Fig. 122). Often, the only opening into the mesotympanum lies between the incus body and medial tympanic wall (see Fig. 66). Aeration can be improved by removal of the superior-mallear and/or tensor folds, thus opening into the anterior mesotympanum and protympanum. If the drumhead is adherent to the long crus of the incus and the malleus head is firmly fixed by new bone formation or firm fibrous adhesions, the otologist might consider cutting the long crus free from the incus body and discarding the incus body and short crus plus the malleus head and neck. The maneuver would open widely into the mesotympanum. In the same manner, the incus and malleus head can be removed and a prosthesis inserted between the stapes and malleus handle to reconstruct an ossicular chain and yet obtain adequate aeration into the antrum and mastoid air cell system.

Second, improved aeration of the mastoid is obtained by performing a posterior tympanotomy. That portion of the dense bony styloid complex lying between the facial nerve in its descending canal and the chorda tympani nerve is carefully removed (see Figs. 59, 60). This will permit wide aeration directly into the posterior tympanum, hypotympanum, and round window niche. To describe this concept in another way, the posterior wall of the tympanum is a dense solid wall that ends superiorly at the fossa incudis and inferiorly as the styloid process. It is a structure of second branchial arch origin (Reichert's cartilage). The nerve of the second branchial arch lies on its posteromedial aspect (facial nerve). This structure (styloid complex) lies between the tympanic ring and the bony labyrinth. With a posterior tympanotomy, we remove this structure from the mastoid side down to the level where

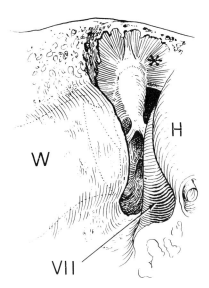

Figure 122. Posterior atticotomy and posterior tympanotomy with preservation of the posterior bony canal wall (*W*). The incus is seen attached by the bifid posterior incudal ligament. Solid bone of the posterior tympanum (styloid complex) was removed inferior to the fossa incudis, and in the interval between the descending facial canal (*VII*) and the thinned out, but intact, posterior bony meatal canal wall. This constitutes the posterior tympanotomy, which exposes the posterior tympanum, round window niche, and posterior hypotympanum. Wide aeration of the mastoid can thus be achieved. Dissection above the fossa incudis constitutes the posterior atticotomy. The lateral incudal fold continues forward and upward as the superior mallear fold to the tensor tendon level. Superior aeration can be greatly improved by removal of persistent folds as the superior mallear and/or tensor folds. *H*, Horizontal canal.

the chorda tympani nerve leaves the trunk of the facial nerve.

Attic-Aditus And The Tympanic Diaphragm

The attic floor (tympanic diaphragm) and the aditus play a very important role in determining the degree to which middle ear suppurations may progress.[17] The pertinent anatomy of the temporal bone at this level will be reviewed, and some of its pathology will be pointed out. The clinical findings in the attic-antrum block were well described recently by Richardson,[33] and will not be included in this discussion.

The tympanic attic (Leidy) or epitympanic recess (Schwalbe) is usually defined as the upper portion of the tympanic cavity above the tympanic membrane. The attic contains the head of the malleus and the body of the incus. Politzer[9] stated that it was bounded above by the tegmen tympani and below by the horizontal portion of the facial canal and the tendon of the tensor tympani muscle.

Careful dissection of fresh temporal bones with preservation of mucosal folds will reveal that the attic is separated from the mesotympanum by a diaphragm (the tympanic diaphragm), made up of the malleus head and neck, the incus body and short crus, the anterior mallear ligament, the posterior incudal ligament, the lateral mallear ligament, the lateral and medial incudal folds, the tensor fold, and even the plica stapedis and the membrana obturatoria when present (See Figs. 91, 104, 113).

The tympanic diaphragm is best seen by removal of the tegmen tympani in fresh temporal bone specimens. The mucosal folds are normally very thin and carry small blood vessels to the ossicles[32] so that they may be considered as mesenteries. Because of their delicate structure, they rapidly dry out and disappear when exposed to dry air. Their embryonic origin has been described by the author in a previous publication.[4]

The tympanic diaphragm always has two small openings that permit aeration between the attic above and the mesotympanum below. They are the anterior tympanic isthmus between the tensor tympani tendon and the stapes, and the posterior tympanic isthmus between the medial incudal fold and the bony posterior tympanic wall (see Fig. 104).

The malleus head and neck and the incus occupy a large share of the attic space (see Figs. 67, 121). The aditus ad antrum is the only communication from the middle ear into the mastoid antrum and air cells. Inflammatory swelling of the mucosa covering the attic and aditus walls, and the mucosa covering the ossicles as well as the mucosa folds, can easily close the tympanic isthmuses and the aditus to aeration, and prevent the normal flow of exudates into the mesotympanum and eustachian tube (see Figs. 117–120).

During the years when a complete mastoidectomy for acute suppurative mastoiditis was common an attempt was always made to enlarge the aditus opening from behind to promote adequate drainage and ventilation into the attic and the mesotympanum. In trying to accomplish this, the incus was sometimes dislodged, causing a disruption of the ossicular chain. We may see the end result of this mishap many years later when the ear is explored to determine the cause of a conductive-type hearing loss.

If blockage of aeration of the antrum and mastoid occurs at the level of the tympanic diaphragm and aditus and persists, it will lead to a persistent effusion of exudates and transudates, progressive organization of these exudates, and transudates, and some degree of permanent adhesive type of otitis media and a chronic conductive-type hearing deficit. Some of these cases can apparently have normal eustachian tube function and normal aeration of the mesotympanum. Long-standing or repeated infections may produce further occlusion of the aditus by concentric healing (tympanosclerotic plaques or new bone formation) until aeration becomes impossible, unless it is surgically relieved.

The tympanic diaphragm will also tend to confine cholesteatomas to the attic. The mucosal folds can sometimes be distinguished as thickened and stretched, in some of these cases, once the cholesteatoma matrix is peeled off. Recognition of this diaphragm may make possible its preservation, since it often seals off a healthy mesotympanum from a cholesteatoma that may completely fill the attic.

Some concepts of possible treatment can be briefly mentioned. If an attic block persists despite conservation treatment, a surgical intervention will usually be indicated. A complete mastoidectomy with restoration of a normal-sized aditus may be helpful in some of the earlier cases. A modified radical mastoidectomy with exteriorization of attic and antrum, along with preservation of the tympanic diaphragm and closure of the isthmuses, will often yield gratifying results. In the younger age group and in large pneumatic mastoids without cholesteatoma, the surgeon might consider performing a mastoidectomy with posterior atticotomy and posterior tympanotomy. This combined procedure would attempt to recreate normal aeration through the aditus and tympanic diaphragm. In the event that occlusion again occurred at the attic floor, the posterior tympanotomy would afford another route of communication between the mesotympanum and mastoid air cell system.

Pneumatization of the Temporal Bone

Air cell tracts expand in various ways into the temporal bone during its development. Since this system of middle ear air cells is susceptible to inflammatory disease, it is important to recognize the various pathways that these cell tracts may take. A system of radiographic studies of the temporal bone will give invaluable information as to the size of the petrosa and the position of perilabyrinthine cells, and give clues to the best method for surgical correction of diseased cell areas.

The extent and arrangement of air cells varies considerably from a minimal air cell system to involvement of most of the temporal bone. The air cell system is divided into:

1. Mastoid pneumatization.
2. Petrous pneumatization.
3. Accessory pneumatization (extending beyond the limits of the mastoid and petrosa).[34]

Mastoid Pneumatization

The anterolateral portion of the mastoid arises from the squamous bone via pneumatization from the saccus superior of the embryonic middle ear (Fig. 94). The posteromedial portion of the mastoid, including the mastoid tip, is derived from the petrosa via pneumatization from the saccus medius. These two parts of the mastoid can be distinguished from each other on the outer surface by the petromastoid fissure and internally by the presence of the petrosquamosal lamina (Körner's septum), which is usually incomplete.

At birth, the mastoid antrum (a large central air cell) is present. The outer antral wall is formed by the squama and is composed of a thin layer of compact bone and an inner layer of small cells, whereas the petrosal portion of the mastoid is usually of a diploic structure or, on rare occasions, sclerotic in nature.

Pneumatization usually begins in late fetal life and progresses during infancy and childhood. Most air cells in the mastoid develop from the antrum; a few may develop directly from the hypotympanum to the mastoid region by passing medial to the vertical portion of the facial canal. Close contact here may result in a dehiscence in the descending facial canal (Figs. 54, 66).

The normal mastoid in the adult may be structured as follows:

1. Pneumatized—most common.
2. Diploic—narrow.
3. Sclerotic—very dense solid bone.
4. Mixed (both marrow and air cells). The mastoid air cells are connected with each other. They communicate with the antrum and then into the tympanum. The mucosa of these cells slowly exude mucus, which flows toward the antrum by a scant system of cilia.

The mastoid air cell system has been divided by Allam[34] as follows:

1. The mastoid antrum, which is connected with the tympanum by way of the aditus.
2. The periantral cell area, which surrounds the antrum and occupies the anterosuperior portion of the mastoid bone.
3. The tegmental cell area, which borders the tegmen and thus lies superiorly in the mastoid bone.
4. The sinodural cell area, which occupies the posterosuperior angle of the mastoid bone and is bounded by the dural plate of bone anterosuperiorly and the sinus plate of bone posterointernally.
5. The perisinus cell area, which lies lateral, medial, and posterior to the lateral venous sinus.
6. The central cell area, which extends from the antrum to the mastoid tip and occupies the middle zone of the mastoid bone.
7. The perifacial cell area, which lies in close relation to the descending portion of the facial canal; these cells empty above the fossa incudis.
8. The mastoid tip area, which is further subdivided into medial and lateral groups by the digastric ridge.

Perilabyrinthine Cell Tracts

The various areas of the petrous bone are pneumatized by extensions from the eustachian tube, middle ear, and mastoid. The petrous bone was divided by Allam[34] into perilabyrinthine and petrous apex regions by a vertical plane passing through the axis of the modiolus of the cochlea. The perilabyrinthine region, which is posterior to this plane, is further divided into supralabyrinthine and infralabyrinthine areas.

Sublabyrinthine Cell Tracts

These cell tracts are quite common. They are found beneath the labyrinth in the space behind the carotid canal. Its importance depends on the size and the structure of the petrosa. Most important is the height of the jugular dome. The jugular dome may be high, and may contact the posterior labyrinthine wall so that the sublabyrinthine area is severely compressed. If the jugular dome is flat or nonexistent, then we may have a wide sublabyrinthine space.

In about 70% of temporal bones, the jugular dome is elevated high in the petrosa and occupies the whole of the posterior region of the sublabyrinthine space, barring the route to the apex for cells that lie behind the mastoid portion of the facial canal and more deeply in the occipitojugular region. The bone with the high jugular dome may have cells under the cochlea, but they infrequently extend to the apex. This subcochlear tract, when it does occur, is long and narrow, leaving the base of the tympanum and passing below the subvestibular part of the cochlea between the carotid canal in front and the jugular dome behind to finally open into the petrous apex below the internal auditory canal (see Fig. 69).

The jugular fossa is absent or nearly so in 30% of temporal bones. Here the route to the apex is largely open, with cells arising from the hypotympanum, the retrofacial area, and the occipitojugular region (see Figs. 69, 123). These cell groups unite under the labyrinth; from there, they extend towards the petrous apex, gliding on the cortex of the inferior wall, passing under the cochlear aqueduct and then under the internal auditory canal, finally skirting in front of the basal region of the cochlea and the upper region of the carotid canal to open into the apex (see Fig. 123). This passage, however, is often closed by a compact mass of bone so that the sublabyrinthine cell tract terminates in a cul-de-sac.

To this group of sublabyrinthine cells may be included the *inferior retrolabyrinthine* cells, which are often encountered in wide petrosas behind the posterior semicircular canal and below the vestibular aqueduct. Girard[35] estimates that the sublabyrinthine cell tracts exists in 16% of temporal bones.

Precochlear or Inferior Prelabyrinthine Cell Tract

This can be called the intercaroticocochlear tract. The cells of its tympanic extremity are known as the peritubal or pericarotid cells. Their point of origin is found in the anterior and inferior region of the tympanum (see Figs. 69,123).

The anterorinferior part of the petrosa, at the level of its middle third, is occupied by the cochlear cone lying on its

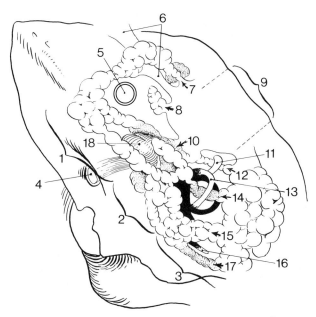

Figure 123.   Pneumatization of the perilabyrinthine and petrous apex regions.[34] 1, Petrous apex region. 2, Perilabyrinthine region, 3, Mastoid region. 4, Internal auditory meatus. 5, Carotid artery. 6, Eustachian tube. 7, Anteroposterior tract. 8, Anterolateral tract. 9, Middle ear. 10, Hypotympanic tract. 11, Facial nerve. 12, Retrofacial tract. 13, Superior semicircular canal. 14, Subarcuate tract. 15, Posterosuperior tract. 16, Vestibular aqueduct. 17, Posteromedial tract. 18, Cochlea.

side with its tip (or apex) in front and a little inferior, and by the carotid canal—which is a large cylindrical canal bent at right angles with a vertical arm, that arises from below the tympanum and a horizontal arm that goes toward the petrous apex. These two structures are superimposed. In very large petrosas, the cochlea lies lightly on top of the carotid canal and makes contact by the most sloped point of its great basal spiral. In the narrow petrosas, on the contrary, the cochlear cone is in intimate contact with the carotid canal by the inferior flank of its three spirals (Fig. 61). In the latter case, there is no room in this region for the development of air cells. In the first case, one can see cells in the bottom of the tympanum occupying the angle between the carotid canal and the superimposed cochlea.

The extent of cellular development is dependent on the relations of the cochlea and carotid canals, with respect to height as well as depth. The elbow of the carotid canal may be superficial and on the same vertical plane as the promontory, or it may be in a deep position with its external surface in a recess that can extend for 5 mm (Figs. 61, 124). When the carotid canal is in a superficial position, the eustachian tube adheres to its anteroexternal surface and there are no air cells between them. However, if the canal is recessed, there exists between the tube and the bend of the carotid canal a space that air cells can occupy (Figs. 57, 125).

It is the same for the canal for the tensor tympani. In contracted petrosas, this canal also adheres to the anteroexter-

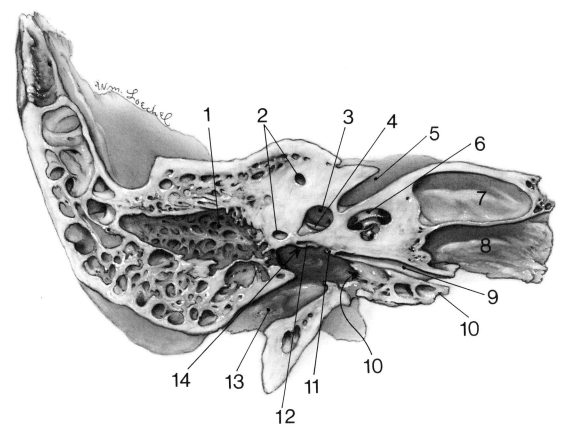

Figure 124. A view of the bottom half of a horizontal cut. 1, Mastoid antrum. 2, Superior semicircular canal. 3, Vestibule. 4, Vestibular crest. 5, Internal auditory canal. 6, Cochlea. 7, Apical cell. 8, Carotid canal. 9, Semicanal for tensor tympani muscle. 10, Eustachian tube. 11, Processus cochleariformis. 12, Facial canal. 13, External auditory canal. 14, Oval window niche.

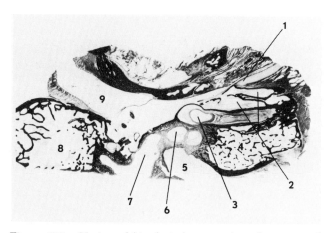

Figure 125. Horizontal histological section through a temporal bone. Note the cartilaginous eustachian tube is separated from the carotid canal by large precarotid cells. Also note how the carotid canal bulges into the tympanum. Note its thinness. Forceful probing from posteriorly placed mastoid antrum for the eustachian tube lumen may instead pass into the precarotid cells. The carotid artery could be endangered. 1, Cartilaginous eustachian tube. 2, Precarotid cells. 3, Carotid canal. 4, Cells in petrous apex. 5, Internal auditory meatus. 6, Cochlea. 7, Vestibule. 8, Antrum. 9, External auditory canal.

nal surface of the horizontal arm of the carotid canal; but in petrosas with a deep carotid canal, the middle region of the muscle canal is found separated from the carotid canal by a space large enough to lodge cells of appreciable size (see Fig. 57).

More anterior and medial, the same cell system may extend past the apex of the cochlea and over the top of the horizontal arm of the carotid canal. At this point, it is covered above by the petrosal cortex, which is grooved for passage of the superficial petrosal nerves. The distance separating the canal for the tensor tympani muscle from the petrosal groove (which indicates the beginning of the apex) is 2 to 3 mm.

At this point, there is a very narrow passage. It is the beginning of the petrous apex, where air cells may enter. Air cells entering the apex are limited externally by the grooves for the petrosal nerves and internally by the external edge of the depression for the Gasserian ganglion just above the carotid canal (see Fig. 2).

The precochlear cell tracts are in relation with the carotid canal along their entire length. Measured from the base of the tympanum to its emergence in the apex, its total length is about 12 mm. It is possible to reach the apex surgically by this route. Kopetzky and Almour followed the

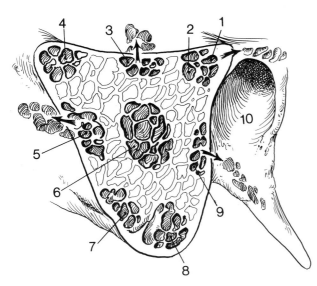

Figure 126. Definitive cell tracts in the mastoid.[34] 1, Antral. 2, Periantral. 3, Tegmental. 4, Sinodural. 5, Perisinus. 6, Central. 7, Lateral tip. 8, Medial tip. 9, Perifacial. 10, External auditory canal.

tract between the cochlea and the carotid canal. Ramadier improved the approach by resecting the superior wall of the carotid canal. In recent years, the middle cranial fossa approach has been developed. It affords easier access to the petrous tip when the apicitis originates via this precochlear route.

Superior Perilabyrinthine Cell Tracts

These cell tracts are in the upper level of the petrosa. They are above a line going from the point where the petrosal cortex is adherent to the cochlea to the vestibular aqueduct posteriorly (see Figs. 69, 123, 126). They pass the labyrinthine barrier by one or more of four possible routes. Once past the labyrinth, these four routes converge, reunite above the internal auditory meatus, and then enter the apex by a unique route. These cell tracts may stop short of the apex ending in a cul-de-sac.

Superior Prelabyrinthine Cell Tracts. These leave from the internal wall of the aditus and enter the triangular superior antelabyrinthine space, which is formed below by the facial canal (anterior fourth of its tympanic portion), in front by the cortex of the anterior slope of the petrosa, and behind by the ampulla of the horizontal semicircular canal and the ampullary arm of the superior canal (see Figs. 69, 123). The cells, extending farther, pass inside the superior canal and go to scatter above the internal auditory meatus, mingling with other superior perilabyrinthine cells. These cells can sometimes be seen as a thin flattened group of cells running under the cortex.

Translabyrinthine Cells Tracts (Subarcuate Cell Tract). This tract leaves the antrum above the horizontal semicircular canal, occupies the trihedral formed by the three canals, and joins the petromastoid canal in the arch of the superior semicircular canal to reach the confluence of the superior perilabyrinthine cells above the internal auditory meatus. This tract is infrequent—perhaps it is present in 2 to 3% of the temporal bones (see Figs 69, 123).

Cell Tracts of the Petrosal Crest. These cells are a prolongation of the periantral cells, which extend along the crest of the petrosa under the cortex (see Fig. 123). They pass over the labyrinth above the junction of the superior and posterior canals, pass behind the superior canal, and end above the internal auditory meatus.

Superior Retrolabyrinthine Cell Tracts (Posteromedial Cell Tract of Lindsay). These cells insinuate between the posterior semicircular canal and the cerebellar cortex of the petrosa. They pass above the vestibular aqueduct and then turn around the posterior aspect of the common crus of the vertical canal to reach the confluence of the superior group of cells above the internal auditory canal. Although this cell tract occupies the posterior region of the petrosa, it has never been seen to pass below the internal auditory canal to reach the apex by the shortest route. It always ascends towards the the crest in order to pass over the internal auditory canal.

Routes to the Apex

There are three main routes for air cells to reach the petrous apex from the middle ear cleft.

1. The *posteroinferior route,* which opens into the apex between the cochlea and the carotid canal in front, the cochlear aqueduct above and behind, the internal auditory canal above the jugular bulb, or the inferior surface of the petrosa below. It is bordering on the sublabyrinthine cells.

2. The *anteroinferior route,* which opens into the apex below the adherent zone of the cochlea to the anterior wall of the petrosa between the cochlea behind, the carotid canal below, and the cortex of the anterior slope of the petrosa in front and above. It is the termination of the antecochlear or intercaroticocochlear cell tracts.

3. The *superior route,* which opens into the crest of the apex above the level of the internal auditory canal and the cochlea. It is the confluence of the four superior perilabyrinthine cell tracts.

In summary, one can encounter air cells and diploic tissue in all parts of the petrosa. Only the labyrinthine capsule, the cortex of the petrous pyramid, and the enclosing of certain structures (facial nerve, internal carotid artery, jugular bulb) are formed by compact bone. Around the adult labyrinth, the compact bone is always thick and forms a block of dense, hard bone in the middle of the petrosa.

5 Canals of the Temporal Bone

The Facial Canal: Normal Anatomy, Variations, And Anomalies[6]

Surgery directed at the skull base has become more frequent due to new diagnostic techniques and the development of microsurgical procedures. The intricate course of the facial nerve through the temporal bone is of vital concern to all otologic surgeons, since it often traverses the surgical field. Therefore, we will review the course of the facial canal through the petrosal portion of the temporal bone from the internal auditory meatus to the stylomastoid foramen, paying particular attention to its relations to adjacent structures.

The facial nerve, along with the intermediate nerve of Wrisberg and the auditory nerve, passes through the internal auditory canal (5 to12 mm) (Figs. 27-129). The facial nerve occupies the anterosuperior segment of the meatus and lies in a shallow gutter (see Fig. 130) that is limited above by the superior wall of the internal auditory canal and below by a barely perceptible crest, which becomes progressively accentuated until it forms a sharp horizontal projection at the bottom (fundus) of the internal auditory meatus, dividing it horizontally into two levels (falciform crest and transverse crest) (Figs. 131-134).

The superior level contains (from front to back) the facial nerve, the intermediate nerve of Wrisberg, the utricular nerve, and the horizontal and superior ampullary nerves (see Figs. 127, 129). The inferior level contains the cochlear, saccular, and inferior ampullary nerves. The latter exists through the singular foramen. These nerves all reach the lateral wall or terminus of the internal auditory meatus. The facial nerve and the intermediate nerve of Wrisberg pass obliquely into the facial canal (Fallopean aqueduct), whereas the remaining nerves (auditory and vestibular) penetrate into the labyrinth.

The facial canal runs a very tortuous course across the petrosa:

1. A first horizontal course, which goes from the internal auditory canal to the site of the geniculate ganglion (Figs. 130, 131, 134, 136).

2. A first turn with an acute angle (Figs. 135-138).
3. A second straight course, which runs along near the top of the tympanum (Figs. 139-144).
4. A second turn, which is a curvature with a large radius and is directed vertically downward (see Figs. 143, 144).
5. A third and last straight portion directed inferiorly and a little posteriorly to end at the stylomastoid foramen (see Figs. 143-149).

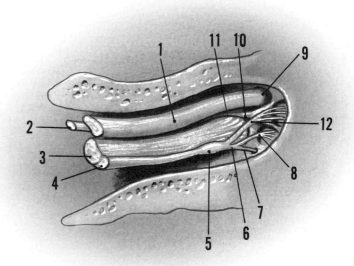

Figure 127. Schema of the internal auditory meatus and its contents. A view looking anteriorly on the right. 1, Facial nerve. 2, Intermediate nerve of Wrisberg. 3, Cochlear nerve. 4, Vestibular nerve. 5, Scarpa's ganglion. 6, Inferior branch of the vestibular nerve. 7, Posterior ampullary nerve exiting through the foramen singulare. 8, Saccular nerve in the saccular fossa. 9, Facial nerve in the fovea facialis at the origin of the facial canal. 10, Falciform or transverse crest. 11, Cochlear nerve in the cochlear fossa. 12, Superior branch of the vestibular nerve in the vestibular fossa.

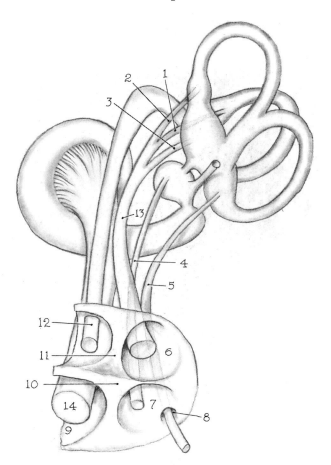

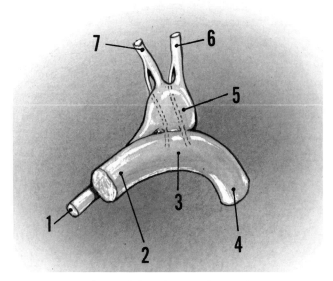

Figure 129.   Schema of the right geniculate ganglion and its connections. 1, Intermediate nerve of Wrisberg. 2, First part of the facial nerve. 3, Genu or first turn of the facial nerve. 4, Second part of the facial nerve. 5, Geniculate ganglion. 6, Lesser superficial petrosal nerve. 7, Greater superficial petrosal nerve.

Figure 128.   Fundus of the internal auditory canal and distribution of the VIII cranial nerve to the membranous labyrinth. 1, External ampullary nerve. 2, Superior ampullary nerve. 3, Utricular nerve. 4, Saccular nerve. 5, Posterior ampullary nerve. 6, Superior foramen of Morgagni. 9, Cochlear fossa. 10, Falciform crest. 11, Vertical crest. 12, Facial nerve. 13, Superior vestibular nerve. 14, Cochlear nerve.

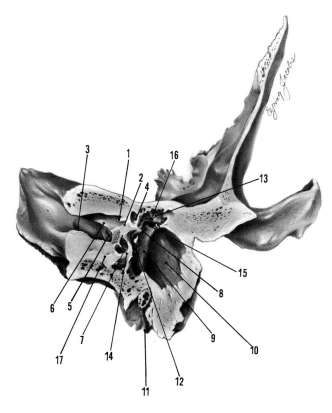

Figure 130.   Vertical cut through the internal and external auditory meatuses showing the anterior wall and internal auditory meatus and the anterior tympanum. 1, Vertical crest with the fovea facialis immediately in front. 2, Utricular fossa above the dot. 3, Internal auditory meatus. 4, Facial canal at the geniculum. 5, Cochlear fossa (spiral cribriform plate of cochlea). 6, Crista transversa. 7, Cochlea. 8, Processus cochleariformis. 9, Sulcus tympanicus. 10, External auditory canal. 11, Styloid process. 12, Protympanum. 13, Pretympanic sinus. 14, Promontory. 15, Glaserian fissure. 16, Canal of Huguier. 17, Cochlear aqueduct.

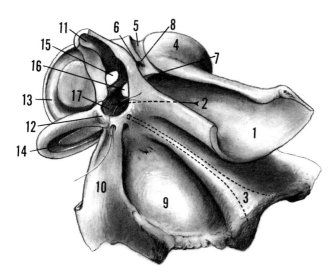

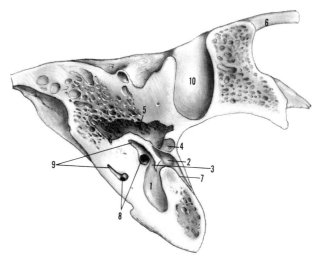

Figure 131. Posterosuperior view of a skeletonized otic capsule of an adult. This shows the cochlear and vestibular aqueducts and their relations, as well as the first part of the facial canal in its intercochleovestibular course. 1, Internal auditory meatus. 2, Arrow in the internal auditory meatus points to the foramen singulare. 3, Cochlear aqueduct. 4, Top coil of cochlea. 5, Geniculate fossa. 6, Superior vestibular foramen. 7, Crista transversa. 8, Vertical crest. 9, Jugular dome. 10, Opened vestibular aqueduct. 11, Superior semicircular canal. 12, Ampullary end of the superior semicircular canal. 13, Lateral semicircular canal. 14, Posterior semicircular canal. 15, Oval window. 16, Round window. 17, Vestibule.

Figure 133. Upper half of a horizontal cut through the internal auditory meatus and geniculate fossa. 1, Roof of the internal auditory meatus. 2, Geniculate fossa. 3, Canal for superior vestibular nerve. 4, Geniculate sinus. 5, Tympanum. 6, Zygoma. 7, Canal and hiatus for greater superficial petrosal nerve. 8, Superior semicircular canal. 9, Lateral semicircular canal. 10, Temporomandibular joint. Note the thin bony wall separating the geniculate sinus from the facial nerve in the geniculate fossa.

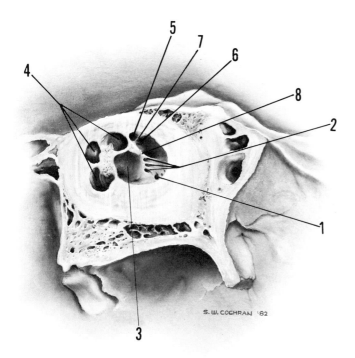

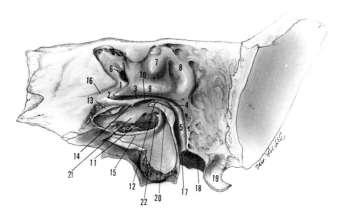

Figure 132. Vertical cut through the temporal bone showing details of the fundus of the internal auditory meatus. 1, Foramen singulare. 2, Saccular fossa. 3, Cochlear fossa. 4, Cochlea. 5, Facial canal. 6, Superior vestibular fossa. 7, Vertical crest. 8, Transverse crest.

Figure 134. The facial canal in its entire length. 1, First part of facial canal (intercochleovestibular). 2, Geniculate fossa with first turn of facial canal. 3, Transverse or second part of facial canal. 4, Second turn of facial canal. 5, Vertical or third part of facial canal. 6, Internal auditory meatus. 7, Superior semicircular canal. 8, Posterior semicircular canal. 9, Lateral semicircular canal. 10, Oval window. 11, Round window niche. 12, Pyramidal eminence. 13, Tensor tympani canal. 14, Processus cochleariformis. 15, Sulcus tympanicus. 16, Facial hiatus. 17, Stylomastoid foramen. 18, Digastric groove. 19, Mastoid tip cell. 20, Posterior wall of external auditory canal. 21, Promontory. 22, Chorda tympani nerve.

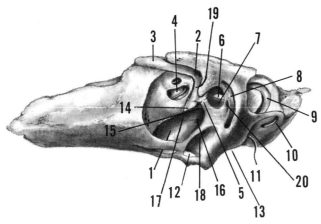

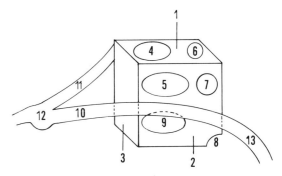

Figure 135. A dissection of the bony labyrinth from the posterior fossa showing relations of the facial nerve canal. Note the proximity of the first part of the facial canal to the basal turn of the cochlea, and to the anterior wall of the vestibule. 1, Internal auditory meatus. 2, Geniculate fossa. 3, Canal for greater superficial petrosal nerve. 4, Cochlea. 5, Canal for superior vestibular nerve. 6, Oval window. 7, Vestibule. 8, Superior semicircular canal. 9, Horizontal semicircular canal. 10, Posterior semicircular canal. 11, Vestibular aqueduct. 12, Termination of cochlear aqueduct at the pyramidal fossa. 13, Arrow points to jugular dome. 14, Transverse crest (falciform crest). 15, Saccular fossa (inferior vestibular area). 16, Foramen singulare. 19, First part of facial canal. 20, Petromastoid canal.

Figure 137. Schema showing relations of the vestibule with the facial canal (left side). Actually, the corners of the vestibule are all rounded, and the walls are convex externally except the superior wall. 1, Superior wall of the vestibule. 2, External wall of the vestibule. 3, Anterior wall of the vestibule. 4, Ampullary orifice of the superior semicircular canal. 5, Ampullary orifice of the lateral semicircular canal. 6, Nonampullary orifice of superior semicircular canal. 7, Nonampullary orifice of lateral semicircular canal. 8, Ampullary orifice of posterior semicircular canal. 9, Oval window. 10, Tympanic or second part of the facial canal. 11, First part of facial canal. 12, Geniculate fossa. 13, Second turn of facial canal.

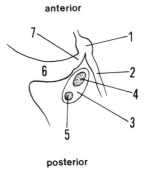

Figure 138. Schema showing divergence of the tympanic part of the facial canal with the external wall of the vestibule. 1, Geniculate fossa. 2, Tympanic (second) part of the facial canal. 3, Superior wall of the vestibule and its external border. 4, Ampulla of superior semicircular canal. 5, Non-ampullated arm of superior semicircular canal. 6, Internal auditory meatus. 7, First part of facial canal.

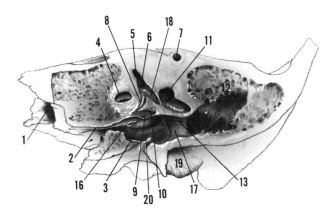

Figure 136. Horizontal cut with an anterior inclination at the upper level of the internal auditory meatus showing the first part of the facial canal and its relations to the cochlea, vestibule, and middle ear. 1, Carotid canal. 2, Tensor tympani canal. 3, Promontory. 4, Cochlea. 5, Internal auditory meatus. 6, Transverse crest. 7, Superior semicircular canal. 8, First part of facial canal. 9, Geniculate fossa. 10, Beginning of second part of facial canal. 11, Vestibule at ampullary end of lateral semicircular canal. 12, Mastoid antrum. 13, Facial sinus. 16, Processus cochleariformis. 17, Fossa incudis. 18, Utricular canal. 19, External auditory meatus. 20, Sulcus tympanicus. The second part of the facial canal and the lateral semicircular canal overhang the oval window and the posterior tympanic sinus to a remarkable degree.

First Part of the Facial Canal (Labyrinthine Segment)

The orifice of the facial canal in the internal auditory meatus measures 0.68 mm in diameter.[36] It opens on the anterosuperior wall of the meatus very near the fundus of the meatus. Above the facial canal, we have the ceiling of the internal auditory meatus; below it is the falciform crest (transverse crest), and externally is a vertical crest (Bill's bar) that separates it from the superior vestibular area. The latter contains several small openings of canals that conduct branches of the upper terminal ramus of the ves-

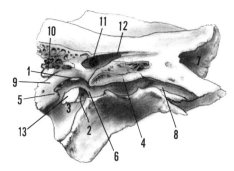

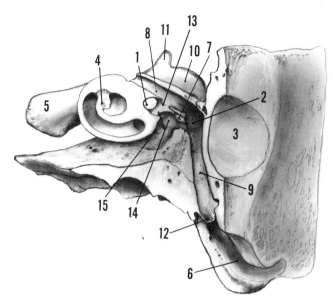

Figure 139. Medial wall of tympanum. Shows a large dehiscence over the geniculate fossa, which extends to the hiatus fascialis, as well as one over the jugular dome. 1, Oval window. 2, Arrow points to round window niche. 3, External auditory meatus. 4, Groove for tensor tympani muscle. 5, Pyramidal orifice. 6, Promontory. 7, Carotid canal. 8, Protympanum. 9, Facial canal. 10, Lateral semicircular canal. 11, Dehiscence over the geniculate fossa. 12, Hiatus fascialis. 13, Dehiscence over the jugular dome.

Figure 141. Medial wall of tympanum showing details at the second turn of the facial canal. 1, Oval window. 2, Facial canal at the second turn. 3, External auditory canal. 4, Helicotrema of the cochlea. 5, Skeletonized wall of internal auditory meatus. 6, Diagastric groove. 7, Pyramidal eminence. 8, Second part of facial canal. 9, Third part of facial canal. 10, Lateral semicircular canal. 11, Vertical semicircular canal. 12, Stylomastoid foramen. 13, Dehiscence in facial canal. 14, Sinus tympani and ponticulus. 15, Subiculum.

tibular nerve through the lamina cribrosa to the superior cribrosa macula, the utricle, and the ampullae of the lateral and superior semicircular canals. The facial canal crosses the petrosa in an anterior direction and almost perpendicular to the petrosal axis to empty into the geniculate fossa.

This first horizontal part (portion) of the facial canal contains the facial nerve and the intermediate nerve of Wrisberg. Its length varies from 3 to 5 mm. It is slightly inclined from above, below, and from behind forward, paralleling the zygomatic line. It describes a curve with internal con-

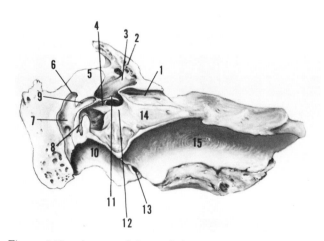

Figure 140. A view of the medial tympanic wall, with a high jugular dome and a high stylomastoid foramen. The pyramidal eminence is a shell. Note the small geniculate cells in the anterior tympanum. 1, Tensor tympani canal. 2, Geniculate cells. 3, Facial canal (second part). 4, Large ponticulus. 5, Lateral semicircular canal. 6, Second turn of the facial canal. 7, Third part of facial canal. 8, Lateral tympanic sinus. 9, Stapedius muscle canal. 10, Jugular dome. 11, Stapes. 12, Promontory. 13, Opening of cochlear aqueduct. 14, Protympanum. 15, Carotid canal.

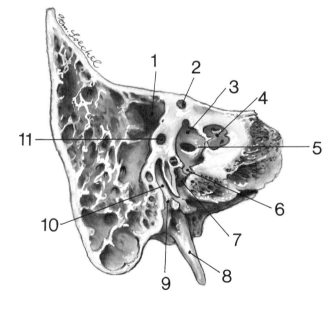

Figure 142. Vertical cut through mastoid and descending facial canal. 1, Antrum. 2, Superior semicircular canal. 3, Vestibule. 4, Cochlea. 5, Oval window. 6, Round window. 7, Tympanum (sinus tympani). 8, Styloid process. 9, Stylomastoid foramen. 10, Descending facial canal. 11, Horizontal semicircular canal.

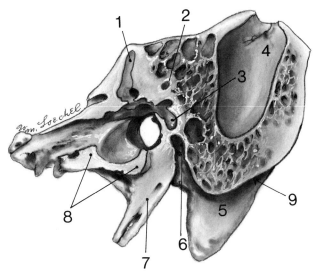

Figure 143. Vertical cut looking laterally through the temporal bone at the level of the styloid complex. 1, Superior semicircular canal. 2, Horizontal semicircular canal. 3, Facial sinus. 4, Lateral sinus groove. 5, Mastoid tip. 6, Facial canal. 7, Styloid process. 8, Tympanic bone. 9, Digastric groove.

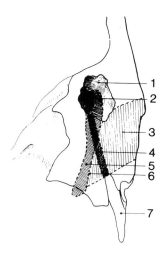

Figure 145. Projection of a vertical-transverse cut of the temporal bone (passing through the mastoid antrum) of the tympanum, external auditory canal, and third part of the facial canal.[92] 1, Superior wall of mastoid antrum. 2, Aditus ad ontrum. 3, External auditory canal. 4, Third part of facial canal. 5, Tympanum. 6, Tympanic membrane. 7, Styloid process.

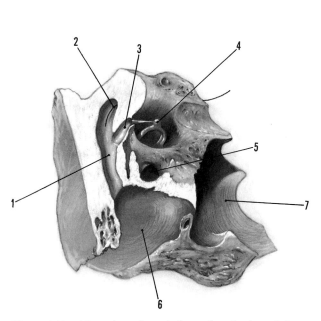

Figure 144. Vertical cut through descending facial canal showing it exiting high in the jugular dome. 1, Vertical portion of the facial canal. 2, Second turn of facial canal. 3, Channel for stapedius muscle in the pyramidal eminence. 4, Stapes. 5, Round window niche. 6, High jugular dome. 7, Carotid canal.

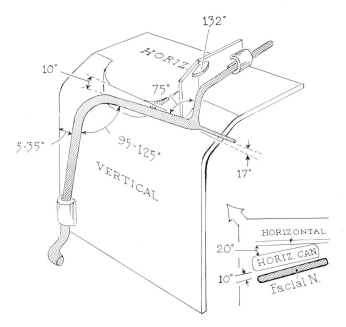

Figure 146. Schematic course of the facial canal. The length of the facial nerve in the internal auditory meatus varies from 5 to 12 mm. Upon entering the facial canal, there is an immediate angulation forward of 132°, as well as a downward inclination for 3 to 5 mm reaching the geniculate fossa. The canal then makes a turn of 75° and continues posteriorly for 10 to 12 mm. At the same time, it is directed outward 17° and inclined inferiorly 7 to 10° from the plane of the lateral semicircular canal, which in turn is inclined 20 to 25° below the true horizontal plane. At the second turn, the curve formed between the second and third parts of the facial canal varies from 95 to 125°. The third part of the facial canal (13 mm) deviates posteriorly as well as laterally from the vertical plane by 5 to 35°.[37]

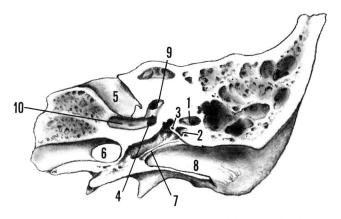

Figure 147. Horizontal cut near the floor of the internal auditory meatus. 1, Descending facial canal. 2, Facial sinus. 3, Pyramidal foramen. 4, Round window. 5, Internal auditory meatus. 6, Carotid canal. 7, Sulcus tympanicus. 8, External auditory meatus. 9, Vestibule. 10, Basal turn cochlea.

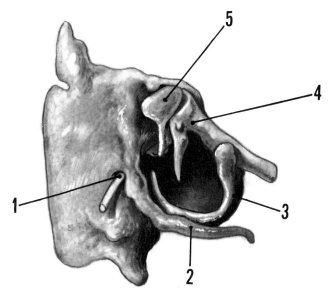

Figure 148. Temporal bone of a premature infant showing the high level at which the stylomastoid foramen is located. 1, Facial nerve at the stylomastoid foramen. 2, Styloid process (Reichert's cartilage). 3, Tympanic ring. 4, Malleus with large anterior mallear process (Meckel's cartilage). 5, Incus.

Bony Dehiscences in Falloppian Canal

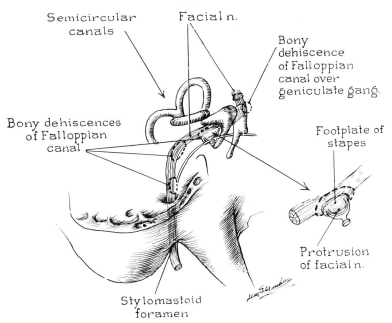

Figure 149. Locations of the congenital dehiscences encountered in the facial canal.

cavity that arrives at the geniculate fossa with a direction—if prolonged following its curvilinear movement—that would go toward the facial hiatus (i.e. anteriorly). It passes in the intervestibulocochlear groove.

At the very beginning of the first portion of the facial canal (see Fig. 136), there is a slight constriction from the vertical crest. The periosteum of the internal meatus is thicker than that in the facial canal, so that the facial nerve is more constricted at this point than in the remainder of the canal. If decompression of the facial nerve is carried out in the labyrinthine segment of the nerve for Bell's palsy, this constricting ring of periosteum should be cut.

As the facial nerve enters the facial canal, three morphologic peculiarities are to be noted.[6]

1. Whereas the nerves have an individual sheath of pia mater in the internal auditory meatus, this sheath curves up as the nerve enters the facial canal and continues with the arachnoid. This arachnoid-pia mater-dura mater junction generally lies in the fundus of the meatus, but it can occur in the neighborhood of the foramen or even far into the facial canal.
2. There is a slight constriction (0.68 mm) of the nerve. This normal stricture must not be confused with a pathologic stricture.
3. There is a change in the direction of the nerve that produces a 132° angle that is open anteriorly and medially (see Fig. 149).

Relations

As it leaves the internal auditory canal, the facial canal is in relation with the canaliculi of the utricular and the superior and lateral ampullary nerves, as well as with the vestibule in its anterior, medial, and superior region—immediately adjacent to the elliptic or utricular fossa.

When surgery is performed on the vestibule, gentle manipulations are necessary to avoid penetration into the internal auditory meatus and facial canal. The party wall between vestibule and internal auditory meatus is very thin (see Figs. 131, 135, 136). It is further weakened by passage of the numerous nerves into the vestibule.

The facial canal (only 3 to 5 mm long in the first first portion) quickly leaves the region of the vestibule and approaches the geniculate fossa. The first portion of the facial canal constitutes the internal arm of the first turn whose external arm becomes the tympanic portion of the facial canal. The two arms of the turn form an acute angle between them of 74° on a nearly horizontal plane,[37] and are separated from each other by a small triangular space filled with compact bone whose base rests against the vestibule and whose summit projects like a wedge into the acute turn in the facial canal (see Figs. 134, 137, 139).

Medially, the first portion of the facial canal includes in its curvature, with internal concavity, the top of the first cochlear turn (see Figs. 134–136).

Inferiorly, near the internal auditory canal, the facial canal rests on the superior external flank of this first spiral in the intervestibulocochlear groove. Near the geniculate

fossa it rests on the second spiral and on the cupula (see Figs. 135, 141).

Superiorly, it is in relation to the petrosal space covered by the petrosal cortex stretched from the top of the arch of the semicircular canal to the cupula of the cochlea (see Fig. 135). This space is frequently pneumatized by cells belonging to the superior prelabyrinthine tract.

First Turn of the Facial Canal and the Geniculate Fossa

The geniculate fossa is the crossroad of four nerve canals: the central and peripheral extremeties of the facial canal, the conduit for the greater superficial petrosal nerve, and the conduit for the lesser superficial petrosal nerve. The geniculate fossa is usually quadrilateral in shape, with sides of 2 or 3 mm when both petrosal nerves are large. However, the canaliculus for the lesser superficial petrosal nerve is often minute; in this case, the crossroads take a triangular form whose base faces the anterior wall of the vestibule and whose apex corresponds medially to the facial hiatus (see Figs. 129, 134). The latter opens on the anterior surface of the petrosa for passage of the superficial petrosal nerves. These run from the surface of the petrosa in two small grooves directed toward the anterior lacerated foramen. More often, the geniculate fossa is completely encased in bone, but sometimes the canaliculus for the greater superficial petrosal nerve does not form; then the facial hiatus is carried back to the geniculate fossa itself, so that it is covered directly by the dura mater (see Fig. 134).

If such a situation is encountered in doing a middle fossa approach to the internal meatus, there is danger of injury to the exposed facial nerve. Care must be taken in elevating the dura from the petrosa whenever the dura penetrates through the petrosal cortex to contact venous lacunae, as shown by Walker.[38]

Relations

Externally, the geniculate fossa contacts the anterior and superior angle(s) of the tympanum in front of the chochleariform process. A bed of small cells conceals it from view (see Figs. 134, 139, 141).

Inferiorly, the geniculate fossa rests on the cupula of the cochlea, which it overhangs to a considerable degree on the medial wall of the tympanum (see Figs. 136, 141).

Internally, it is in relation with the compact tissue that unites the cupula of the cochlea to the cortex of the anterior petrosal wall (see Fig. 136).

Superiorly, the geniculate fossa is in contact with the cortex of the anterior wall of the petrosa; but, in some cases, there is a space of as much as 3 mm that contains air cells of the superior labyrinthine tract (see Figs. 130, 133, 139, 140).

Posteriorly, the geniculate fossa is in relation to the anterior wall of the vestibule—from which it is separated by 2 to 3 mm of compact bone (see Figs. 134-136).

The geniculate fossa contains the geniculate ganglion. It is a bulbous enlargement of the facial canal. The intermediate nerve of Wrisberg terminates in the ganglion, but emerges from the ganglion as the greater superficial petrosal nerve passing through the facial hiatus (see Fig. 129). A portion continues on for about 1 mm and emerges as the lesser superficial petrosal nerve. Running parallel to the greater superficial petrosal nerve, it passes through the accessory facial hiatus.

The first portion of the facial canal is directed anteriorly. At the geniculate fossa, however, its course is abruptly changed; it courses posteriorly and slightly laterally, thus forming an acute angle of variable degree, but usually at an angle of 75° (see Figs. 134, 136–138.

Anterior to the turn, the facial canal is anterior to the vestibule; but once it turns, its course is along the side of the vestibule. Thus, the two arms of the facial canal embrace the anterior portion of the vestibule (see Figs. 134, 136, 137). It is at this point where the facial canal passes the labyrinthine barrier after leaving the cranial cavity.

The external relations of the geniculate fossa have been studied in some detail in recent years. The anterior epitympanic sinus was studied by Wigand and Trillsch.[13] This sinus lies between the bony compartment of the tensor tympani muscle and the floor of the middle cranial fossa, which slopes down to meet it anteriorly. The length, height, and width of this space vary from 1.8 to 5 mm. Its medial wall is in contact with the geniculate ganglion and may be dehiscent. A preferred nomenclature for this sinus, when present is *geniculate sinus* to indicate its position. This same area was studied by Hawke et al.,[18] who reported frequent nonlamellar new bone formation in the sinus in the absence of ear or systemic disease. This appeared to be a normal anatomic feature for this sinus.

A tiny bony plate extending down (1.5 to 3 mm) from the epitympanum in front of the malleus head and extending from the facial canal to the scutum was described by Hoshino and Suzuki.[39] This structure is not uncommon. It represents the anterior bony wall of the attic. Anteriorly, the space (supratubal recess) is in communication with the protympanum.[4] This same structure was reported by Gacek,[19] who uses it as a surgical landmark when seeking the facial nerve at the geniculate ganglion level. He shows the temporal bone of a four-month-old fetus in which this structure forms the outer wall of the facial canal in its tympanic or second part.

Second Part or Tympanic Portion of the Facial Canal

The tympanic portion of the facial canal is straight and measures 10 to 12 mm in length. It extends from the geniculate fossa to the posterior wall of the tympanum, running the length of the superior edge of the internal wall of the tympanum. Sometimes, its course is parallel to the plane of the horizontal semicircular canal; but more often, it is slightly inclined inferiorly, and forms an angle of less than 10° with the plane of the horizontal canal (see Fig. 146).

The longitudinal axis of the petrous pyramid forms an angle of 50° to 53° with the sagittal plane, whereas the tympanic course of the facial canal forms an angle of 35° to 40° with the same sagittal plane. If one were to extend the plane of the tympanic portion of the facial canal anterior to the geniculate fossa, the line would follow the gutter for the superficial petrosal nerves into the facial hiatus. Passing through the facial hiatus, we find the greater superficial petrosal nerve, the artery of the geniculate ganglion, and especially the homonymous veins, whose diameter is five times that of the nerve—all passing in a common fibrous sheath.[37]

The tympanic (second) part of the facial canal forms an angle of 37°, with the horizontal plane opening posteriorly with the anteroposterior axis—but this time opening laterally, so that its anterior part is deep and its posterior part superficial.

Relative positions of the tympanic facial canal are indicated below.

1. Anteriorly, it lies above and medial to the cochleariform process.
2. In its middle portion, it runs over the oval window forming the roof of the posterior tympanic sinus (Fig. 54).
3. It then runs under the lateral semicircular canal.
4. The lateral semicircular canal forms an angle of 30° with the horizontal plane. Therefore, the second part of the facial canal forms a backward and downward opening angle of 7°.
5. The facial nerve forms a backward and outward opening angle of 17° with the labyrinthine wall of the tympanic cavity.

Relations

The principal relations are established externally with the tympanum and internally with the vestibule.

External Surface. This faces the tympanum. It is free, except at its two extremities: (1) at its exit from the geniculate fossa, where it is concealed by small air cells (see Figs. 139, 140) and (2) at the level of the pyramid, where it enters the bony mass of the styloid complex (Reichert's cartilage) (Fig. 64).

Between these two extremities, the external wall of the facial canal is made up of a very thin bony lamella that is easily fractured at surgery if delicate techniques are not used. In such instances, the facial nerve may be seriously damaged even by a tiny bone spicule.

At the level of the aditus, the facial canal forms a semicylindrical projection running from front to back on the floor of the aditus passage, thus constituting its threshold; below, it is the tympanum and above, it is the aditus and antrum or passage into the antrum (see Fig. 136). This portion of the canal, which is 3 mm long, is usually seen clearly at surgery. If not, its position may be indicated by its relation to the anterior extremity of the projection of the lateral semicircular canal, below which it can be localized—or by finding it directly across the oval window niche from the projecting cochleariform process.

The tympanic portion of the facial canal lies medial to the attic; its contents from front to back are the malleus head, the incudomallear joint, and the incus body and its horizontal or short process.

Inferior Surface   The inferior surface of the tympanic portion of the facial canal can be divided into three parts: anterior, middle, and posterior.

The anterior part goes from the geniculate fossa to the extremity of the cochleariform process, which advances up over the anterior border of the oval window niche. It has a length of 3 to 4 mm (see Figs. 134, 136, 139, 140). Its internal border rests on the superior and external side of the cochlear cone, and its external border overhangs the promontory and adheres to the superior lip of the cochleariform process (see Fig. 134).

The middle part of the inferior surface of the facial canal goes from the cochleariform process to the pyramidal apex and measures 3 to 4 mm. It is made up of a very thin bony lamella and is often dehiscent. Thus, the facial canal in the middle part of its tympanic course is covered by very thin and fragile bone that overhangs the oval window. It may conceal the top of the oval window, so that in order to see the top of the oval window, one must look at it from below (see Figs. 134, 136, 139, 141).

The posterior part of the inferior surface of the facial canal is about 2 mm long. It adheres closely to the pyramid and overhangs the posterior tympanic sinus or the upper portion of the tympanic sinus (see Figs. 134, 136, 139, 141).

Superior Surface.   The superior surface of the tympanic portion of the facial canal is, at first, in relation with the small prelabyrinthine air cells in front of the projection of the semicircular canal (see Figs. 133, 139, 141); then, exactly at the point where it passes above the anterior commissure of the oval window, the facial canal engages under the ampulla of the horizontal semicircular canal. Its superior surface enters in very intimate contact with the inferior surface of the ampulla for a length of about 2 mm (see Figs. 134, 139). The bony plate separating the cavity of the horizontal ampulla and the facial canal is often less than 1 mm thick (see Fig. 141). More posterior, the facial canal passes under the horizontal canal until it reaches the middle of the arch of the canal. It then begins its second turn in order to assume a vertical direction downward (see Figs. 134, 141). The facial canal slopes slightly downward in relation to the plane of the horizontal canal. If only 1 mm separates it from the anterior edge of the ampulla, there is often 2 mm at the level of the arch of the canal.

The horizontal canal covers the superior surface of the facial canal to a variable degree. If the facial canal takes a more transverse direction in its relation to the petrosa, it engages deeply under the semicircular canal (see Fig. 136). On the other hand, if it tends to become parallel to the longitudinal axis of the petrosa, the facial canal is only slightly engaged under the anterior arm of the horizontal canal.

Internal Surface.   On leaving the geniculate fossa for 2 to 3 mm, the internal surface of the facial canal corresponds to the triangular space separating the two arms of its first turn in front of the vestibule (see Fig. 134). It then arrives at the anteroexternal angle of the vesibule just above the anterior commissure of the oval window and just below the anterior edge of the ampulla of the external canal (see Fig. 134). This is the point where the facial canal and the vestibule are the closest to each other. Only the labyrinthine capsule separates their cavities by 1 mm or less of bone (see Figs. 137-139, 141).

At this level, the facial canal passes in a sort of groove formed above by the ampulla of the horizontal canal and, medially, by the portion of the vestibular wall that extends from the ampulla to the superior edge of the oval window. This section of the wall rarely has more than 1 mm of height in the middle of the window. It is a little wider at the level of the commissure because of the rounded shapes of the ampulla and of the lintel of the window, which it faces on their convexity. That is why the facial canal, which often has nearly a 2 mm diameter, including cavity and walls, cannot lodge comletely in the groove; instead, it hangs over the lintel of the oval window below. That is why the top of the oval window is often found concealed by the facial canal (see Figs. 134, 136-137, 139).

The facial canal is closest to the ampulla of the horizontal canal, the external wall of the vestibule, and the oval window at the level of the anterior commissure of the oval window. At that point, the facial canal is equidistant from the ampulla above, the vestibule medially, and the oval window below. The distance is usually less than 1 mm.

Posterior to this point, the facial canal tends to swerve externally, while the external wall of the vestibule is inclined toward the interior (see Fig. 138). That is why the relations of these structures at the level of the posterior commissure of the oval window are no longer the same as before. Here the facial canal can be 2 mm from the window and a lesser distance from the vestibule. The facial canal would be even more separated if the external wall of the vestibule did not present an external convexity.

On leaving the posterior commissure of the oval window, the external wall of the vestibule turns medially, while the facial canal goes externally—so that at the level of the posterior edge of the vestibule, the two structures can be found separated from each other by 3 or 4 mm (see Figs. 134, 138).

It is possible for the facial canal to lose contact with the bony labyrinth because an assessory cavity of the tympanum, the tympanic sinus, or the posterior tympanic sinus is insinuated between them while occupying the angle formed by the posterior half of the external wall of the vestibule medially, the posterior semicircular canal posteriorly, and the horizontal semicircular canal above.

Second Turn of the Facial Canal

The second turn of the facial canal is a curvature with a wide, graceful radius that starts in the horizontal plane and then becomes almost vertical. Sometimes this curvature is double—not only bending inferiorly, but also a bit posteriorly and medially to approach the posterior semicircular canal and the vestibule.

The angle formed by the second and third portion(s) of the facial canal is never a right angle, but varies from 95° to 125°. The curvature presents various forms; sometimes it is short, and at other times very large, with the inflexion beginning at the level of the posterior commissure of the oval window and ending at the inferior third of the vertical portion of the facial canal.

In the newborn and young child, the second turn appears to stretch backward like a loop. This disposition can also be found in the adult and then represents an anomaly in its course.

The tympanomastoid course of the facial canal is extremely variable; hence, descriptions vary considerably.

Relations

The concavity of the second turn corresponds to the posterosuperior region of the tympanum. It is divided by the pyramidal eminence for the stapedius muscle, which is seen at the bottom of the bend (Fig. 14). The concavity faces the rounded eminence of the promontory separating the oval and round windows. The bend of the facial canal is 3 to 4 mm from the posterior commissure of the oval window and 3 mm from the tympanic sulcus. The latter distance is fairly constant, and represents the thickness of the styloid complex, which is derived from Reichert's cartilage.

The convexity of the second turn of the facial canal has relations posteriorly with the posterior semicircular canal and the posterior cranial fossa. In large pneumatized petrosas, 10 to 12 mm separate the turn from the posterior fossa (see Fig. 134), and in small, narrow petrosas, the distance may be only 4 mm. In the first case, the ampullary arm of the posterior canal is 3 to 4 mm from the turn; but in the second, the facial canal and posterior canal contact each other, and their cavities are separated only by the thickness of the labyrinthine capsule and the facial canal wall—a distance of 1.5 mm.

The distance separating the turn of the facial from the summit of the angle formed by the horizontal semicircular canal and the posterior vertical canal is at most 3 to 4 mm from the turn; but in the second, the facial canal and posterior canal contact each other, and their cavities are separated only by the thickness of the labyrinthine capsule and the facial canal wall—a distance of 1.5 mm.

The distance separating the turn of the facial from the summit of the angle formed by the horizontal semicircular canal and the posterior vertical canal is at most 3 to 4 mm (see Fig. 134).

Above the second turn of the facial canal lies the arch of the horizontal semicircular canal, but the turn in the facial canal quickly separates from it as it proceeds posteriorly and inferiorly (see Fig. 134).

Medially, the second turn of the facial canal is separated from the ampulla of the posterior semicircular canal by 4 to 5 mm of compact bone or cells in large petrosas (se Fig. 134) and by only 2 mm of compact bone in contracted petrosas. In the first case, the tympanic sinus often separates it from the posterior ampulla. This does not occur in the second case.

Externally, on leaving the posterior third of its tympanic portion, the facial canal immediately encounters progressively thickening bone on its external and superior surface. This heavy bone separates the posterior tympanum from the mastoid cells up to the level of the fossa incudis, which is the floor of the mastoid antrum. It is referred to as the posterior buttress and as the "massif du facial" by French otologists. It is of second branchial arch origin (Reichert's cartilage). The facial nerve is the nerve of the second branchial arch. It takes a position on the posterior and medial portion of this extension up into the complex posterior tympanum of the styloid complex. The term *styloid complex* is applied to the styloid process, posterior wall of the tympanum up to the fossa incudis, pyramidal process, ponticulus, and sibiculum and chordal eminence.[5] The facial canal keeps this relationship until it emerges at the stylomastoid foramen.

From the surgeon's view, the facial canal and the posterior limb of the horizontal canal are suddenly covered by this styloid complex. If one dissects carefully through this mass of bone, one can uncover the facial sinus (see Fig. 64) which is a recess descending along the external surface of the facial canal as far down as the level of the canal for the chorda tympani nerve.[5] Once this sinus is uncovered laterally, it is usually possible to see the descending facial canal beneath its thin, smooth medial wall. Laterally, the styloid complex fuses with the tympanic bone.

Third Part or Vertical Portion of the Facial Canal

The vertical portion of the facial canal extends from the second turn to the stylomastoid foramen (13 mm). It is nearly rectilinear. It forms an angle of 95° to 125° with the tympanic portion of the facial canal (Figs. 134, 140-143, 145, 146). It deviates from the vertical posteriorly. It runs through the mastoid process, and thus merits the name *mastoid portion.*

The vertical portion of the facial canal tends to swing laterally (Fig. 145); at the level of the stylomastoid foramen, the nerve is found more external than at the level of the last turn. This lateral deviation may reach 2 or 3 mm. In some individuals, however, the canal may be found to have deviated medially instead of laterally.

The superior half of the third portion of the facial canal rarely deviates from its vertical course except for a minimal external shift. The second turn lies beneath the posterior portion of the horizontal canal. Therefore, the facial canal is very rarely external to the projection of the horizontal canal. If the surgeon remains 1 or 2 mm external to the horizontal canal, there is no risk of injury to the facial nerve.

Posteriorly, the vertical portion of the facial canal is separated from the posterior fossa by a distance of 4 to 12 mm. This retrofacial space is usually occupied by the retrofacial air cells. The inferior third of the descending mastoid portion of the lateral sinus lies directly behind the facial canal at a distance varying form 3 to 10 mm. The mastoid portion of the facial canal deviates posteriorly from the vertical by 5° to 35°—a point to always remember when operating in the mastoid (see Fig. 146).

Medially, the vertical portion of the facial canal enters in relation to the jugular bulb (Figs. 140, 144). These relations are very variable. When the jugular fossa is high, the facial canal is accessible from the posterior via the retrofacial space, or anteriorly via the tympanum. The facial canal can be found 8 mm external to the jugular dome; at other times (rarely), its thin bony shell can adhere to the dome along its entire vertical length. The facial canal may even be dehiscent in the jugular bulb, which remains below the level of the stylomastoid foramen.

When the facial canal is not in contact with the jugular dome (this is the usual case), the space that separates them is filled with compact bone separating the tympanum from the occipitojugular region. However, this endofacial region can be filled by air cells, the jugular fossa may be absent, and the sublabyrinthine space is found to be pneumatized. In such a case, the tympanum, occipitojugular cells, and sublabyrinthine spaces can form a very large pneumatic area, which could be difficult to eradicate in cases of infection. The tympanic sinus often passes medial to the facial canal as far up as the inferior arm of the posterior canal (see Fig. 57).

The third portion of the facial canal is in relation anteriorly with the tympanum and the external auditory canal. In its superior region, it is in relation to the posterior wall of the tympanum, which is made up of the styloid complex (see Fig. 64) and varies from 2 to 4 mm in thickness. At the level of the round window, it crosses the tympanic bone in an "X" and is found hereafter behind the external auditory canal (see Figs. 140, 145). This crossing results form the fact that the tympanic membrane is more or less strongly inclined from above to below and from externally to internally, while the facial canal is nearly vertical.[40] The tympanic ring is thus a good landmark for the facial canal, with 3 mm constantly separating it. Further down, the posterior wall of the external auditory canal and the facial canal deviate a little more from each other. The external auditory canal is horizontal and the facial canal is vertical; their relationships are measured by the height of the external canal and cease completely at the level of its floor, which corresponds to the junction of the middle and inferior thirds of the facial canal.

Stylomastoid Foramen

The stylomastoid foramen opens at the base of the petrosa between the mastoid process and the styloid. It is always very close to the styloid process, and is often contiguous to its base and lies on its posteroexternal surface. Viewed from the profile of the head, it is projected on the suture of the tympanic bone and the mastoid (tympanopetrosal suture). At the time of mastoid surgery, the stylomastoid foramen can be localized by following the middle of the digastric groove forward to the base of the styloid process. The foramen lies immediately posterior to the styloid process (Figs. 134, 140, 141). To avoid injury to the facial nerve at the stylomastoid foramen, the surgeon should limit the surgery to the anterior extremity of the digastric groove or to the anterior edge of the base of the mastoid process.

In the newborn, the stylomastoid foramen (Fig. 148) is at a very high level, with the facial nerve emerging at the level of the floor of the mastoid antrum. With the growth of the squamosal portion of the mastoid, the facial canal is displaced downward while adhering to the styloid process. The position of the facial nerve in the newborn must be noted whenever surgery is done in this area.

Extensive studies of the anatomy of the facial canal have been made by Bellocq,[11] Girard,[35] and Paturet.[41] Further information may be obtained from these sources.

Anatomic Variations and Anomalies Involving the Facial Canal

All portions of the temporal bone are subject to variations and anomalies. They concern the formation of the components that constitute the temporal bone, the extent of pneumatization, the configuration of the middle ear cavity, the differentiation of the middle ear structures, and the development of the otic and vestibular capsule.[6] They also involve the anatomy of the facial canal, the architecture of the internal and external auditory meatuses, the position of the endolymphatic sac, the location of the major blood vessels, and the persistence of certain embryonic vascular structures.

The facial canal, as it traverses the temporal bone, may display congenital bony dehiscences, variations, and anomalies of its natural course, and (in a rare instance), may include a large persisting embryonic artery or vein. Each of these features may have clinical and surgical significance.

The otologic surgeon must be familiar with these variations and anomalies, and must suspect them and identify them presurgically whenever indicated, so that he or she can adjust his or her surgical approach or leave them undisturbed in order to avoid an injury to the facial nerve.

Congenital Bony Dehiscenses in the Facial Canal

It is not surprising that the facial canal can be defective, since it is made from two separate embryologic structures

—the primordial otic capsule and Reichert's cartilage from the second branchial arch.[42] In the 10-week-old fetus, the *facial canal* is a deep sulcus in the canalicular portion of the primordial otic capsule. The otic capsule is, at that time, entirely cartilaginous. Reichert's cartilage becomes attached to the otic capsule and provides the remaining cartilaginous circumference to the labyrinthine and tympanic segments of the facial canal. Its ossification begins at that time. This contribution from Reichert's cartilage persists as a readily identifiable histologic structure through the first postnatal year. By the end of the year, ossification is generally completed. In some instances, closure of the facial canal is never fully accomplished; and in localized areas or dehiscences, the canal remains open to mucoperiosteum of the middle ear, just as the tissue of the facial sulcus in fetal life was continuous with the mesenchyme beneath the epithelium of the expanding tympanic cavity.[42]

A gap in the continuity of the osseous wall may be observed in any portion of the facial canal; the majority, however, are observed along the tympanic segment (Fig. 149). Such dehiscences may involve the inferior, lateral, and medial walls. They are most frequently located above and posterior to the oval window, and occasionally at the cochleariform process over the lateral apsect of the geniculate ganglion. The remaining gaps are found along the mastoid segment, and very rarely over the superior aspect and medial to the geniculate ganglion. Their greatest width varies from 0.5 to 3 mm. As a rule they are less numerous and smaller in a well-pneumatized temporal bone; and they are regularly observed bilaterally and symmetrically in location and extent. The presence of more than one gap is not unusual.

The most accurate information concerning their incidence, size, and location has been derived from histologic examination of serially sectioned temporal bones. Baxter[43] examined 535 temporal bones from 332 individuals from the collection of the Massachusetts Eye and Ear Infirmary. His observation revealed an incidence of 55%. Ninety-one percent of dehiscences were located in the tympanic segment, and 9% in the mastoid segment. Of all dehiscences in the tympanic segment, 83% were located adjacent to the oval window involving the lateral, inferior, and medial portion of the canal, with the facial nerve protruding from its canal in 26%. Their greatest diameter ranged from 0.5 to 3.1 mm. In less than 1% (0.8%) did a dehiscence involve the entire length of the tympanic segment. Of all the dehiscences in the mastoid segment, 79% opened into the facial sinus and 21% into the tympanic sinus or the retrofacial cells, with the nerve protruding from its canal in 12%. Their greatest diameter ranged from 0.4 to 2 mm. Baxter's findings are very similar to those of Dietzel's,[44] who had examined 211 temporal bones and found an incidence of 57%, identical predilective sites, and comparable dimensions. The frequency of dehiscences in the facial canal is therefore sufficient to regard them as a variation rather than an anomaly. Guild[45] emphasized the clinical and surgical significance. Since Politzer[46] wrote about them in his textbook in 1894, numerous aural surgeons have reported their observations.

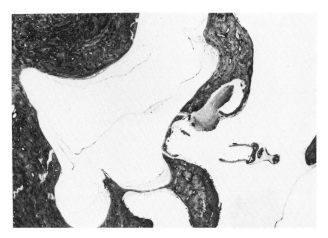

Figure 150.   Vertical section through the (L) temporal bone at the level of the vestibular and cochlear fenestra in an adult. The facial nerve partially protrudes through a congenital dehiscence in the inferior wall of the tympanic segment of the facial canal (H & E stain; × 16).

Dehiscences in the tympanic segment of the facial canal may lead to an inferior protrusion of the nerve from its canal (Fig. 149). This protrusion may vary from a slight bulge of the nerve through a small opening to a situation in which the greater portion of the nerve has emerged from the facial canal and has come to lie upon the superior aspect of the crural arch, and upon a portion of the footplate of the stapes (see Figs. 150-154). Occasionally, the entire lateral and inferior circumferences of the facial canal may be missing around the posterior crus of the stapes, leaving the facial nerve widely exposed (Fig. 155). That such an exposed nerve has a higher risk to become involved in an inflammatory process (Figs. 156, 157) or any other form of in-

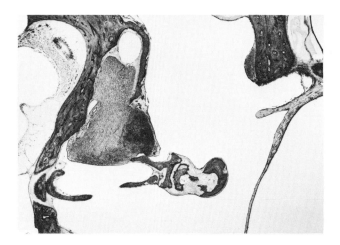

Figure 151.   Vertical section through the (L) temporal bone at the posterior end of the stapes foot plate in an adult. An abnormal vein (a persistent lateral capital vein) occupies one third of the facial canal. The major portion of the facial nerve lies outside the canal on the posterior crus of the stapes. Its lateral portion reveals an early asymptomatic schwannoma (H & E stain; × 12).

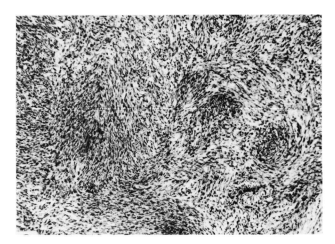

Figure 152. Same section as in Figure 151. The tumor is composed of interwoven bundles of long bipolar spindle cells with ovoid or rod-shaped central nuclei containing variable amounts of chromatin and inconspicuous nucleoli (type A tissue of Antoni) (× 250).

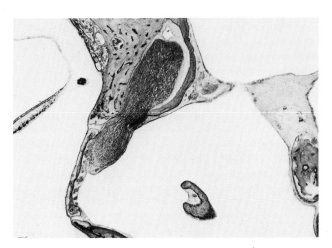

Figure 154. Same section as in Figure 153. The extracanalicular portion of the facial nerve covers the cranial half of the stapes foot plate in its entire length. There is no separation between the epineurium of the nerve and the mucoperiosteum of the foot plate (× 30).

jury is readily understandable. Similarly, a facial nerve injury may result, for example, from elevation of the middle cranial fossa dura during an approach to the trigeminal nerve in a patient with a bony dehiscence in the labyrinthine segment of the facial canal, above or just medial to the geniculate ganglion (Figs. 152-159). The observation that, in a dehiscence, the mucoperiosteum of the middle ear is in direct apposition with the epineurium may explain the potential effect upon the facial nerve of a local anesthetic in the middle ear. The inferior sagging of the VII nerve through a bony defect above the oval window (see Fig. 149) should not be confused with an aberrant course of the facial canal in that particular area.

A dehiscence in the lateral wall of the facial canal of the geniculate ganglion exposes the nerve to the anterior epitympanic recess. Care must therefore be exercised when eradicating disease from that area.[47] Similarly, the aural surgeon must be aware of the frequent occurrence of dehiscences in the lateral, inferior, and medial walls of the facial canal above and posterior to the oval window.[45,48] A dehiscence over the vestibular fenestra may be large enough to permit the facial nerve to slide out of its bony canal and rest on the stapedial arch, where it may produce a conductive hearing loss. Marked protrusions of an exposed facial nerve have been observed by many surgeons

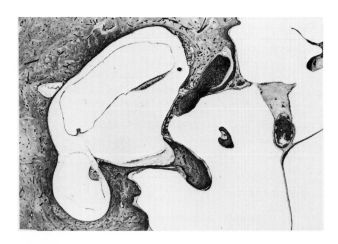

Figure 153. Vertical section through the (L) temporal bone at the center of the stapes foot plate of an adult. Almost half of the facial nerve protrudes into the oval window niche through a congenital dehiscence in the floor of the facial canal (H & E stain; × 15).

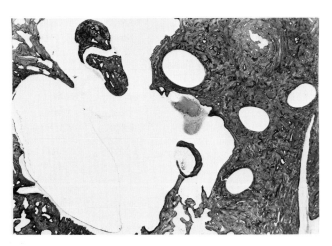

Figure 155. Vertical sections through the (R) temporal bone at the junction of the tympanic with the mastoid segment of the facial canal in an adult. The congenital absence of the lateral, inferior, and part of the medial portions of the bony canal wall resulted in an almost total exposure of the facial nerve in that location (H & E stain; × 12).

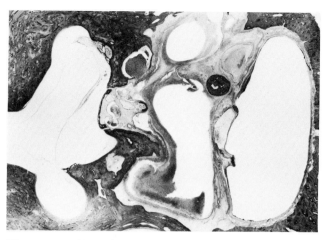

Figure 156. Vertical sections through the (L) temporal bone at the level of the oval window in a child with a congenital dehiscence in the tympanic segment of the facial canal, and an acute bacterial otitis media. Purulent exudate occupies most of the middle ear cavity and drains through a central perforation in the inferior tympanic membrane into the external auditory canal (H & E stain; × 12).

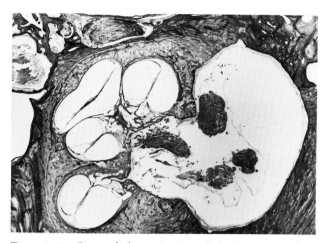

Figure 158. Paramodiolar section through the (R) temporal bone at the level of the geniculate ganglion and the origin of the greater superficial petrosal nerve in an adult (H & E stain; × 14).

and reported in the literature. Their occasional presence in middle ear dysplasias is well recognized.[49] Many years ago, a small asymptomatic schwannoma was discovered in a herniated facial nerve in this location in the left temporal bone (see Figs. 151, 152). A subsequent report of a tumor-like herniation of the tympanic portion of the right facial nerve in a 17-year-old girl[50] raises the question of a possible causal relationship. Of interest in this respect are the observations by Babin et al.[51] of a "traumatic" neurinoma of the facial nerve in such a herniation in two patients with a history of long-standing chronic otitis media.

Anatomic Variations in the Course of the Facial Canal

The labrinthine segment of the facial canal extends from the fundus of the internal acoustic meatus to the geniculate ganglion across the axis of the petrous pyramid. It varies in length between 2.5 and 6 mm.[52] The tympanic segment runs from the geniculate ganglion posteriorly to the lateral semicircular canal in a more or less inclined plane parallel to the axis of the pyramid. As it courses along the medial wall of the tympanic cavity above the oval window, it follows an oblique direction from inside out. It varies in length from 7 to 11 mm.[52] The mastoid segment generally

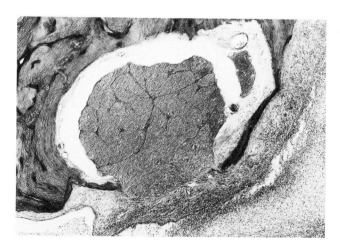

Figure 157. Same section as in Figure 156. An acute cellulitis involves the mucoperiosteum covering the facial canal, and extends through the dehiscence in the bony canal into the exposed underlying facial nerve (× 75).

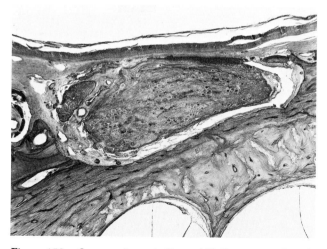

Figure 159. Same section as in Figure 158. Due to complete absence of the superior bony wall of the labrinthine segment of the facial canal, the geniculate ganglion is exposed and has become firmly attached to the overlying dura of the middle cranial fossa (× 50).

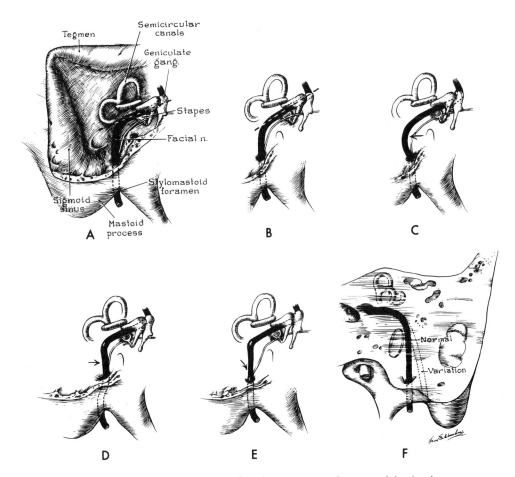

Figure 160.   The variations encountered in the intratemporal course of the facial nerve.

runs straight downward from the posterior margin of the oval window to the stylomastoid foramen. Its length varies between 9 and 16 mm.[53] It may form a slight anterior, posterior, or medial curve when viewed laterally (Fig. 160 C-E). In most cases, its course is straight downward. In some patients, however, the stylomastoid foramen is located more laterally when viewed from behind; and in such instances, the mastoid segment of the facial canal follows,—instead of a vertical,—an outward oblique direction (Fig. 160 F). Rarely does the mastoid segment follow and inward oblique course.

Anatomic Anomalies of the Course of the Facial Canal

In addition to the variations, there are a number of recognized anomalies involving the course of the facial canal. These anomalies are seldom encountered in the normally developed temporal bone, but they are frequently observed in its malformations. Fowler[54] collected the most pertinent forms from the literature and depicted them in a diagrammatic manner. Whereas the observations involving the mastoid segment may be found in a normally developed temporal bone, the ones involving the tympanic segment are frequently associated with a dysplasia of the stapes, lack of differentiation, or agenesis of the oval window. Severe dysplasias of the middle and inner ear are—with few exceptions—regularly accompanied by an aberrant course of the facial canal.

The anomalies of the course of the facial canal may be conveniently classified according to either the level at which they involve the facial nerve or the segment of the facial canal in which they are encountered.

Canalicular Segment of the Facial Canal

In an exceptional instance, the facial nerve may enter the petrous pyramid instead of via the internal acoustic meatus through the subarcuate fossa, and may run through the center of the superior semicircular canal to the stylomastoid foramen, bypassing the middle ear cavity[55] (Fig. 161A). In a rare situation, a bifurcation of the nerve may be encountered within the internal auditory canal.

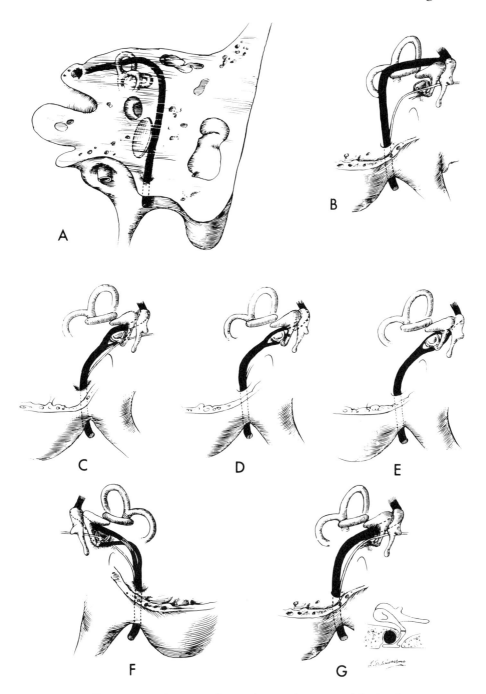

Figure 161.   Anatomic abnormalities in the course of the facial nerve.

Labyrinthine Segment of the Facial Canal

Rare cases of a bifurcation of the facial nerve within the labyrinthine segment of the facial canal were described by Altmann[56] and Miehlke and Partsch.[57]

Tympanic Segment of the Facial Canal

Aberrations in the course of the facial canal can be subdivided into the following categories:

1. Facial nerve coursing along the superior aspect of the lateral semicircular canal (see Fig. 161B).
2. Bifurcation of the facial nerve anterior or proximal to the oval window (see Figs. 161C-P).
3. Facial nerve coursing horizontally over the oval window (see Fig. 161G).
4. Facial nerve coursing through the stapedial arch (Fig. 162 H).
5. Facial nerve coursing posteriorly between the oval and round windows (see Fig. 162).
6. Facial nerve coursing posteriorly inferior to the round window (see Fig. 162K).
7. Facial nerve coursing from the geniculate ganglion straight downward over the promontory (see Fig. 162L).
8. Hypoplasia of the facial nerve (Fig. 163N, 164X, Y).

House (personal communication) has seen the facial nerve coursing along the superior aspect of the lateral semicircular canal in two instances (see Fig. 161(B). One observation was in a cadaver; the other was in a patient scheduled for a fenestration procedure.

Bifurcations of the facial nerve anterior to the oval window are commonly associated with developmental anomalies of the vestibular fenestra and stapes, whereby the greater or lesser portion of the nerve may run above or below the totally or partially undifferentiated oval window. This form of bifurcation has been observed on many occasions (see Fig. 161C-F).[54, 58]

A transcrural course of a facial nerve has been observed on several occasions,[56] (see Fig. 162,H). Marquet[59] reported a patient in whom one portion of a bifid facial nerve passed through the center of the stapedial arch (see Fig. 162). Butler,[60] during the removal of a cholesteatoma, found an exposed facial nerve passing through the stapedial arch almost totally occupying its lumen. The facial nerve reentered a bony facial canal that continued its course downward posterior to the round window (see Fig. 162,H).

Fowler[54] observed a facial nerve crossing the promontory in a patient with congenital fixation of the footplate and a persistent stapedial artery. Martin and Martin[61] reported a bilateral course of the facial nerve below the oval window in association with bilateral congenital fixation of the footplate and ossification of the stapedius tendon. Mayer and Crabtree[62] added three additional patients and reviewed nine previous cases from the literature. All 12 patients had a congenital conductive hearing loss, and the facial canal was dehiscent in that segment. The exposed nerve appeared normal in nine patients, but as a "boggy mass" in three patients. In 10 instances, the stapedial arch was markedly anomalous, and the stapedial footplate lacked differentiation. In one of these author's three patients, the lateral semicircular canal and vestibule were abnormally large.

Durcan et al.[58] discussed three patients in whom the facial nerve ran over the promontory between the oval and round window. The nerve appeared slightly larger than normal and overlaid the oval window from below. Leek[63] and Henner[64] made a similar observation in one patient with an otosclerotic process, and in another with a dysplasia of the stapedial arch and oval window. Jahrsdoerfer[49] observed anomalies of the facial nerve in 13 of 54 ears (24%) operated on for minor malformations of the ear (patent outer ear canal and identifiable tympanic membrane). The most frequent abnormalities were an exposed facial nerve devoid of any bony cover (10 of 13 patients), and an abnormal position of the facial nerve. The position of the tympanic segment of the facial nerve was normal above the oval window in two patients. In two, it was impinging the stapedial arch from above. In four patients, it was covering the oval window, in four it was below the oval window, and in one the exposed nerve segment was suspended in midair. In these 13 patients, the anomaly of the facial nerve was associated with a normal stapes in three patients, with a malformed stapes in eight, and with an absent stapes in two. The oval window was present in four patients but absent in nine. The round window was present in seven patients, absent in two, and not visualized in three.

A facial nerve, descending over the promontory anterior to both windows and leaving the temporal bone through the hypotympanum, was associated with an empty facial canal in a normal position as reported by Dickinson et al.[65] (See Fig. 162,L). Angell-James (personal communication to Fowler[54]) described a patient in whom the facial nerve ran through the anterior wall of the external auditory canal wall (see Fig. 162M).

Kodama et al.[68] discussed the histologic findings in the left temporal bone of a 9-year-old girl born with a deformed left auricle and left facial nerve paralysis. The extremely hypoplastic left facial nerve ran together with a large persisting stapedial artery within a bony canal downward over the promontory anterior to the oval and round window (see Fig. 163 N). The stapedial artery entered the middle cranial fossa at the facial hiatus. Failure of certain portions of the branchial arch cartilages to develop, and nonunion or a delayed union between these branchial arch elements and the primordial otic capsule, may permit the developing facial nerve to assume the abnormal forward position in these malformations. Similarly, a delay in the fusion of the stapedial crura with the lamina stapedialis of the primordial otic capsule may be responsible for a partial or total transcrural course of the facial nerve.[67,68]

Mastoid Segment of the Facial Canal

Aberrations in the course of the facial canal in this segment can be subdivided into the following three categories:

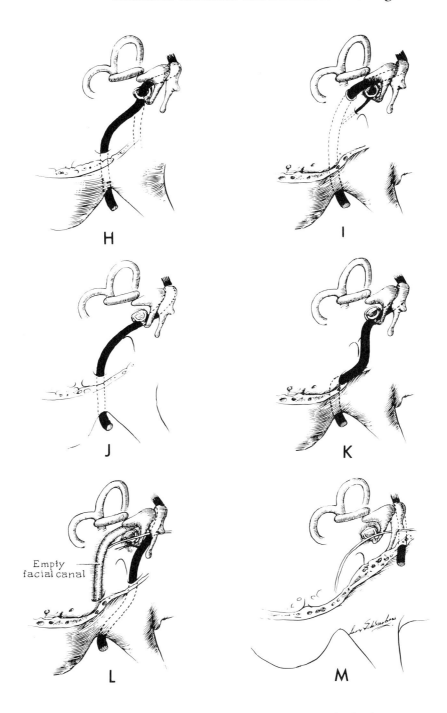

Figure 162. Anatomic abnormalities in the course of the facial nerve.

1. Facial nerve following an abnormal posterior, lateral, or anterior course (see Figs. 163R, 164S,T).
2. Bifurcation and trifurcation of the facial nerve posterior or distal to the oval window (see Figs. 164U-W).
3. Hypoplasia of the facial nerve (see Figs. 164,X, Y).

The most frequent anomaly observed thus far is the one characterized by a distinct posterior and lateral bulge ("*dorsal hump*") of the canal just beneath the prominence of the lateral semicircular canal (see Fig. 163 O).[54, 69] In that instance, the nerve is in a more lateral postion than usual and closer to the operator. Fowler[54] and Angell-James (personal communication to Fowler[54]) both had observed seven patients with that anomaly. Wright[70] reported seeing vascular prominences in that location. They represent anastomoses between the descending superficial petrosal

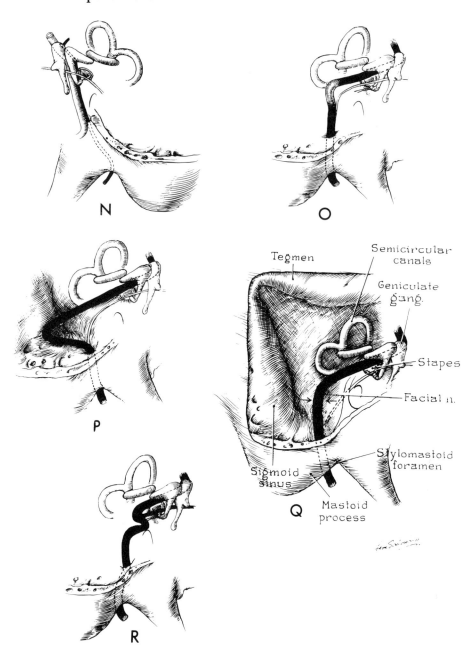

Figure 163. Anatomic abnormalities in the course of the facial nerve.

vessels and the ascending pharyngeal vessels. Their usual location is just above the level of the pyramidal process of the facial canal.

Fowler[54] and Kettel[71] described an abnormal posterior position of the mastoid segment, with the nerve overlying the anterior wall of the lateral sinus. This situation may be associated with an unusual lateral displacement of the nerve[54,72] (see Fig. 163P).

The entire mastoid segment of the facial nerve may be in an abnormal posterior location[69] (see Fig. 163,Q).[71] In such a situation, it may course 2 to 4 mm posterior to its usual location, which is posterior to the posterior wall of the tympanic cavity. The mastoid segment is therefore located between the external meatus and the sigmoid sinus.

Glasscock[73] reported an S-shaped anomaly of the right mastoid segment of the facial canal in a 5-year-old girl with a history of two episodes of right facial palsy preceded, in each instance, by acute otitis media. An abnormally large chorda tympani nerve joined the facial nerve at the level of the pyramidal process (see Fig. 163,R).

Pou[74] reported an infant with agenesis of the mastoid segment of the facial canal. In its absence, the facial nerve

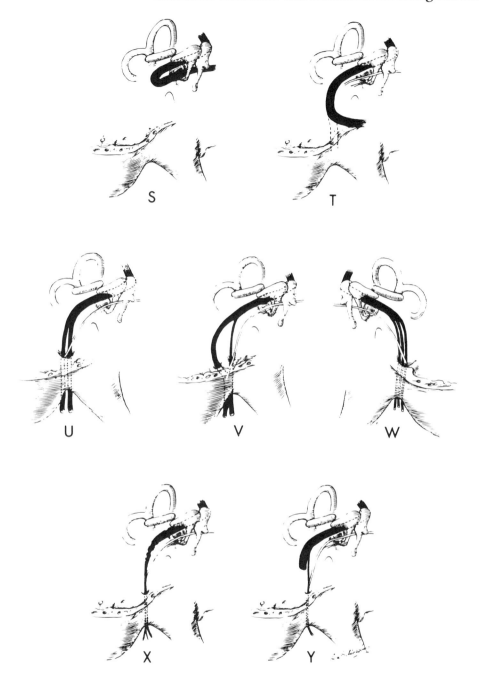

Figure 164. Anatomic abnormalities in the course of the facial nerve.

made an anterior turn somewhat anterior and lateral to the level where normally the second turn of the facial canal would be encountered, to follow the chorda tympani nerve (see Fig. 164,S).

Bellucci[77] noted that in 9 of 71 patients with congenital aural dysplasia, the facial nerve followed an abnormal course in the hypotympanum, turning anteriorly at the level of the round window instead of continuing downward toward the stylomastoid foramen (see Fig. 164T).

During the removal of the atresia plate in congenital aural dysplasia, Pracy,[75] on two occasions, observed the facial nerve taking a lateral turn below the short process of the incus, passing forward at this level to leave the temporal bone at the height of the temporomandibular articulation.

The tympanic segment of the facial nerve is formed by the 35th week of gestation. The posterior opening of the canal is located at the end of the second turn. This aperture is referred to as the primitive mastoid foramen. The formation of the mastoid portion of the facial canal occurs during the subsequent development of the mastoid process. Any disturbance in the development of that segment of the canal may result in an abnormal location or division of the nerve. Harpman[76] presented an X-ray film of the mastoid process of a patient in whom the facial nerve emerged from the lateral surface of the mastoid—about 1.27 cm (0.5 in) above the tip.

A bifurcation of the facial nerve posterior or distal to the oval window, with the two branches continuing in separate canals and leaving the mastoid process through individual foramina, was mentioned by several otologists (see Figs. 164,U, V).[52, 74, 78] The separate branches may cross on their way to individual stylomastoid foramina, or reunite either at or just outside the stylomastoid foramen into a single trunk again.[52,70] The lateral of the two trunks is usually the larger and the one that received the chorda tympani nerve (Fig. 164,U, V). Basek[79] found bifurcations in 3 of 500 individuals (0.6%). A trifucation of the facial nerve in the same location and with identical characteristics (separate canals and separate stylomastoid foramina) was reported by Botmann and Jongkees[80] and Heermann.[81]

Miehlke,[72] Hawley,[82] and Tobeck[83] found that the main trunk of the facial nerve ended in a blind pocket of the mastoid process, while only a very small branch continued the normal course of the nerve (see Fig. 164,Y). Marquet[59] reported a similar dysplasia of the facial canal and nerve (see Fig. 164,X).

The most severe malformations of the facial canal and nerve, including their total agenesis, have been observed in the thalidomide embryopathy.[72]

Anatomic Variations of the Chorda Tympani Nerve

The chorda tympani nerve may exhibit variations and aberrations in relation to its origin from the facial nerve, as well as its course through the mastoid process.[84] Its origin may vary from 1 mm distal to 11 mm proximal to the stylomastoid foramen. On the average, the chorda arises 5 mm above the stylomastoid foramen. In the rare situation of an extratemporal origin (2%), the chorda travels in its own separate bony canaliculus parallel to the facial canal. In an exceptional middle ear malformation, the chorda may join the facial nerve in its tympanic segment at the cochleariform process.[54] Three instances of a bifurcation of the chorda tympani nerve have been described by Durcan et al.[63]

Abnormal Artery and Vein

Occasionally, a persisting stapedial artery may be encountered entering the tympanic segment of the facial canal through the stapedial arch. It is a remnant of the dorsal end of the second aortic arch, which usually disappears early in fetal life. The persisting stapedial artery arises from the internal carotid artery, traverses the floor of the hypotympanum, ascends along the promontory within its own

bony canal, passes through the stapedial arch, and enters the facial canal above the oval window. It accompanies the facial nerve upward and supplies the outer surface of the dura in a fashion similar to the middle meningeal artery.[57]

In a rare instance, a large vein of equal size or larger than the facial nerve may be observed joining the nerve in the facial canal near the geniculate ganglion, and accompanying it to the stylomastoid foramen. This vessel represents a persisting lateral capital vein (Figs. 165-167). During early embryonic life, it provides the main venous drainage from the anterior and middle portions of the brain. It normally undergoes involution in later fetal life, when the anterior and middle cerebral veins begin to drain into the posterior cerebral vein.

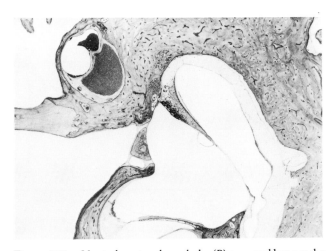

Figure 165.   Vertical section through the (R) temporal bone at the level of the cochleariforme process in an adult. An abnormally large vein (a persistent lateral capital vein) occupies half of the lumen of the tympanic segment of the facial canal (H & E stain; × 10).

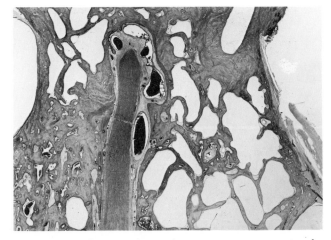

Figure 166.   The same abnormal vein is seen accompanying the (R) facial nerve in the mastoid segment of the facial canal (H & E stain; × 10).

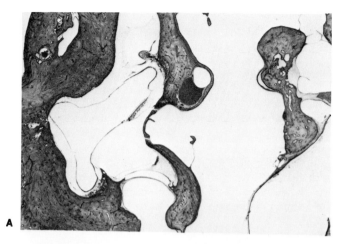

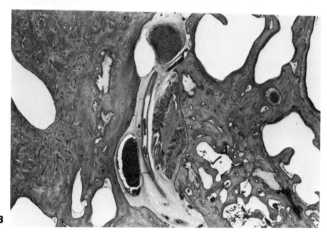

Figure 167A. Vertical section through the (L) temporal bone of the same patient at the level of the oval and round window. The abnormal vein, accompanying the facial nerve, is well recognized (H & E stain; × 12).

Figure 167B. The same abnormal vein accompanies the (L) facial nerve and stylomastoid artery in the mastoid segment of the facial canal (H & E stain; × 16).

Summary

The regional and surgical anatomy of the facial canal, as it traverses the temporal bone and relates to important adjacent structures, has been reviewed in detail.

Congenital bony dehiscences in the facial canal are encountered in about 55% of temporal bones. They result from incomplete closure of the canal wall during its development. Dehiscences may be observed in any portion of the facial canal. The majority (about 90%) are located in the tympanic segment, and about 10% are situated in the mastoid segment. In the tympanic segment, about 80% are located adjacent to the oval window, involving the lateral, inferior, and medial portions of the canal—with the facial nerve protruding in about 25%. In the mas-

toid segment, about 80% of the dehiscences open into the facial sinus, and about 20% communicate with the tympanic sulcus or with the retrofacial cells, with the nerve protruding in about 12%.

The variations of the facial canal may involve the length and direction of each segment, the angular relation between the tympanic and the mastoid segment, and the downward course of the mastoid segment.

Anomalies of the facial canal are seldom encountered in the normally developed temporal bone, but are frequently observed in its malformations. They include (1) aberrations of the course of a single or of all segments of the canal; (2) an abnormal relation to the oval and round window; (3) bifurcations and trifurcations of the nerve; and (4) associations with dysplasias of the stapes, oval window, external ear canal, and auricle. In a rare instance, the facial nerve may be severly hypoplastic or totally absent.

Two abnormal vessels may occasionally accompany the facial nerve in the facial canal: a persistent stapedial artery and a persistent lateral capital vein.

Axioms and Conclusions

1. Always look for the facial nerve.
2. Know exactly where you are at all times. Being careful is not enough.
3. If the surgical procedure involving the facial nerve makes corrective surgery difficult, then the procedure should not be pursued to the point where facial paralysis is a possibility.
4. Anticipate dehiscences all along the course of the facial canal.
5. If the facial canal is opened without injury to the nerve, there is no need to do a decompression.
6. If a soft tissue mass involves the promontory and hypotympanum, check the facial nerve at the geniculate and follow it peripherally before curetting soft tissue. A boggy mass on the promontory can be the facial nerve.[65]
7. When cholesteatoma obscures the course of the facial nerve, identify the nerve in an uninvolved area; using important landmarks (promontory, lateral semicircular canal, cochleariform process), follow the nerve into and through the diseased tissue.
8. Remove the matrix if it is present on the facial nerve—even if there is a dehiscence.
9. If in doubt, probe the facial nerve gently with a blunt probe.
10. Never avulse the stapedial muscle or tendon, but rather cut it with a sharp scissors or knife—it may be firmly attached to the facial nerve.
11. Polytomography is essential when anomalies are suspected.
12. Look for minor anomalies (preauricular cysts, etc.) that may indicate other anomalies.
13. A birfucated facial nerve can easily be cut accidentally—the two parts are usually unequal and the small part is overlooked.

14. Beware of any soft tubular structure in the middle ear regardless of its location.
15. If an anomaly is evident, do not cut a large chorda tympani nerve—it may have facial nerve fibers.
16. Never ligate the stapedial artery—it may compromise cerebral circulation.
17. Abnormalities should be carefully documented and reported.

The Extratemporal Facial Nerve

The facial nerve is the motor nerve to the muscles of facial expression, to those in the scalp and external ear, and to the buccinator, platysma, stapedius, stylohyoideus, and posterior belly of the digastricus. The sensory part supplies the anterior two thirds of the tongue with taste, and parts of the external acoustic meatus, soft palate, and adjacent pharynx with general sensation. The parasympathetic part supplies secretomotor fibers for the submandibular, sublingual, lacrimal, nasal, and palatine glands.

As it emerges from the stylomastoid foramen, the nerve runs anteriorly in the substance of the parotid gland, crosses the external carotid artery, and divides at the posterior border of the ramus of the mandible into two primary branches: a superior branch (the temporofacial) and an inferior branch (the cervicofacial) from which numerous offsets—in a plexiform arrangement called the *parotid plexus*—are distributed over the head, face, and upper part of the neck, supplying the superfacial muscles in these regions.

A plan for finding the facial nerve as it leaves the stylomastoid foramen is essential for preservation of the nerve when surgery is indicated for removal of parotid and other tumors in the area, as well as for repair of injured or severed facial nerves. The normal parotid gland abuts the facial nerve trunk as soon as it leaves the stylomastoid foramen. The parotid gland fills the parotid space (Figs. 168-178) which on cross-section is somewhat quadrilateral in shape with a lateral cutaneous surface (see Fig. 168) an anterior mandibular surface (see Fig. 174) posterior surface (see Figs. 169-173) and a smaller medial surface (see Figs 169, 173).

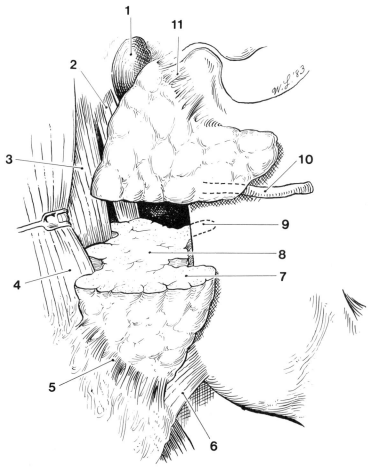

Figure 168.   External aspect of parotid gland. 1, External auditory canal. 2, Stylohyoid muscle. 3, Digastric muscle. 4, Sternomastoid muscle. 5, Adherent area. 6, Sternomandibular ligament. 7, Superficial lobe. 8, Deep lobe. 9, Internal extension. 10, Stensen's duct. 11, Adherent area.

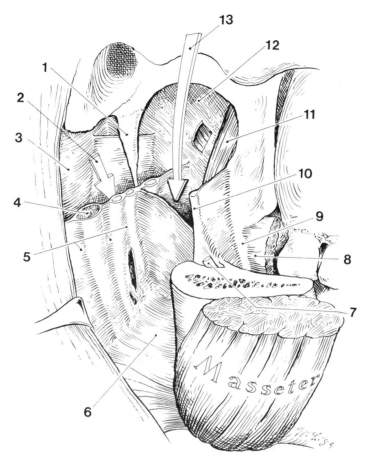

Figure 169. Parotid space, limited behind by the styloid diaphragm and inferiorly by the paroticomandibular fascia. 1, Styloid process. 2, Posterior parapharyngeal space. 3, Prevertebral fascia. 4, Digastric muscle. 5, Styloid diaphragm. 6, Paroticomandibular fascia. 7, Inferior alveolar nerve. 8, Buccopharyngeal fascia. 9, Pterygomandibular ligament. 10, Sphenomandibular ligament. 11, Internal pterygoid muscle. 12, Superior constrictor muscle. 13, Peritonsillar space.

The anterior surface lies medial to the ascending ramus of the jaw and masseter (see Figs. 173, 174). It extends to the medial pterygoid muscle, where it contacts the interpterygoid aponeurosis—the reinforced posterior edge of which forms the sphenomandibular ligament. Superiorly, we find two pouches. One is extracondylar, where a venous plexus passes; and the other is intracondylar—the pouch of Juwara (see Fig. 175) which lies between the neck of the condyle and the sphenomandibular ligament. Here we find a prolongation of the parotid gland and a neurovascular pedicle formed by the auriculotemporal nerve and the internal maxillary artery and vein.

The posterior surface is called the *styloid diaphragm* (see Figs. 169, 173, 176). Superficially, at this level are found the mastoid process and the posterior belly of the digastric muscle (see Fig. 170). At a deeper level is a large quadrilateral limited externally by the posterior belly of the digastric and internally by the styloid process and styloid diaphragm (see Fig. 169). This quadrilateral is crossed diagonally by the stylohyoid muscle and anteriorly by the

stylohyoid ligament. It is then subdivided into two triangles (see Fig. 170).

1. A retrostylohyoid triangle with a superior base traversed superiorly by the facial nerve emerging from the stylomastoid foramen.
2. A prestylohyoid triangle with an inferior base through which enters the external carotid artery.

The medial surface lies between the stylomandibular ligament behind and the sphenomandibular ligament in front (see Figs. 170-173). Its thin aponeurosis is often distended by a pharyngeal prolongation of the parotid gland into the peritonsillar space, where it contacts the styloglossus muscle and the glossopharyngeal nerve (see Figs. 175, 176).

The superior pole of the parotid gland extends upward between the external auditory meatus and the temporomandibular joint up to the skull base at the Glaserian fissure (see Fig. 168). Posteriorly, it is easily separable from

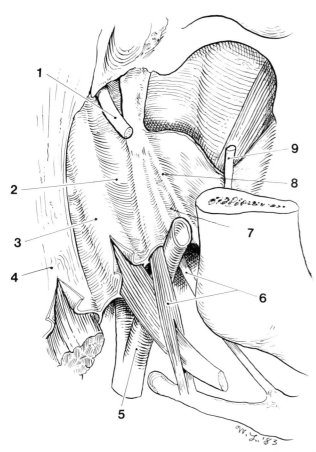

Figure 170.   Posterior wall (styloid diaphragm). 1, Facial nerve. 2, Retrostylohyoid triangle. 3, Digastric muscle. 4, Sternomastoid muscle. 5, External carotid artery. 6, Stylohyoid muscle and ligament. 7, Prestylohyoid triangle. 8, Stylomandibular ligament. 9, Sphenomandibular ligament.

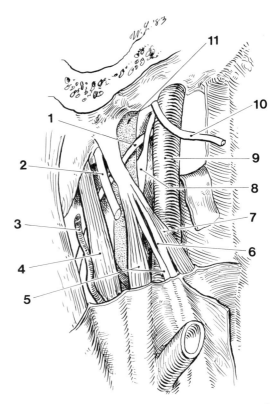

Figure 171.   Relations behind the styloid diaphragm. 1, Spinal accessory nerve. 2, Facial nerve. 3, Occipital artery. 4, Digastric muscle. 5, Stylohyoid muscle and ligament. 6, Stylomanidibular ligament. 7, Styloglossus muscle. 8, Vagus nerve. 9, Internal carotid artery. 10, Glossopharyngeal nerve. 11, Internal jugular vein.

the meatus; but anteriorly, it is firmly fixed to the joint surface (see Fig. 168).

The inferior pole of the parotid gland is supported on a fibrous hammock—the *sternomandibular ligament* (see Figs. 168, 169, 172, 175-177) which merges medially with the styloid diaphragm via the paroticomandibular fascia. This fascial hammock separates the parotid from the submaxillary gland. It is a thickened band of the superficial layer of the deep cervical fascia that runs from the anterior border of the sternocleidomastoid muscle at its midportion to the angle of the jaw.

Intrinsic Relations of the Parotid

Neural Plane

This lies superficial to the vasculature. It is constituted essentially of the facial nerve, which issues from the stylomastoid foramen in the deepest and most posterior part of the parotid space (see Figs. 170, 172, 176, 177) and crosses the

most superior part of the retrostyloid triangle. After crossing the lateral surface of the styloid process, it penetrates the parotid gland and rapidly ascends within it to become more superficial (see Fig. 178). At its bifurcation it is on the lateral surface of the external jugular vein (see Figs. 177, 178). Between the two main divisions of the facial nerve is a neural space, usually without branches, called the *triangle of Friteau* (see Fig. 178).[85] The division of the facial nerve is highly variable, both in the number of divisions and the level of branching, so that it creates difficulties in parotid surgery.

The auriculotemporal nerve issuing from the cleft of Juwara is situated above the internal maxillary vessels (see Figs. 174, 177). This is the deepest element of the parotid at this level. It crosses horizontally on the deep surface of the superficial temporal pedicle and ascends at its posterior edge, which it follows until leaving the region at the superior pole. It anastomoses with the facial nerve.

Venous Plane

This a venous plexus formed by the union of numerous veins (internal maxillary, superficial temporal, posterior auricular, occipital, extracondylar venous plexus, and

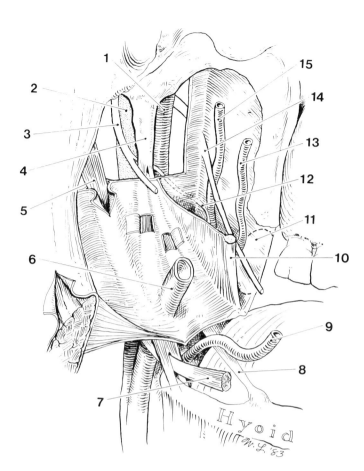

Figure 172. Medial wall and peritonsillar space. 1, Internal carotid artery. 2, Internal jugular vein. 3, Facial nerve. 4, Styloid process. 5, Digastric muscle. 6, External carotid artery. 7, Anterior belly of digastric muscle. 8, Stylohyoid ligament. 9, Facial artery. 10, Sphenomandibular ligament. 11, Projection of the tonsil. 12, Lingual branch of facial nerve (inconstant). 13, Ascending palatine artery. 14, Glossopharyngeal nerve. 15, Ascending pharyngeal artery.

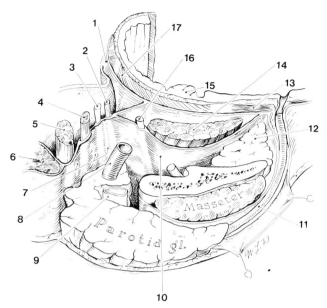

Figure 173. Anterior wall (horizontal cut). 1, Buccopharyngeal fascia. 2, Stylomandibular ligament. 3, Stylohyoid ligament. 4, Stylohyoid muscle. 5, Digastric muscle. 6, Sternomastoid muscle. 7, Styloid diaphragm. 8, External carotid artery. 9, Posterior facial vein. 10, Interpterygoid fascia. 11, Stensen's duct. 12, Fat pad of Bichat. 13, Buccinator muscle. 14, Internal pterygoid muscle. 15, Tonsil. 16, Sphenomandibular ligament. 17, Superior constrictor muscle of pharynx.

parotid veins). This venous plexus is drained essentially by the external jugular vein (see Fig. 177). The latter is oblique inferiorly and posteriorly, leaving the region to run along the lateral surface of the sternomastoid muscle. Earlier, it gave off the communicating intraparotid vein, which perforates the mandibular fascia to joint the facial vein (see Fig. 177).

Arterial Plane

Within the parotid space, the external carotid artery is the deepest element (see Fig. 177). It penetrates the flat inferior part of the space in the prestyloid triangle, while passing between the stylohyoid muscle and ligament after having crossed beneath the deep surface of the digastric muscle. At first, it forms a groove on the medial surface of the gland; then it tends to swerve superficially to penetrate the parotid gland. It gives off the posterior auricular and parotid branches. It bifurcates at the level of the posterior

edge of the ascending ramus, about 4.5 cm above the angle of the mandible, into the internal maxillary artery, which enters the cleft of Juwara and the superficial temporal artery.

Lymph Nodes

These are found in several planes:

1. Subcutaneous plane.
2. Subaponeurotic plane such as the pretragal node.
3. Deeper intraglandular nodes in the interlobar cellular tissue.
4. Along the great vessels.

Parotid Space

On emerging from the stylomastoid foramen, the facial nerve immediately enters the parotid space. The posterior wall of this space is limited by the styloid diaphragm, which is a fascial structure enclosing the posterior belly of the digastric muscle, the stylohyoid muscle, the stylohyoid ligament, and the stylomandibular ligament (see Figs. 169, 173, 176). Medial (internal) to the stylohyoid diaphragm lies the posterior infratemporal or parapharyngeal space, which contains the stylopharyngeus and styloglossus muscles, the internal jugular vein, the internal carotid artery, and the spinal accessory nerve (see Figs. 169, 176, 177).

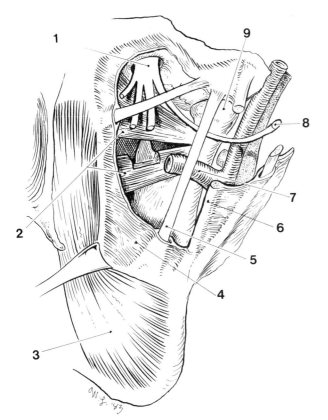

Figure 174. Internal part of the anterior wall viewed from behind. 1, Mandibular nerve emerging from foramen ovale. 2, External pterygoid muscle. 3, Internal pterygoid muscle. 4, Interpterygoid fascia. 5, Sphenomandibular ligament. 6, Stylomandibular ligament. 7, Internal maxillary artery. 8, Auriculotemporal nerve. 9, Condyle of mandible.

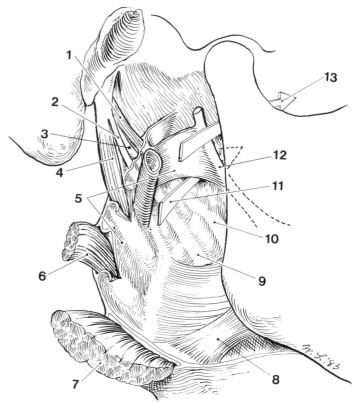

Figure 175. Inferior wall: 1, Styloglossus muscle. 2, Stylohyoid ligament. 3, Stylomandibular ligament. 4, Stylohyoid muscle. 5, Styloid diaphragm. 6, Digastric muscle. 7, Sternomastoid muscle. 8, Sternomandibular ligament. 9, Stylomandibular ligament. 10, Mandibular head of styloglossus muscle. 11, Pharyngeal extension of parotid gland. 12, Sphenomandibular ligament. 13, Retrocondylar pouch of Juwara.

The styloid diaphragm presents three *thin* areas:

1. Between the sternocleidomastoid and digastric muscles (see Fig. 170).
2. Between the digastric and stylohyoid muscles (the retrostyloid triangle—the superiorly placed base of which has the facial nerve entering the parotid space (see Figs. 170, 173.
3. Between the stylohyoid and stylomandibular ligaments (the prestyloid triangle).

The facial nerve is directed obliquely in an inferior, anterior, and external direction for a very short but important distance (1.5 cm), because it is here that the nerve must be sought. The facial nerve crosses the styloid diaphragm at the summit of the retrostyloid triangle, between the digastric muscle externally and the stylohyoid muscle internally. The facial nerve immediately penetrates the parotid, which at this level is separated from the parotid aponeurosis by a loose or cellular tissue.

The facial nerve is related to three arteries in this parotid space:

1. The occipital artery, which ascends the length of the inferior border of the posterior belly of the digastric muscle (see Figs. 176, 177).
2. The posterior auricular artery, which emerges from the parotid and climbs the length of the superior border of the digastric muscle (see Figs. 176, 177).
3. The stylomastoid artery, which arises from either one of the two perceding vessels and accompanies the nerve back into the cranium.

Branches of the facial nerve in the parotid space are as follows (see Figs. 176, 177):

1. The ansa of Haller, which is inconstant, arises immediately below the stylomastoid foramen and anastomoses with the glossopharyngeal nerve while passing lateral to the jugular vein (see Fig. 176, 177):
2. The posterior auricular branch arises 1 to 2 mm below (see Fig. 176) winds around the digastric muscle, and extends posteriorly and up on the anterior surface of the mastoid. Here it is joined by a filament from the auricular branch of the vagus and communicates with

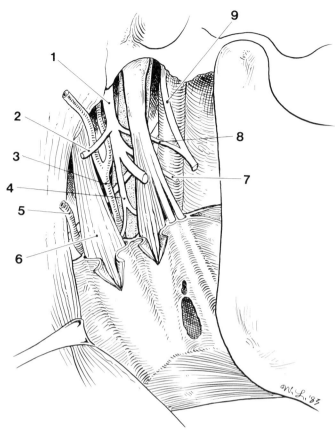

Figure 176. Facial nerve relations at entrance into the parotid. 1, Facial nerve. 2, Auricular branch. 3, Posterior auricular artery. 4, Nerve to stylohyoid and posterior belly of digastric muscles. 5, Occipital artery. 6, Digastric muscle. 7, Lingual branch of facial nerve. 8, Anastomosis of facial nerve to glossopharyngeal nerve. 9, Glossopharyngeal nerve.

the posterior branch of the greater auricular and with the lesser occipital. Between the external auditory meatus and the mastoid process, it divides into auricular and occipital branches. (a) The auricular branch supplies the posterior auricular muscle and the intrinsic muscles on the cranial surface of the auricle. (b) The occipital branch, which is larger, passes backward along the superior nuchal line of the occipital bone and supplies the occipitalis muscle.
3. The stylohyoid branch frequently arises in conjunction with the digastric branch (see Fig. 176). It is long and slender and enters the styloid muscle in its midportion.
4. The posterior belly of the digastric branch (several filaments (see Fig. 176).
5. The lingual branch (inconstant) follows the styloglossus muscle and replaces the ansa of Haller (see Fig. 176). It passes inferiorly and medially to the medial side of the styloglossus and stylopharyngeus muscles, and then pierces the superior constrictor muscle of the pharynx, Fine sensory filaments go into the vicinity of the base of the tongue.

Facial Nerve in the Parotid Gland

The penetration of the facial nerve into the parotid gland is made at variable levels; but, on the average, it is at a point slightly medial and posterior to the junction of the upper third with the lower two thirds of the posterior border of the mandible (see Fig. 177). This is fairly near the middle of a line uniting the superior border of the tragus to the angle of the jaw.

The nerve enters the gland accompanied by a descending branch coming from the stylomastoid artery. It is the satellite facial artery of Friteau, which follows it to its termination.

The facial nerve presents a curvilinear course with anterior concavity. It courses inferiorly, anteriorly, and externally, so that it rapidly becomes superficial (see Fig. 178). At its bifurcation, it is situated very near the external wall of the parotid space, from which it is separated only by a thin glandular bed.

The terminal portion of the facial nerve, within the substance of the parotid gland, divides into a temporofacial division (horizontally directed and larger) and a cervicofacial division (vertically directed, longer, and smaller) that in turn—either within the gland or after leaving it—break up into a plexus and supply the facial muscles (see Figs. 177, 178).

The facial nerve branches pass forward over the masseter muscle, pass deep to the superficial lobe of the parotid gland, and even run in tunnels in the fascia over the masseter muscle. The principal motor nerves lie in furrows, but do not penetrate the gland.

Temporofacial Division

The temporofacial division (see Fig. 177) lies between the superficial and deep lobes of the parotid gland and above the isthmus connecting the two lobes. The branches of this part of the facial nerve are complex and variable, and are in close relation to the superficial lobe of the parotid gland.

1. The *temporal branches* cross the zygomatic arch to the temporal region supplying the *anterior* and *superior auricular muscles.* They communicate with the zygomaticotemporal branch of the mandibular division of the trigeminal nerve. The more anterior branches supply the *frontalis,* the *orbicularis oculi,* and the *corrugator,* and join the supraorbital and lacrimal branches of the ophthalmic nerve.

2. The *zygomatic branches* run across the face in the region of the zygomatic arch to the lateral angle of the orbit, where they supply the *orbicularis oculi* and communicate with filaments from the lacrimal nerve of the ophthalmic division and the zygomaticofacial branch of the maxillary division of the trigeminal nerve. The lower zygomatic branches commonly join the deep buccal branches and assist in forming the infraorbital plexus.

3. The *buccal branches,* of larger size than the rest, pass horizontally rostralward to be distributed inferior to the orbit and around the mouth. The superficial branches run

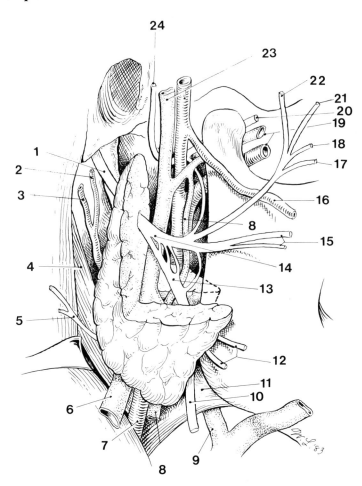

Figure 177.   Intraglandular relations (vessels). 1, Facial nerve. 2, Stylomastoid artery. 3, Posterior auricular artery. 4, Digastric muscle. 5, Auriculoparotid branch from cervical plexus. 5, External jugular vein. 7, External carotid artery. 8, External carotid vein. 9, Intraparotid communicating vein. 10, Cervical branch of facial nerve. 11, Sternomandibular ligament. 12, Buccal and mental branches of facial nerve. 13, Cervicofacial division of facial nerve. 14, Temporofacial division of facial nerve. 15, Superior buccal nerves. 16, Transverse facial artery. 17, Suborbital branch. 18, Palpebral branch. 19, Internal maxillary artery and vein. 20, Auriculotemporal nerve. 21, Frontal branch. 22, Temporal branch. 23, Superficial temporal vein and artery. 24, Auriculotemporal nerve. 19,20, Retrocondylar pedicle.

beneath the skin and superficial to the muscles of the face, which they supply. Some are distributed to the *procerus*, communictating at the medial angle of the orbit with the infratrochlear and nasociliary branches of the ophthalmic nerve. The deep branches, commonly reinforced by zygomatic branches, pass deep to the *zygomaticus* and the *levator labii superioris*, supplying them and forming an infraorbital plexus with the infraorbital branch of the maxillary division of the trigeminal nerve. These branches also supply the small muscles of the nose. The more inferior deep branches supply the *buccinator* and *orbicularis oris*, and communicate with filaments of the buccal branch of the mandibular division of the trigeminal nerve.

Cervicofacial Division

4. The *mandibular branch* passes rostralward deeply to the *platysma* and *depressor anguli oris*, both supplying the muscles of the lower lip and chin and communicating with the mental branch of the inferior alveolar nerve.

5. The *cervical branch* runs rostralward deeply to the platysma, which it supplies and forms a series of arches across the side of the neck over the suprahyoid region. One branch joins the cervical cutaneous nerve from the cervical plexus (auriculoparotid branch). The cervicofacial division is usually longer and more distinct than the temporofacial division. Sometimes the buccal branch of one or

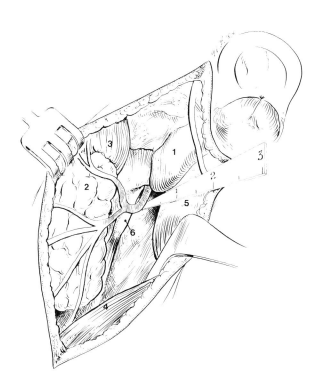

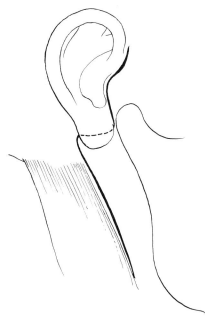

Figure 179. Surgical exposure of the facial nerve by dissecting the parotid sheath from the external auditory meatus. The skin incision begins from the root of zygoma (see text for succeeding steps).

Figure 178. Uncovered facial nerve found 2 inches (5 cm) below skin incision. It crosses on the lateral surface of the styloid process. The sternomastoid muscle is retracted posteriorly just below the attachment to the mastoid. The meatal cartilage narrows and points to the facial nerve. The tympanomastoid fissure also points to the nerve. The facial nerve rapidly ascends the posterior surface of the parotid gland, which is retracted forward so that it quickly approaches the skin of the face. 1, Cartilaginous external auditory meatus. 2, Parotid gland. 3, Masseter muscle. 4, Sternomastoid muscle. 5, Mastoid tip. 6, Styloid process.

both main divisions form(s) a medial horizontal trunk. According to Guerrier,[37] this occurs in 50% of the cases.

A constant anastomosis between the temporofacial and cervicofacial divisions crosses on the external surface of Stensen's duct. The temporofacial division often anastomoses above with the auriculotemporal nerve.

All the branches may anastomose by numerous filaments and with great variability to form the parotid plexus, which may be very extensive.

The facial nerve trunk and its branches are superficial to the blood vessels. The posterior facial vein often comes off the superficial temporal vein higher up in substance of the gland—and after picking up the internal maxillary vein it courses along near the mandibular division of the facial nerve. It may serve as a guide to this nerve.

The external carotid artery and its terminal branches (internal maxillary and superficial temporal arteries) lie deep in the intraparotid structures and deep to the posterior belly of the digastric muscle. At a more superficial level are

found the external jugular vein and its branches of origin, which are accompanied by some lymph nodes (intraparotid nodes).

When dissecting in the deep portions of the parotid gland, it is very helpful to have an assistant insert a finger into the mouth and push laterally while working against the finger from the outside. This minimizes the danger of entering the mouth, and aids in freeing the gland from the veins and the terminal branches of the external carotid artery.

Surgical Exposure of Facial Nerve

1. The preferred method of surgically exposing the facial nerve is to dissect the parotid sheath from the external auditory meatus, because it provides the best exposure. The incision begins from the root of the zygoma (Fig. 179), and extends vertically downward a little in front of the anterior edge of the foot of the helix and in the groove separating the helix from the tragus.[85] It follows the free edge of the tragus to the anterior edge of the lobule; then it proceeds along the attachment of the lobule to the anterior border of the mastoid in the retroauricular groove. The incision is then directed vertically to descend along the anterior border of the mastoid process, and then along the anterior border of the sternomastoid muscle. If necessary, the incision can be carried forward while staying one finger's breadth below the ramus of the mandible to avoid the mandibular branch of the facial nerve.

Returning to the upper end of the incision, the parotid

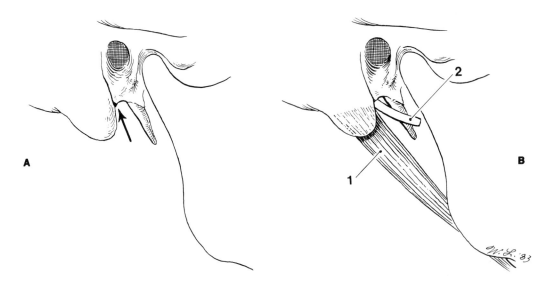

Figure 180.   A, Tympanomastoid suture. The medial course points to the stylomastoid foramen and emerging facial nerve. B, Digastric groove. Anterior end of the digastric groove is in very close relationship with stylomastoid foramen. Dissection is carefully carried forward and only slightly medially once the anterior border of the digastric muscle is identified and cleared. 1, Digastric muscle. 2, Facial nerve.

fascia is separated from the cartilage of the external meatus. Since the parotid fascia is firmly attached to the external meatus, sharp dissection is ususaly required here. The knife strokes must closely follow the curvature of the meatus. Then with blunt dissection, the cartilage of the external meatus is separated from the capsule of the parotid gland medially until the firm, bony resistance of the styloid process is felt at a distance of 1.5 to 2 inches (4 to 5 cm) from the skin incision (see Fig. 178). This distance, of course, is much shorter in an infant or child. Below, at the level of the inferior vertical incision, one exposes the anterior border of the mastoid and the sternomastoid muscles, whose anterior edge should be separated in front from the adherence to the parotid fascia (see Fig. 168). Some small vessels, such as the external jugular vein, should be tied. The great auricular nerve's anterior branch is sectioned. If at all possible, the posterior branch should be saved, since it supplies sensation to the lobule. One must remember to stay high, just under the root of the zygoma, so that the base of the styloid process is the first important structure to be identified.

With gentle traction on the capsule of the parotid anteriorly and inferiorly, and on the sternomastoid posteriorly, the facial nerve is brought into view, emerging from the posterolateral aspect of the styloid process (see Fig. 178). The digastric muscle in the depth is exposed at this time, and its superior edge is dissected free (Fig. 180 B).

The facial nerve is covered by a dense cellular and fibrous tissue that impedes the dissection. At this point, in exposing the nerve, one can take advantage of the fact that

the deep extension of the auricular cartilage tapers as it approaches the bony meatus and points in the direction of the facial nerve, which lies only a few millimeters beneath (see Fig. 78).

2. Another method of exposing the facial nerve is to use the fact that the digastric notch on the medial side of the mastoid tip always points to the stylomastoid foramen, which lies immediately anterior to the notch. The anterior border of the sternomastoid near the mastoid tip is retracted posteriorly. The *anterior border of the posterior belly of the digastric muscle above the level of the transverse process of the atlas is defined.* The transverse process of the atlas can be palpated through the thickness of the digastric muscle. By blunt dissection, the nerve can be exposed between the anterior border of the mastoid process and the styloid process (see Fig. 180 B).

3. A third method is *via the tympanomastoid fissure* (see Fig. 180 A). This fissure is practically subcutaneous. When followed medially, the fissure points the way to the facial nerve as it lies inferior to the stylomastoid foramen. Inspection of a dried skull will convince one of the logic of this approach.

4. A fourth method is *by tracing termimanl branches of the facial nerve to the point of origin.* Usually, the mandibular branch is sought; when found, it is followed up to the cervicofacial division, and then on the to the trunk of the facial nerve.

The landmark is formed by the posterior facial vein. This vein is formed by the junction of the superficial temporal and internal maxillary veins; at first deep, it crosses the parotid gland, leaves the inferior pole of the gland (see Fig. 177), and traverses the sternomandibular ligament to go forward to join the facial vein near the thyrolinguofacial trunk. The mandibular nerve or the cervicofacial division of the facial nerve is found just medial to it.

The proper technique is as follows:

1. The incision follows the anterior border of the sternomastoid from the mastoid to 4 to 5 cm below the angle of the jaw.
2. The anterior border of the sternomastoid muscle is freed above from the posterior surface of the parotid.
3. The inferior parotid pole is freed from the posterior pole of the submaxillary gland following the fascial plane. The freeing of the deep surface of the inferior parotid lobe is then followed from behind and forward, and the communicating intraparotid vein is found at its emergence from the sternomandibular ligament (see Fig. 177).
4. Having been found, the vein is freed and the inferior pole of the parotid gland is raised; and on the medial side of the vein, one finds the facial nerve, which likewise emerges from the sternomandibular ligament.
5. The mandibular nerve is dissected retrograde to the bifurcation of the facial nerve, and then on to its trunk.

The mandibular nerve may be sought in the submaxillary region. Unfortunately, the mandibular nerve has a variable course. The incision should aways be at a distance at least 2 cm from the mandible. Two features must be recognized: (1) the nerve is under the skin; and (2) the nerve crosses the facial artery near the edge of the mandible. The artery is located near the inferior edge of the mandible just in front of the masseter muscle. The external surface of the artery is dissected clear until the mandibular nerve is identified. Next, the crossing of the nerve on the external surface of the facial vein is picked up by dissecting of the vein from below, upward.

The Petromastoid Canal

The petromastoid canal was described by Mouret and Rouviere[86] in 1904 as a straight, inconstant, translabyrinthine conduit that connects the mastoid antrum with the cranial cavity. The petromastoid canal has also been called the *antrocerebellar canal of Chatellier* and the *subarcuate canaliculus* (Figs. 181,182).[35] It is partially a vestige of the voluminous subarcuate fossa, which one sees in the fetus (Fig. 18). It contains a prolongation of the dura mater and the subarcuate blood vessels (Fig. 183).

The petromastoid canal begins in the subarcuate fossa above and lateral to the internal auditory canal, and at the level of the midportion of the superior rim of the petrosa (Fig. 184). It continues externally, while describing a curve with a posterointernal concavity (Figs. 183,185,186). It passes successively in the arcade formed by the superior semicircular canal; then it passes above the horizontal semicircular canal, and opens directly into the antrum by

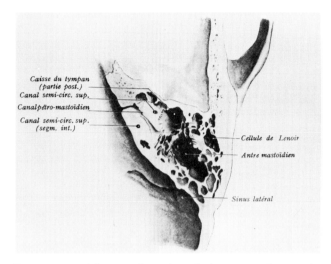

Figure 181. A horizontal cut through the petrosa showing the connection between the mastoid cavity and the petromastoid canal. Also note the large cell of Lenoir found equidistant from the external wall of the antrum and the corresponding area on the mastoid cortex.[41]

the intermediary of an internal mastoid cell (Figs. 183, 185, 187). This opening lies just above the second turn of the facial canal. the length of the petromastoid canal varies from 6 to 10 mm.

In the fetus and in the newborn, the petromastoid canal does not exist as such. It is superseded by a large pit,—the *subarcuate fossa,* which is situated on the posterior surface of the petrosa above and external to the internal auditory canal and within the projection of the superior and posterior semicircular canals (Figs. 18,187). The bottom of this fossa reaches the internal wall of the mastoid antrum. the orifice of this fossa is concealed by the dura mater. In the newborn, the subarcuate fossa does not appear to communicate with the petrosal antrum,[41] being separated by a variable thickness of spongy bone (Fig. 188).

In the course of development of the petrosa, the subarcuate fossa narrows and stretches out transversely, thus becoming the petromastoid canal, which can persist in the adult (see Figs. 183, 197-191).

The internal surface of the superior semicircular canal looks topward the petrous apex. In the newborn, it is free and rises on the side of the petrosa at the entrance of the subarcuate fossa like the vault that forms the entrance of a tunnel (see Fig. 18). In the adult, the tunnel is filled, its entrance is leveled, and the slope of the petrosa is no longer uneven at this level (see Fig. 184).

The medial surface of the superior semicircular canal is in relation with the bone overlying the roof of the internal auditory canal. Here one finds the intracranial orifice of the petromastoid canal, which opens into the posterior cranial fossa 5 mm from the superior semicircular canal. Air cells of the superior labyrinthine cell tracts may be found here. More distant still, in the posterior fossa, we find the open-

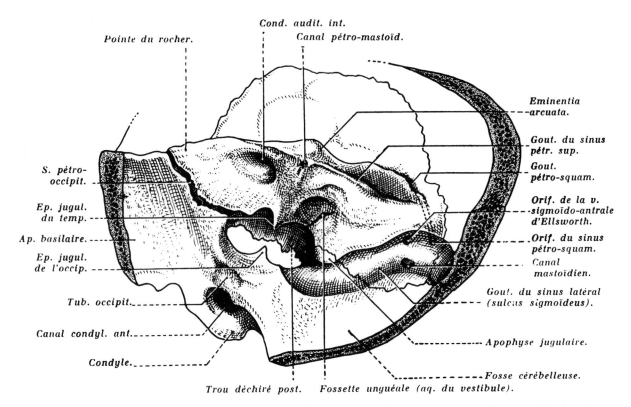

Cond. audit. int.

Pointe du rocher.

Canal pétro-mastoïd.

Eminentia arcuata.

Gout. du sinus pétr. sup.

Gout. pétro-squam.

S. pétro-occipit.

Orif. de la v. sigmoïdo-antrale d'Ellsworth.

Ep. jugul. du temp.

Orif. du sinus pétro-squam.

Ap. basilaire.

Canal mastoïdien.

Ep. jugul. de l'occip.

Gout. du sinus latéral (sulcus sigmoïdeus).

Tub. occipit.

Apophyse jugulaire.

Canal condyl. ant.

Fosse cérébelleuse.

Condyle.

Trou déchiré post.   *Fossette unguéale (aq. du vestibule).*

Figure 182. A posterosuperior view of the petrosa, petrooccipital suture, posterior lacerated foramen, and groove of the lateral sinus. Note the orifice of the petromastoid canal. The stippled duct is the course of the petrosquamosal sinus of Krause—Luschka or aqueduct of Verga.[92]

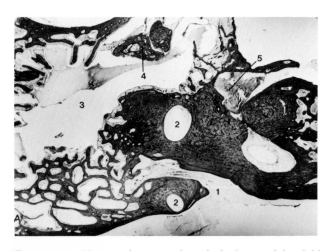

Figure 183. Horizontal sections through the bones of the child dying of acute otitis media and meningitis—left temporal bone. Shown are mastoid cells in direct contact with the large petromastoid canal containing a dural extension. 1, Dura in the petromastoid canal. 2, Superior semicircular canal. 3, Antrum. 4, Incus. 5, Geniculum.

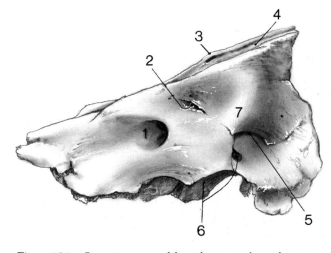

Figure 184. Posterior aspect of the right petrous bone showing internal orifice of the petromastoid canal. 1, Internal auditory meatus. 2, Internal orifice of petromastoid canal. 3, Superior semicircular canal. 4, Groove for superior petrosal sinus. 5, Vestibular aqueduct. 6, Jugular dome with dehiscence. 7, Prominence of posterior semicircular canal.

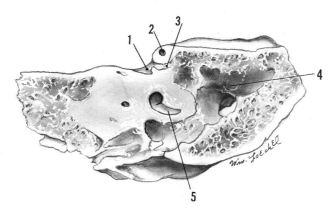

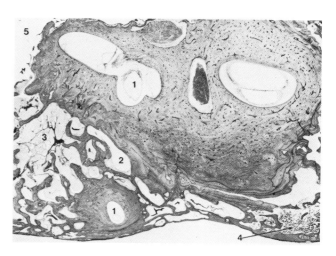

Figure 185. Vertical cut along long axis of the petrosa. 1, Subarcuate fossa. 2, Superior semicircular canal. 3, Petromastoid canal. 4, Mastoid antrum. 5, Horizontal semicircular canal.

Figure 187. Horizontal section through the left temporal bone of a young adult who died with otitis media and pneumococcus meningitis. The subarcuate cell tract is well developed. The posterior wall of the petrous bone is very thin. Most anterior cells of the posteromedial cell tract appear to come in direct contact with dura of the posterior cranial fossa. 1, Superior semicircular canal. 2, Subarcuate cell tract. 3, Mastoid air cells. 4, Marrow in petrosa. 5, Middle ear.

ing of the internal auditory meatus at a distance of 10 to 15 mm from the superior canal (see Fig. 184).

The external orifice of the petromastoid canal is found when one excavates the inner wall of the antrum above the horizontal semicircular canal in the direction of the petrosal crest, and in front of the posterior arm of the superior semicircular canal. The orifice usually is found in a periantral cell (see Fig. 185) but in 5% of cases, it opens directly into the antrum itself.[35] It then passes beneath the arch of the superior semicircular canal, nearer the nonampullary arm than the ampullary arm, and proceeds to open into the posterior fossa 5 mm external to and above the internal auditory meatus,—sometimes on the petrosal ridge, or sometimes 4 to 5 mm below by a slit-like orifice or even a depression.

The presence of the dura mater in the petromastoid canal is explained by the fact that in the lower apes (lemur to gibbon), the subarcuate fossa is occupied by a lobule of the cerebellum,—the *flocculus.* In higher apes, the flocculus is retracted and the cavity is narrowed; but the dura mater continues to adhere to the wall of the canal, turned into a recess where it fulfills its usual functions,—periosteal and vascular.[35]

In a human fetus at five months gestation, the subarcuate fossa is relatively large in the pyramid, and is as large as the internal auditory meatus. The superior semicircular canal approaches to within 1 mm of the squama, so that the depth of the subarcuate fossa is in intimate contact with the primitive middle ear cleft.

In a human fetus at seven months gestation, the subarcuate fossa is seen in the form a cylindrical cavity 5 mm in diameter and 7 to 8 mm in depth.[35]

In the newborn, the subarcuate fossa is reduced in size by new bone formation around its periphery and on the interior of the superior canal arch narrowing the hiatus (see Fig. 188). At six months of age, the subarcuate fossa is usually an ovoid cavity 7 mm long and 4 mm wide. The subarcuate hiatus still has a diameter of 2 mm.[35]

Toward the age of five years, the subarcuate fossa has been transformed into a simple canal. The subarcuate hiatus is now very narrow, and is no longer found under the arch of the superior semicircular canal, but has been carried back 3 to 4 mm medially by the development of the petrous ridge. With development of membranous bone, the subarcuate fossa narrows, lengthens, and is transformed into a true canal containing several vessels that pass from the subdural space to the pneumatic mucosa of the mastoid antrum.

Extension of the mastoid air cell system into the petrous pyramid begins shortly after birth, and may be well

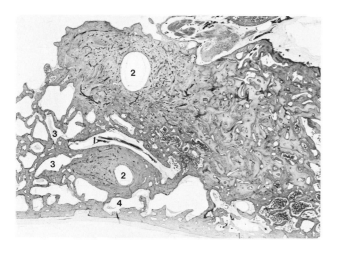

Figure 186. 1, Petromastoid canal. 2, Superior semicircular canal. 3, Mastoid air cells. 4, Posteromedial cell tract. Note proximity of the petromastoid canal with a subarcuate vessel to the mastoid air cells and the posteromedial cell tract.

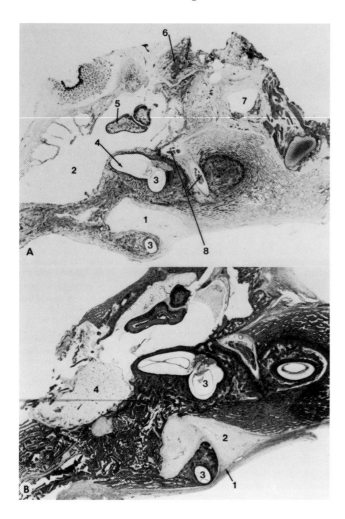

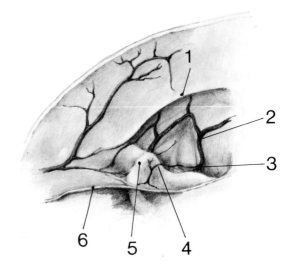

Figure 189. View into the fetal middle fossa. 1, Petrosquamosal suture. 2, Middle meningeal artery. 3, Foramen spinosum. 4, Subarcuate vein. 5, Arcuate eminence. 6, Tentorium.

Figure 188. Horizontal sections through left temporal bone of the newborn. A, Petromastoid canal (1) is wide and contains loose fibrous tissue. 2, Antrum. 3, Superior semicircular canal. 4, Horizontal semicircular canal. 5, Incus. 6, Condyle. 7, Middle fossa. 8, Facial nerve. B, Extension of connective tissue from the dura through subarcuate fossa approaching primitive nonpneumatized mastoid antrum. 1, Dura. 2, Subarcuate fossa. 3, Superior semicircular canal. 4, Antrum.

were pneumatized directly from the epitympanum plus a cell tract through the subarcuate region; and in 3%, pneumatization arose solely from the mastoid antrum and through the subarcuate region. Girard[35] and Bellocq[11] also reported that subarcuate cell tracts occur in 3% of temporal bones.

Subarcuate Blood Vessels

The subarcuate artery (or arteries) always arises either directly from the internal auditory artery, or from its parent

developed by the age of four years. Cells from the internal (medial) antral wall extend into the dihedral angle formed between the semicircular canals. These cells sometimes extend into the loop of the superior semicircular canal. Thus, the mucosa of the antrum is in direct relationship to the vascular connective tissue that fills the subarcuate canal. The most frequent site of pneumatization is the posterior-superior angle of the pyramid, which is medial to the superior semicircular canal, where a large block of membranous bone is deposited to fill out the subarcuate fossa after birth.

In his pneumatization studies, Lindsay[15] found that pneumatization of the petrosa was via the superior or petrosuperior route in 36% of specimens. Of these, 4%

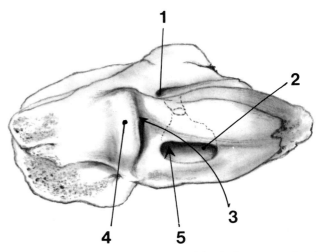

Figure 190. Intracranial cavity view of the fetal petrosa. 1, Facial hiatus and groove for the greater superficial petrosal nerve. 2, Internal auditory meatus. 3, Subarcuate foramen. 4, Superior semicircular canal. 5, Arrow points toward facial canal.

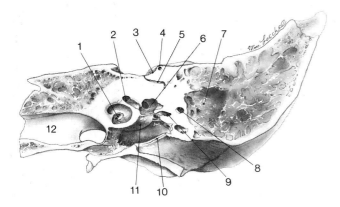

Figure 191. The petromastoid canal. 1, Cochlea. 2, Internal auditory meatus. 3, Subarcuate pit. 4, Superior semicircular canal. 5, Petromastoid canal. 6, Vestibule. 7, Mastoid antrum. 8, Horizontal semicircular canal. 9, Facial canal. 10, Sulcus tympanicus. 11, Promontory. 12, Carotid canal.

vessel (the basilar or the anterior-inferior cerebellar artery). Usually, the subarcuate artery arises from the internal auditory artery outside the internal auditory canal, courses laterally and superiorly, and enters the temporal bone at the subarcuate fossa. Occasionally, the branching occurs after the parent artery is in the internal auditory canal. It may then pass out through the porus to reach the subarcuate fossa, or pass directly through the posterior meatal wall to the subarcuate canal.

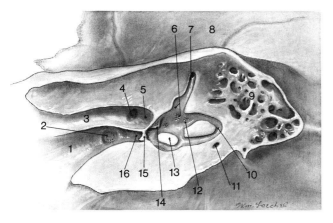

Figure 192. Anterior wall of the internal auditory canal and anterior and external walls of the vestibule (× 3). 1, Internal auditory canal. 2, Cochlear fossa. 3, Facial gutter. 4, Facial fossa. 5, Superior vestibular fossa. 6, Ampulla superior semicircular canal and its cribriform area. 7, Anterior arm of superior semicircular canal. 8, Temporal fossa. 9, Periantral cells. 10, Horizontal semicircular canal. 11, Posterior semicircular canal. 12, Ampulla of the horizontal canal and its cribriform area. 13, Oval window. 14, Pyramid of the vestibule and its utricular cribriform area. 15, Wall separating the depth of the internal auditory canal from the vestibule. 16, Inferior vestibular fossa.

Occasionally, there are two or three subarcuate arteries arising from the internal auditory artery and from the anterior inferior cerebellar artery.

The subarcuate artery or arteries may receive a large anastomotic branch from the superficial petrosal artery. In its course from the subarcuate fossa to the mastoid antrum, the subarcuate artery has small anastomotic connections with dural branches of the posterior meningeal artery.

The first branch of the subarcuate artery passes through the bone above the internal auditory canal into the petrous apex. Several small branches arise from the subarcuate artery in its course through the arch of the superior semicircular canal; they supply the otic capsule in the region of the three semicircular canals and the posterosuperior wall of the vestibule.[87, 90, 91]

The terminal branches reach the anteromedial wall of the tympanic antrum. One passes downward, supplies bone and mucosa of the anterior part of the mastoid region, and anastomoses with branches of the stylomastoid artery; the other branch passes posterolaterally to supply the mucosa and bone of the superomedial region of the mastoid antrum and the postantral cells. This branch also sends branches to the wall of the superior petrosal sinus, and may anastomose with branches of the mastoid branch of the occipital artery.[91, 92]

Clinical Significance

The petromastoid canal and its accompanying cell tracts may be the route for infections to pass from the tympanum to the meninges, to the superior petrosal sinus, and to the cerebellum.[41, 92] This is particularly true in children. In 125 autopsy specimens of cerebellar abscesses, Eagleton (cited in Girard[35]) reported that the route of propagation of infection was through the subarcuate hiatus in four cases.

The internal orifice of the petromastoid canal can vary considerably in position and size. When elevating the dura along the posterior fossa surface of the petrosa, the surgeon may have difficulty in elevating the dural extension into the petromastoid canal, particularly if it is in close approximation to the aperture of the vestibular aqueduct (see Fig. 184). A dural tear at this point may result in a troublesome cerebrospinal fluid leak and fistula.

If the subarcuate vessels are large, they may be of some surgical significance when removing acoustic nerve tumors.

Finally, the facial nerve may be anomalous in its course and pass through the petromastoid canal instead of through the internal auditory meatus.[6] The motor fibers of the facial nerve arise from the facial nucleus situated in the basal plate of the myelencephalon. These fibers grow outward and enter the internal auditory canal very early in embryonic life, (i.e., before five weeks). On rare occasions, these fibers may enter the subarcuate fossa,—following the subarcuate vessels instead of the internal auditory meatus,—and enter the middle ear cleft via the petromastoid canal.

Temporal Canals

The cavities of the inner ear contain cribriform areas by which nerve fibers and vessels reach the membranous labyrinth. Upon following the canalicules from these orifices, we reach the depth of a large conduit,—the *internal auditory canal.*

The petrosa also contributes to shape the middle ear, carrying conduits by which muscles, vessels, and nerves penetrate into this middle ear. The tensor tympani muscle is contained in the canal for the tensor tympani, and the stapedius muscle is contained in an elongated cavity,—the *canal for the stapedius muscle,* whose anterior extremity corresponds to the summit of the pyramid. The petrous canals, by which vessels or nerves go to the middle ear or leave it, are *Jacobson's canal* and the *carotico-tymapnic canal.*

The petrosa is crossed: (1) by the facial canal, its hiatus and the canaliculus for the auricular branch of the vagus, and (2) the carotid canal.

Finally, the brain, which influences the development of the petrosa, modifies its endocranial form and converts the large *subarcuate fossa* of the newborn into a delicate canal,—the *petromastoid canal.*

Petrous Canals Annexed to the Internal Ear and to the Middle Ear

These include the internal auditory canal for the inner ear, the muscular canals for the tensor tympani and the stapedius, and Jacobson's canal and the carotico-tympanic canal for the middle ear.

Internal Auditory Canal.

The internal auditory canal drives in like a wedge between the cochlea (which is internal) and the vestibule (which is external). The canal is directed externally and forms with the external auditory canal (placed lower than it) a very open, obtuse angle whose opening looks posterior and inward.

Its deep extremity is divided into two parts by a horizontal crest,—the *falciform crest.* The upper part is divided into two orifices by a vertical ridge. The anterior orifice, which is smaller, is the *fovea facialis* (facial fossa or fossette) and indicates the entrance of the facial canal.

The posterior orifice, which is larger, is called the *superior vestibular fossa* and is in relation with the vestibule. More often, one finds the superior vestibular fossa partially or completely divided into two canals corresponding, respectively, to the vestibular pyramid and to the ampullas of the external and superior semicircular canals. This fossa crosses the capsule of the vestibule obliquely, and corresponds to the superior cribriform plate. It stops opposite the vestibular pyramid.

The inferior part of the bottom of the internal auditory canal is, in large part, occupied by the *cochlear fossa,* which corrresponds to the base of the cochlea. This fossa is per-forated by very numerous orifices, which together constitute the *spiral sieve* or *perforated spiral lamina* of the cochlea. It is by this sieve, which extends down and out up to the level of the external wall of the internal auditory meatus, that the vessels and nerves penetrate into the modiolus, and from there are the spiral lamina to the membranous cochlea.

The external part of the sprial sieve, which arrives against the external wall of the auditory canal after having followed the inferior wall of this auditory duct, leaves between it and the falciform crest a small space in which is located a fossa pierced by several orifices,—the *inferior vestibular* fossa (Figs. 132, 192). This fossa separated from the vestibule by a very thin wall, corresponds to the middle cribriform plate (Fig. 193).

A little behind the bottom of the internal auditory canal, one finds on its external wall[93] which is (see Fig. 132) an orifice,—the *foramen singulare of Morgagni,* the beginning of a canal leading to the inferior cribriform plate. (Fig. 194).

We see from what precedes that each of the zones, from which the acoustic fibers reach the interior of the cavities of the inner ear, correspond to a particular zone at the bottom of the internal auditory meatus. Also, the top of this canal presents a zone,— the *facial fossa,*—that is not related to the inner ear. The internal auditory canal is not only a neurovascular canal for the internal ear, but also a canal for passage of certain structures (facial nerve, intermediate nerve of Wrisberg, and stylomastoid artery) that leave the cranium or penetrate it.

Muscular Canals.

The muscular canals contain the tensor tympani and stapedius muscles. The canal for the stapedius in its vertical portion corresponds to the posterior wall of the tympanum at the upper end of the styloid complex.

Jacobson's Canal.

This rises on the posterosuperior surface of the petrosa, enters the jugular fossa and the inferior orifice of the carotid canal, and opens at the level of the inferior part of the internal labyrinthine wall of the tympanum (see Fig. 4). It permits passage for an important nerve branch,—the *nerve of Jacobson* and the *inferior tympanic artery and vein.*

Carotico-tympanic Canal

The internal wall of the tympanum is traversed by several conduits that go from this cavity to the carotid canal. They permit tympanic veins to empty into the carotid sinus (contained in the canal with the same name). They also provide for passage of nerve filaments originating from the carotid plexus surrounding the internal carotid artery. The largest of these conduits is called the carotico-tympanic canal. It gives passage for the carotico-tympanic nerve (branch of Jacobson's nerve).

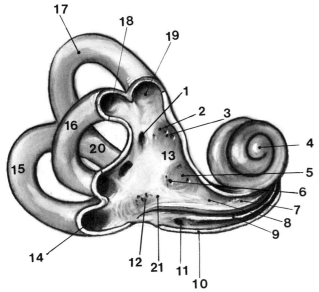

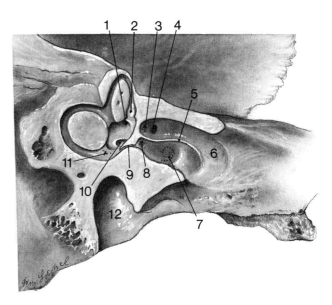

Figure 193. Lateral wall of the vestibule and basal coil of the cochlea removed (× 6).[103] 1, Internal orifice of the vestibular aqueduct and sulciform gutter. 2, Elliptical recess. 3, Superior macula cribrosa. 4, Apex of the cochlea. 5, Spherical recess. 6, Medial macula cribrosa. 7, Osseous spiral lamina. 8, Scala vestibuli. 9, Secondary spiral lamina. 10, Otic capsule. 11, Internal aperture of the cochlear aqueduct. 12, Inferior macula cribrosa. 13, Crista vestibuli. 14, Posterior ampulla. 15, Posterior semicircular canal. 16, Horizontal semicircular canal. 17, Superior semicircular canal. 18, Horizontal ampulla. 19, Superior ampulla. 20, Common crus. 21, Cochlear recess.

Figure 194. The internal auditory canal and the vestibular apparatus with its partition of separation. 1, Ampulla of the horizontal canal and its cribriform area. 2, Ampulla of superior canal and its cribriform area. 3, Superior vestibular fossa (canaliculi for the utricular nerve and for nerves to superior and horizontal ampullae). 4, Orifice of facial canal. 5, Falciform crest. 6, Anterior wall of internal auditory meatus. 7, Spiral sieve of the modiolus. 8, Inferior vestibular fossa (saccular nerve). 9, Foramen singulare of Morgagni and canal for the inferior ampullary nerve. 10, Oval window. 11, Ampulla of the posterior semicircular canal and its cribriform area. 12, Jugular fossa.

Petrous Canals for Neurovascular Elements Crossing the Cranial Wall

Carotid Canal.

The carotid canal is a large elbowed canal that occupies the internal part of the petrosa. It arises at the level of the posteroinferior surface of the petrosa (see Figs. 4, 7), is directed vertically upward, elbows on itself and goes horizontally inward (see Fig. 61). This horizontal portion which is longer than the preceding one, leads to an orifice with an irregular contour adjoining the petrous tip (see Fig. 2). The carotid canal is successively in relation with the tympanum and the eustachian tube, at the level of which it often makes a projection (Figs. 44, 61, 125, 195).

This canal is also almost always in intimate relation with the cochlea, either placed immediately medial to it or more often partly overlapping it (see Fig. 125).

Canals Reaching the Interior via Sutures

There are two such canals. One proceeds at the level of the posterior tympanosquamosal suture, and the other assumes the course of the anterior tympanopetrosal suture.

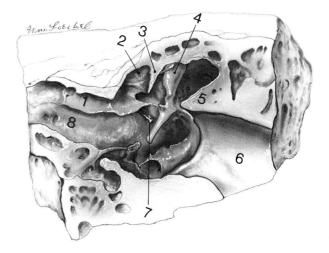

Figure 195. Vertical cut through external meatus, tympanum, and eustachian tube to illustrate the attic. 1, Canal for tensor tympani muscle with remnant of its tendon inserting on malleus neck. 2, Anterior compartment of the attic (supratubal recess). 3, Transverse bony septum dividing the attic. 4, Malleus head. 5, Scutum. 6, External auditory canal. 7, Stapes. 8, Eustachian tube.

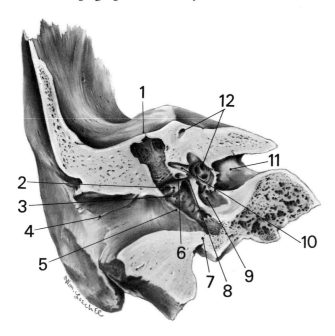

Figure 196.   Vertical cut through external and internal auditory meatus. 1, Petrosquamosal suture. 2, Pyramidal eminence. 3, Chordal canal. 4, Tympanomastoid suture. 5, Sulcus tympanicus. 6, Facial canal. 7, Tympanopetrosal suture. 8, Oval window. 9, Basal coil of cochlea. 10, Horizontal semicircular canal. 11, Internal auditory meatus. 12, Superior semicircular canal.

The first corresponds to the *posterior canal of the chorda tympani,* by which this nerve penetrates into the tympanum. It could be called the *tympanosquamosal canal.* The second is disposed in a Y or V shape. Its internal branch is the anterior canal for the chorda tympani, by which this nerve leaves the tympanum. This can be called the *tympanopetrosal canal.*

Posterior Canal for the Chorda Tympani or Tympanosquamosal Canal

The posterior canal for the chorda tympani has its orifice of entry either on the posteroinferior surface of the petrosa,—anterior and external to the stylomastoid foramen—or on the anteroexternal wall of the facial canal (see Fig. 143) a little above and occasionally very much above the stylomastoid foramen.

From there, it proceeds obliquely, superiorly, anteriorly, and externally, and emerges at the level of the posterior surface of the tympanum between the styloid complex and the tympanic bone (Figs. 50, 110, 196).

Tympanopetrosal Canal.

This opens at the level of the external wall of the tympanum by a large orifice located above and in front of the tympanic bone. At first, we have a large and short external canal, and then a long, narrow inner canal.

The *external canal,* directed obliquely inferiorly, anteriorly, and internally, quickly ends at the level of the posterior branch of the Glaserian fissure (Figs. 14-16). It gives passage to the anterior mallear ligament and to the anterior tympanic vessels.

The *internal canal,* carrying the chorda tympani, is more oblique internally and ends at the level of the internal part of the Glaserian fissure by an orifice that is often difficult to find (see Fig. 142).

6   Topographic Anatomy and Relations
of the Bony Labyrinth

General Considerations

The previous chapters in this book have been concerned primarily with descriptive anatomy of the temporal bone. We will now correlate important structures as they are related to adjacent structures. This will enable us to better understand the pathologic sequence of events in disease states, and also to help plan surgical interventions should they be required.

Situations of the Labyrinthine Capsule in the Petrous Pyramid

The bony labyrinth occupies the middle third of the petrous bone. It is longer than it is wide, and projects into the petrosa. From the aspect of the middle ear and mastoid, it presents its different parts in the following order:

1. The cochlea is in front and below.
2. The vestibule is in the middle.
3. The semicircular canals are posterior and cover the vestibule with their arches.

The tiering of the three parts of the labyrinth is not vertical but rather oblique from within outwards and from below upwards. The rolled portion of the cochlea is on a deeper plane than the vestibule. The arch of the horizontal semicircular canal wholly, and the posterior canal partially, overlap the vestibule externally so well that it appears as if the cochlea leads the vestibule and semicircular canals towards the petrous apex.

From the anterior extremity of the cochlear to the most external region of the posterior semicircular canal, the bony labyrinth, including the capsule, measures 18 to 20 mm long. The anterior cochlear end adheres intimately with the cortex of the anterior petrosal surface; the posterior end (posterior semicircular canal) borders on the posterior slope of the petrosa, and enters in direct relation with the posterior fossa by the intervening of the vestibular and cochlear aqueducts.

The axis of the inner ear is not parallel to the axis of the petrosa. Girard[35] quotes Chatellier, who stated that the axis of the petrosa forms, with the sagittal plane of the cranium, an angle that is open behind of 52° to 53°, while the axis of the inner ear forms an angle of only 42° to 43° with the same sagittal plane. The labyrinth is found interposed between the tympanum and the fundus of the internal auditory canal. If one passes a stylet through the external auditory canal into the oval window, it can cross the vestibule, break its internal wall, and penetrate directly into the internal auditory canal.

Variability of the Form and Composition of the Petrosa

The labyrinthine capsule does not change in form and dimension after five months gestation. Its position remains fixed, and the petrosa develops and expands around it. If the petrous pyramid is small, its cortex may hug the otic capsule very intimately, so that the otic capsule is found in very compact bone. If the petrous pyramid is large, its cortex is raised in all directions by pneumatic cells; and the capsule is covered with a multitude of air cells. In other cases, the petrosal mass is made up entirely of spongy bone with a rich marrow, especially in the young, which may filter out cells or microbes from the circulating blood.[94] Various combinations of the above three types are commonly encountered.

The compact type is most frequently encountered (70%). The petrosa is small, and dense bone surrounds the otic capsule. The middle and posterior fossa dural plates project into the middle ear cleft. The cellular (or spongy) types of petrosa, in which air cells and/or marrow are interposed between the labyrinth and the walls of the pyramid, are less numerous (30%). However, these are the ones that present the most unexpected forms, with air cells distending and displacing the cortical bone of the petrosa. Finally, the variability of the vascular spaces—carotid, sigmoid, and jugular—further contributes to the great variety of forms in the petrosa.

Relations of the Labyrinthine Capsule With the Petrosal Walls

The portion of the petrosa that contains the labyrinth presents three walls for consideration:

1. The inferior wall—called *jugulocarotid,* because it is in almost exclusive relationship with the carotid canal and jugular dome.
2. The anterior wall, which is in relationship to the middle cerebral fossa.
3. The posterior wall, which is in relationship to the posterior fossa.

Relations of the Labyrinth With the Inferior Petrosal Wall

The labyrinth viewed from below presents the inferior side of the cochlear cone, the posterior third of the floor of the vestibule, and the ampullary crus of the posterior semicircular canal. The subjacent petrosal region (sublabyrinthine) is very uneven. In front, we find the carotid canal; and posteriorly, we find the jugular dome in the anterior of the petrosa. The intervening spaces are variable in size and made up of bone that is either compact, spongy, or cellular.

Relations With the Carotid Canal

The carotid canal is a cylindrical conduit 6 to 7 mm in diameter. Its vertical arm rises from the base of the petrosa towards the cochlea. There it bends, contacting the inferior side of the cochlear cone, to extend with a horizontal arm to the petrous apex.

The cochlear cone is superimposed on the carotid canal. In very large petrosas, the cochlea barely contacts the carotid canal by the lowest point of its large basal spiral. In the small petrosa, the cochlear cone is in intimate contact with the carotid canal by the inferior edge of its three spiral turns. The relationships of the cochlea with the carotid canal vary in the direction of height, but they are equally variable in the direction of depth. If one looks at the promontory, the vertical arm of the carotid canal is now found in a superficial position, with its external surface on the same vertical plane as the promontory (contracted petrosa) in a deep position, its external surface forms a recess of 5 mm below the cochlea (large petrosa).

The cochlea is thus separated from the inferior surface of the petrosa by the height of the vertical arm of the carotid canal, which is about 5 mm.

The presence of the internal carotid canal in the floor and medial wall of the tympanum is a surgical hazard. The fixed and consistent landmark is the oval window, which also indicates the position of the facial nerve. Most often, the carotid canal is found 7 mm below and slightly in front of the anterior commissure of the oval window. This distance can extend to 9 mm on very large petrosas, or it can be reduced to 4 to 5 mm on narrow petrosa.

Relations With the Jugular Dome

In about 30% of temporal bones, the jugular dome is small and creates only a very slight depression on the inferior surface of the petrosa. It may be found separated from the labyrinth by a distance of 8 to 10 mm. This absence of a jugular fossa creates a large space under the posterior labyrinth that extends from the carotid canal in front to the posterior fossa behind, and where one usually finds numerous air cells (see Fig. 69).

More often, the jugular bulb hollows a fossa that rises in the sublabyrinthine space. When viewed at the bottom of a petromastoidectomy, the jugular fossa appears as a dome that rises in the petrosa medial to the descending portion of the facial canal and posterior to the ascending arm of the carotid canal (see Figs. 139, 140, 144).

The jugular dome and the carotid canal rise in the petrosa, separate from each other; the first rise posteriorly, and the second anteriorly. Thus, they form the sides of a triangular space whose summit is below and whose base is above, where it forms the subvestibular portion of the cochlea. This is the *subcochlear space,* which is made up of sublabyrinthine cellular tracts. The jugular dome sometimes fills all of the posterior sublabyrinthine space as far as the round window (up to the floor of the vestibule), up to the ampullary crus of the posterior semicircular canal, which sometimes indents the jugular dome. On rare occasions, it may go higher.

In summary, the jugular fossa is very variable. It can be totally absent or so developed that it contacts the internal carotid artery in front and the facial nerve externally, and that it presses the subvestibular part of the cochlea against the floor of the vestibule—the ampullary arm of the posterior semicircular canal. It can insinuate between the vestibule and the posterior fossa, where it embraces the vestibular aqueduct and rises toward the petrous crest between the lateral sinus externally and the internal auditory meatus internally.

Relations of the Labyrinth With the Anterior Wall of the Petrosa (Middle Cerebral Fossa)

The cortex of the anterior slope of the petrosa always contacts the otic capsule at two points: (1) at the level of the cochlea; and 2) at the level of the arch of the superior semicircular canal. In between these two points of contact, there exist between the cortex and the labyrinth some remaining spaces filled by compact or cellular bone.

The cochlea contacts the anterior petrosal wall by its anterosuperior region. The superior edge of the cupula of the cochlea is found under the pit of the geniculate ganglion. Cells or diploic tissue are never interposed at this level. The otic capsule addheres to the cortical petrous wall at the level of the Fallopian hiatus, which it overlaps a little posteriorly and medially, but never externally.

Anterior to this point of contact, the cortex of the petrosa extends to cover the carotid canal. In doing so, it forms (with these two structures) a *precochlear triangular space* or *intercarotico-cochlear* space. This space is usually very small (see Fig. 125), at times, however, it is filled with air cells that can extend into the petrous apex while following the carotid canal.

The petrosal cortex also adheres to the summit of the arch of the superior semicircular canal to form the *arcuate eminence.* Between these two sites of adherence, the petrosal cortex is separated from the labyrinth (vestibule and ampullae of the external and superior semicircular canals) by a space called the *superior prelabyrinthine space* (see Fig. 69). This space, which creates a pneumatized channel between the middle ear and petrous apex, has pathologic and surgical significance.

In performing a petromastoidectomy, the facial canal can be seen at the threshold of the aditus. Between the threshold of the horizontal semicircular canal and the petrosal cortex above, one sees a small space 3 to 6 mm wide made up of small bony trabeculae. If one excavates this space, one finds as a floor the first turn of the facial canal, with its two arms and the space of the geniculate ganglion, and at a deeper level is found the superior flank of the cochlear cone. Posteriorly, one finds the ampullary branch of the superior semicircular canal, which towards the middle of its ascending course rejoins the petrosal cortex in order to fuse with it. Anteriorly, we have the anterior wall of the petrosa. In this way, a triangular passage can be made that goes from the aditus to the petrous apex (see Figs. 69, 123).

The anterior petrosal cortex adheres to the bow of the superior semicircular canal to a variable extent. This plate of bone varies in thickness, but it is usually thin. Dehiscences into the canal have been reported. The bow or arch of the superior semicircular canal raises the petrosal cortex to form a ridge perpendicular to the petrosal axis that is called the *arcuate eminence.*

In newborn and very young infants, the arcuate eminence surrounds the intracranial orifice of the *subarcuate fossa.* In the adult, the subarcuate fossa is obliterated by bone, leaving only a fine canaliculus. At times, however, a pneumatized tract develops that extends to the petrosa—the *subarcuate tract.* In such cases, where there is extensive pneumatization, the arcuate eminence is much less apparent and may even disappear completely. In some petrosas, particularly when well pneumatized, a transverse bulge may be seen external to the superior semicircular canal and parallel to it. This is produced by adjacent air cells elevating the petrosal cortex.

Relations of the Vertical Semicircular Canals With the Petrosal Crest

The petrosal crest, along which runs the superior petrosal sinus, corresponds in general with the junction of the vertical canals. The petrosal crest, usually with a sharp edge, is found 4 to 5 mm from the point of junction of the canals (see Figs. 123, 194). The crest, however, may be flat and ac-

tually grooved by the superior petrosal sinus, so that the crest and sinus may be within 2 mm of the point of junction of the vertical canals. The petrosal cortex may even adhere to the superior edge of the arch of the posterior canal. In certain large petrosas, the petrosal crest may be more posterior (6 to 7 mm) due to the extension of air cells into the petrosa via the posteromedial route.

Relations of the Labyrinth With the Posterior Wall of the Petrosa (Cerebellar Wall)

The labyrinth enters in relation with the posterior cerebral fossa by its posterior semicircular canal, by the posterior wall of the vestibule, by the internal auditory canal, and by the vestibular and cochlear aqueducts.

In the narrow petrosa, its posterior fossa cortex is applied directly on the posterior semicircular canal. One normally sees, in the young infant and sometimes in the adult, the superior crus of this canal projecting into the cranial cavity, where it may even be dehiscent. The inferior crus of the canal is always within the petrosa, which widens at this level. The posterior wall of the vestibule may be as close as 2 mm from the posterior fossa. In large, well-pneumatized petrosas, its cerebellar cortex may be separated from the labyrinth as much as 12 mm. In such instances, a well-developed posteromedial cell tract is present, which we will discuss later.

1. *The internal auditory canal* opens on the cerebellar surface of the petrosa at an average of 3 mm below the crest and at a depth of 38 to 46 mm when measured from the mastoid cortex.
2. *The cochlear aqueduct* opens on the posteroinferior angle of the petrous pyramid, below the level of the orifice of the internal auditory meatus. Its position obstructs the advance of sublabyrinthine air cells into the petrosa.
3. *The vestibular aqueduct* is short in narrow petrosas and long in well-pneumatized ones. It opens into the posterior fossa by a fissure called the *endolympathic meatus.* With the internal auditory canal and the cochlear aqueduct, it restricts the size of the retrolabyrinthine space (see Fig. 69).

Perilabyrinthine Cellular Tracts

Air cell tracts expand in various ways into the petrosa when the temporal bone is being pneumatized. Since this system of middle ear air cells is susceptible to inflammatory disease, it is important to recognize the various pathways that these cell tracts may take. A system of radiographic studies of the temporal bone will give invaluable information on the size of the petrosa, the position of perilabyrinthine cells, and the best method for surgical correction of diseased cell areas. The following cell tracts will be described:

1. A sublabyrinthine cell tract.
2. A precochlear or inferior prelabyrinthine cell tract.
3. Superior perilabyrinthine cell tracts. (a) Superior pre-labyrinthine cell tracts. (b) A translabyrinthine tract (sub-arcuate). (c) A tract of the petrosal crest. (d) A superior retrolabyrinthine tract.

Sublabyrinthine Cell Tract

This is the most common cell tract. It is found beneath the labyrinth in the space behind the carotid canal. Its impor-tance depends on its size and the structure of the petrosa. Most important is the height of the jugular dome. The jugular dome may be high and contact the posterior labyrinthine wall, so that the sublabyrinthine area is severe-ly compressed. If the jugular dome is flat or nonexistent, then we may have a wide sublabyrinthine space.

In about 10% of the temporal bones, the jugular dome is elevated high in the petrosa, and occupies the whole of the posterior region of the sublabyrinthine space, barring the route to the apex for cells lying behind the mastoid portion of the facial canal and more deeply in the occipitojuglar region. The bone with the high jugular dome may have cells under the cochlea, but they infrequently extend to the apex. This subcochlear tract, when it does occur, is long and narrow, leaving the base of the tympanum to pass below the subvestibular part of the cochlea between the carotid canal in front and the jugular dome behind, and finally opening into the petrous apex below the internal auditory canal (see Fig. 123).

The jugular fossa is absent or only faintly present in 30% of temporal bones. Here the route to the apex is largely open, with cells arising from the hypotympanum, the ret-rofacial area, and the occipitojugular region (see Fig. 123). These cell groups, separated at first by the facial canal, unite under the labyrinth; from there, they extend towards the petrous apex, gliding on the cortex of the inferior wall, passing under the cochlear aqueduct (then under the in-ternal auditory canal), and skirting in front of the basal region of the cochlea and the upper region of the carotid canal to finally open into the apex (see Fig. 123). This passage, however, is often closed by a compact mass of bone, so that the sublabyrinthine cell tract terminates in a cul-de-sac. To this group of sublabyrinthine cells may be added the *inferior retrolabyrinthine cells,* which are often encountered in wide petrosas behind the posterior semi-circular canal and below the vestibular aqueduct. Girard[35] estimated that the sublabyrinthine cell tract exists in 16% of temporal bones.

Precochlear or Inferior Prelabyrinthine Cell Tract

This can be called the intercarotic-cochlear tract. The cells of its tympanic extremity are known as *peritubal* or *pericarotid cells* (see Fig. 125). Their point of origin is found in the anterior and inferior region of the tympanum.

The anteroinferior part of the petrosa, at the level of its middle third, is occupied by the cochlear cone lying on its side with its tip (or cupula) in front and a little inferior—and by the carotid canal, which is a large, cylindrical canal bent at right angles with a vertical arm arising from below the tympanum and a horizontal arm going toward the pet-rous apex. These two structures are superimposed. In very large petrosas, the cochlea lies lightly on top of the carotid canal and makes contact by the most sloped point of its great basal spiral. Conversely, in the narrow petrosas, the cochlear cone is in intimate contact with the carotid canal by the inferior flank of its three spirals. In the latter case, there is no room in this region for the development of air cells. In the first case, one can see cells in the bottom of the tympanum occupying the angle between the carotid canal and the superimposed cochlea.

The extent of cellular development is dependent on the relations of the cochlea and carotid canals, with respect to height as well as depth. The elbow of the carotid canal may be superficial and on the same vertical plane as the prom-ontory, or it may be in a deep position with its external sur-face in a recess that can extend for 5 mm (see Fig. 57). When the carotid canal is in a superficial position, the eu-stachian tube adheres to its anteroexternal surface, and there are no air cells between them. However, if the canal is recessed, there exists between the tube and the bend of the carotid canal a space that air cells can occupy (see Fig. 118).

It is the same for the canal for the tensor tympani. In con-tracted petrosas, this canal also adheres to the anteroexter-nal surface of the horizontal arm of the cochlear canal; but in petrosas with a deep carotid canal, the middle region of the muscle canal is found separated from the carotid canal by a space large enough to lodge cells of appreciable size (see Fig. 118).

More anteriorly and medially, the same cell system may extend past the cupula of the cochlea and over the top of the horizontal arm of the carotid canal. At this point, it is covered above by the petrosal cortex, which is grooved for passage of the superficial petrosal nerves. The distance separating the canal for the tensor tympani muscle from the petrosal groove, which indicates the beginning of the apex, is 2 to 3 mm. At this point, there is a very narrow passage. It is the beginning of the petrous apex, in which air cells may enter. Air cells entering the apex are limited externally by the grooves for the petrosal nerves, and inter-nally by the external edge of the depression for the Gas-serian ganglion just above the carotid canal.

The precochlear cell tracts are in relation with the car-otid canal along their entire length. Measured from the base of the tympanum to its emergence in the apex, its total length is about 12 mm. It is possible to reach the apex surgically by this route. Kopetzky and Almour followed the tract between the cochlea and the carotid canal. Ramadier improved the approach by resecting the superior wall of the carotid canal. In recent years, the middle cranial ap-proach affords easier access to the petrous tip when the apicitis originates via this precochlear route.

Superior Perilabyrinthine Cell Tracts

These cell tracts are in the upper level of the petrosa. They are above a line going from the point where the petrosal cortex is adherent to the cochlea posteriorly to the vestibular aqueduct (see Figs. 69, 123). They pass the labyrinthine barrier by one or more of four routes. Once past the labyrinth, these four routes converge and reunite above the internal meatus, and then into the apex by a unique route. These cell tracts may stop short of the apex, ending in a cul-de-sac.

Superior Prelabyrinthine Cell Tracts

These leave from the internal wall of the aditus and enter the triangular superior antelabyrinthine space, which is formed below by the facial canal (anterior quarter of its tympanic portion), in front by the cortex of the anterior slope of the petrosa, and behind by the ampulla of the horizontal semicircular canal and the ampullary arm of the superior canal. The cells extending further, pass inside the superior canal and scatter above the internal auditory meatus, mingling with other superior perilabyrinthine cells. These cells can sometimes be seen as a thin, flattened group of cells running under the cortex.

Translabyrinthine Cell Tracts
(subarcuate cell tract)

This tract leaves the antrum above the horizontal semicircular canal, occupies the trihedral formed by the three canals, and joins the subarcuate canal in the arch of the superior semicircular canal to reach the confluence of the superior prelabyrinthine cells above the internal auditory meatus. This tract is infrequent. Perhaps it is present in 2 to 3% of the temporal bones.

Cell Tracts of the Petrosal Crest

These cells are a prolongation of the periantral cells extending along the crest of the petrosa under the cortex. They pass over the labyrinth above the junction of the superior and posterior canals, pass behind the superior canal, and end above the internal auditory meatus.

Superior Retrolabyrinthine Cell Tracts
(posteromedial cell tract of Lindsay)

These cells insinuate between the posterior semicircular canal and the cerebellar cortex of the petrosa. They pass above the vestibular aqueduct, and turn around the posterior aspect of the common crus of the vertical canal to reach the confluence of the superior group of cells above the internal auditory canal. Although this cell tract occupies the posterior region of the petrosa, it has never been seen to pass below the internal auditory canal to reach the apex by the shortest route. It always ascends towards the crest in order to pass over the internal auditory canal.

Routes to the Apex

There are three main routes for air cells to reach the apex from the middle ear cleft.

The Posteroinferior Route

This opens into the apex between the cochlea and the carotid canal in front, the cochlear aqueduct above and behind, the internal auditory canal above, and the jugular bulb on the inferior surface of the petrosa below. It is bordering on the sublabyrinthine cells.

The Anteroinferior Route

This opens into the apex below the adherent zone of the cochlea to the anterior wall of the petrosa between the cochlea behind, the carotid canal below, and the cortex of the anterior slope of the petrosa in front and above. It is the termination of the antecochlear or intercarotico-cochlear cell tracts.

The Superior Route

This opens into the crest of the apex above the level of the internal auditory canal and the cochlea. It is the confluence of the four superior perilabyrinthine cell tracts.

In summary, one can encounter air cells and diploic tissue in all parts of the petrosa. Only the labyrinthine capsule, the cortex of the petrous pyramid, and the enclosing of certain structures (facial nerve, internal carotid artery, and jugular bulb) are formed by compact bone. Around the adult labyrinth, the compact bone is always thick and forms a block of dense, hard bone in the middle of the petrosa.

The Antrocerebellar Canal

This is the classic *petromastoid canal*. It has clinical importance. Through it—or with participation of the cell tracts that sometimes accompany it—it can carry antral infection toward the cerebellar fossa. This is particularly important in infants, where the canal is more likely to be patent.

The antrocerebellar canal is found when one dissects the internal wall of the antrum above the horizontal semicircular canal in the direction of both the petrosal crest and the posterior arm of the superior semicircular canal. It originates 8 to 10 mm externally to the posterior crus of the superior semicircular canal—not far from the crest of the petrosa, either in the periantral cells or in the antrum itself (5% of cases). It enlarges as it goes internally to pass under the arch of the superior semicircular canal, closer to the common crus that the ampullary crus, and proceeds to open in the posterior fossa 5 mm outside and above the internal auditory meatus—sometimes on the petrosal ridge, or sometimes 4 to 5 mm below by an orifice in the form of a slit or even a depression. It is the vestige of the subarcuate fossa of the fetus. It contains blood vessels and fibrous tissue that is a prolongation of dura mater.

The presence of the dura mater in the antrocerebellar canal is attributed by Girard[35] to the fact that in lower apes (lemurs to gibbons), the subarcuate fossa is occupied by a lobe of the cerebellum called the flocculus. In higher apes, the flocculus is retracted and the cavity is narrowed, but the dura mater continues to adhere to the wall of the canal, which is now a recess.

In a seven-month-old fetus the subarcuate fossa is seen as a cylindrical cavity 5 mm in diameter and 7 to 8 mm in depth. Its intracranial orifice occupies, in such cases, all of the space circumscribed by the superior semicircular canal. Externally, beyond the superior canal, the bony tissue is spongy and friable as it approaches the lateral sinus. It is filled by very vascular prolongations of the dura mater. In the newborn, the subarcuate fossa is already filled with bony tissue. The hiatus itself is narrowed by new bone applied to the arch of the superior semicircular canal. Girard[35] describes the petrosa of a six-month-old who had an antrocerebellar canal in the form of a ovoid cavity 7 mm long and 4 mm wide. Its external extremity rose toward the petrous ridge just external to the junction of the superior and posterior canals. It is near the age of five years that the subarcuate fossa is finally transformed into a simple canal. The subarcuate hiatus becomes very narrow and is no longer found under the arch of the superior semicircular canal, rather it is found 3 to 4 mm further medially due to development of the petrous ridge.

The veins of the subarcuate fossa and of its vestige—the antrocerebellar canal—are of interest. The venous network appears to originate from the bottom of the subarcuate fossa or from the antral extremity of the canal. It opens into the intracranial cavity by the subarcuate hiatus, and empties into the superior longitudinal sinus by a small veinule.

It appears, furthermore, that there exists direct vascular relations between the subarcuate fossa and the lateral sinus. If, in the fetus, one compresses the continuation of the dura mater of the fossa, one makes the blood gush into the lateral sinus at the level of its superior turn.

Sometimes, in the adult, one encounters a vascular bony canal more than 1 mm in diameter that crosses the petrous pyramid for a length of 2.5 cm from the subarcuate hiatus to the sigmoid sinus groove[35]. In its internal half, it presents the usual course of the antrocerebellar canal; but the course of the external half recalls the course of the sigmoid-antral vein of Ellsworth, like this vein, it pours into the sinus fossa at the level of its superior turn (see Fig. 30).

Anson and Donaldson[8] have pointed out that striking variations of the subarcuate fossa do occur. These may be of surgical consequence where the fossa approaches or actually occupies the customary site of the external aperture of the vestibular aqueduct.

7 *The Vestibule*

View of the Entire Labyrinth

The vestibule is the central part of the bony labyrinth. It is convenient to compare the vestibule to a parallelepiped with six distinct walls. These walls, however, are curved, and all of the angles are rounded or lost in large openings so that the vestibule has an irregular form that is somewhat globular and slightly flattened laterally to medially (Fig. 197).

The walls of the vestibule are:

1. Inferior wall or floor.
2. Superior wall that curves above.
3. External wall—separates it from the tympanic cavity.
4. Internal wall—separates it from the internal auditory canal.
5. Anterior wall in relation with the middle cranial fossa.
6. Posterior wall in relation to the posterior cranial fossa.

These walls present very small surfaces, since they are penetrated by seven relatively large orifices: the oval window, the five orifices of the semicircular canals, and the mouth of the scala vestibuli of the cochlea (see Fig. 137).

The floor and roof of the vestibule are parallel in a vestibular horizontal plane that passes through the center of the vestibular orifices of the external semicircular canal. The posterior and anterior walls, parallel to each other, are perpendicular to the two preceding walls. These four walls form the framework of the parallelepiped whose angles are straight or nearly straight.

The external and internal walls are applied to this rectangular framework, thus completing the paralleledpiped. Their horizontal components are parallel in the horizontal vestibular plane; they form an angle open, in front, of 35° to 40° with the sagittal plane. Their vertical components are not parallel in the sagittal plane, but are slowly oblique from above down and from outward inward, so that the superior border of the vestibule is a little more prominent than the inferior border.

In summary, the vestibule resembles a parallelepiped rectangle, gently tilting outward, whose great anteropos-terior horizontal axis makes an angle, open in front, of 35° to 45° with the sagittal plane.

Its dimensions are:

1. From anterior to posterior wall: 6 to 7 mm.
2. From floor to roof: 5 to 6 mm.
3. From the external to internal wall at the periphery: 1.5 to 2 mm.
4. To the center and below: 3 mm.

The Walls of the Vestibule

The External Wall

It is represented on the medial tympanic wall by a rectangular surface 6 to 7 mm long and 5 to 6 mm high. It is directed externally, anteriorly, and slightly inferiorly. Externally, it is strongly convex (see Fig. 197). These different sectors do not have the same orientation; that of the inferior region faces more towards the base, while that of the anterior region is more external and a little forward. Each of the superior angles of the external wall is occupied by an orifice of the external semicircular canal—the ampullary orifice in front and the nonampullary orifice behind.

The ampullary orifice is elliptical, and its great axis is horizontal. It measures 2 to 2.5 mm long and about 1.5 mm in height. Above, it is contiguous with the ampullary orifice of the superior semicircular canal (Fig. 198). Its inferior border is 1 mm above the oval window. Its anterior border is in continuity with the anterior wall of the vestibule (Fig. 199).

The nonampullary orifice is more nearly circular, its diameter can vary from 1 to 2 mm. Above, it is contiguous to the orifice of the common branch of the superior and posterior canals; its inferior border is 1 to 2 mm above the ampullar orifice of the posterior canal, and its posterior border is in continuous relation with the posterior wall of the vestibule (see Fig. 198).

The two orifices are separated by 3 mm of the external wall of the vestibule (Fig. 200). Immediately below is the

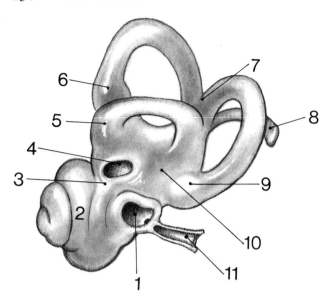

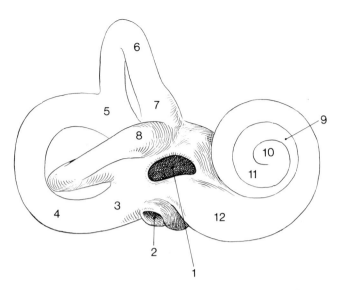

Figure 197.   The external configuration of the bony labyrinth (left side) in a newborn (× 5).[35] 1, Round window. 2, Cochlea. 3, Anterior wall of the vestibule. 4, Oval window. 5, Ampulla of the horizontal semicircular canal. 6, Ampulla of the superior semicircular canal. 7, Common crus of the superior and posterior canals. 8, Vestibular aqueduct. 9, Ampulla of the posterior semicircular canal. 10, External wall of the vestibule. 11, Cochlear aqueduct.

Figure 198.   Right bony labyrinth viewed laterally and anteriorly. 1, Oval window. 2, Round window. 3, Bony ampulla of the posterior canal. 4, Posterior semicircular canal. 5, Common crus. 6, Superior semicircular canal. 7, Bony ampulla of the superior canal. 8, Bony ampulla of the horizontal canal. 9, Middle turn of the cochlea. 10, Cupula of the cochlea. 11, Apical turn of the cochlea. 12, Basal turn of the cochlea.

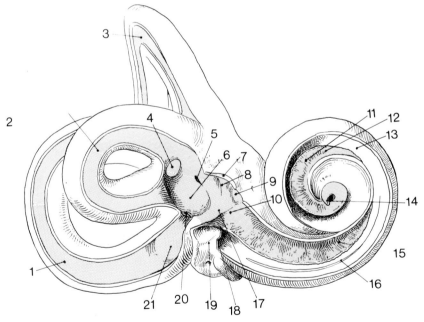

Figure 199.   The left bony labyrinth—frontal view. The vestibule and the cochlea have been opened as far as the cupula. 1, Posterior semicircular canal. 2, Lateral semicircular canal. 3, Superior semicircular canal. 4, Orifice of the common crus in the vestibule. 5, Internal aperture of the vestibular aqueduct. 6, Elliptical recess. 7, Edge of the oval window. 8, Vestibular crest. 9, Spherical recess. 10, Vestibular aperture of the cochlea. 11, Bony spiral lamina. 12, Vestibular scala. 13, Tympanic scala. 14, Modiolar lamina. 15, Bony spiral lamina. 16, Secondary spiral lamina. 17, Cochlear recess. 18, Crest of the cochlear fenestra. 19, Fossula of the cochlear fenestra. 20, Inferior cribriform macula. 21, Posterior osseous ampulla (modified from Sobotta). (From Sobotta, J., *Atlas der deskriptiven anatomie des Menschen*, ed. 3, Vol. III. Munich: J.F. Lehmanns, 1920, pp, 724-732.)

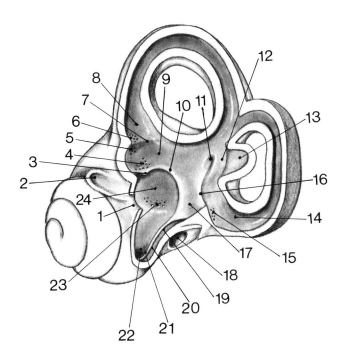

Figure 200. A view of the interior of the vestibule after resection of its external wall, and of the horizontal semicircular canal in the newborn.[35] 1, Anterior commissure of the oval window. 2, Facial canal. 3, Pyramid of the vestibule. 4, Cribriform area of the utricle. 5, Cribriform area of the ampulla of the horizontal canal. 6, Cribriform area of the ampulla of the superior canal. 7, Superior ampullar crest. 8, Ampulla of the superior semicircular canal. 9, Utricular fossa. 10, Vestibular crest. 11, Sulciform gutter. 12, Posterior fossette. 13, Posterior arm of the horizontal semicircular canal. 14, Ampulla of posterior semicircular canal. 15, Cribriform area of the posterior ampulla. 16, Inferior ampullary crest. 17, Cochlear fossa. 18, Round window. 19, Vestibulo-tympanic fissure. 20, Scala tympani. 21, Spiral lamina. 22, Scala vestibuli. 23, Saccular cribriform area. 24, Saccular fossa.

oval window, which opens onto the tympanum and is closed by the stapes footplate. The oval window is 3 mm wide and 1.5 mm high. It is elongated in a horizontal direction. Its great axis is oblique below and horizontal in front. Its superior, anterior, and posterior borders are concave, while its inferior border is straight; or, more often, it is gently convex, which gives this opening a kidney shape.

It is located in the anterior and inferior regions of the external wall of the vestibule. Its anterior commissure is placed on the anterior border of this wall, its posterior commissure reaches the middle of the wall (see Fig. 197), its superior border passes 1 mm below the ampullary orifice of the horizontal canal, and its inferior border is located 1 mm above the mouth of the scala vestibuli of the

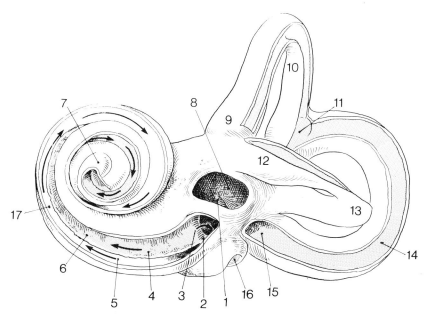

Figure 201. Bony right labyrinth—frontal view. 1, Crista vestibuli. 2, Beginning of the osseous spiral lamina. 3, Vestibular aperture of the cochlear canal. 4, Osseous spiral lamina. 5, Scala tympani. 6, Scala vestibuli. 7, Cupula or apex of the cochlea. 8, Oval window (vestibular window). 9, Bony ampulla superior canal. 10, Superior semicircular canal. 11, Common crus. 12, Bony ampulla horizontal canal. 13, Horizontal semicircular canal. 14, Posterior semicircular canal. 15, Bony ampulla posterior canal. 16, Round window (cochlear window). 17, Spiral cochlear canal.

cochlea (i.e., 1 mm above the floor of the vestibule) (Figs. 199, 201). When looking at the external wall of the vestibule from an external exposure, one notes that the oval window lies in the lower anterior and inferior portions of this wall due to the convexity of the external wall.

Internal Vestibular Wall

The internal vestibular wall has the same dimensions as the external wall, the same general anteroposterior orientation of 35° to 40° on the sagittal plane, and the same gentle inclination from above below and without inwards. It separates the vestibule from the internal auditory canal, and it is pierced by a large number of openings that provide passage for the terminal filaments of the vestibular nerve. It is convex on the side of the internal auditory meatus and concave on its endovestibular aspect (Figs. 202, 203).

On examining this internal vestibular wall, one can detect slight depressions on its surface that are separated by crests (Figs. 200, 204). The depressions, called *fossettes,* are the imprints left on the bone by the membranous labyrinth. There are four fossettes: elliptical, hemispherical, cochlear, and posterior. To these large impressions must be added a deep narrow fissure—the sulciform (sulcus-like) groove.

Semioval Fossette *(elliptical recess, utricular recess)*

It occupies the superior third of the internal wall of the vestibule. Its long axis is horizontal. Anteriorly, its imprint ex-

tends up to the anterior wall of the vestibule (Figs. 200, 204, 205) to the height of the ampullary orifice of the external semicircular canal. Posteriorly, it ends at the sulciform groove. Superiorly, its limits are clear only in the anterior region, where the superior ampullary crest separates it from the ampulla of the superior semicircular canal. Further posteriorly, there does not exist any demarcation between it and the superior wall of the vestibule. Below, it is limited by the crest of the vestibule, which separates it from the spherical recess (*hemispherical fossette*) (see Fig. 200).

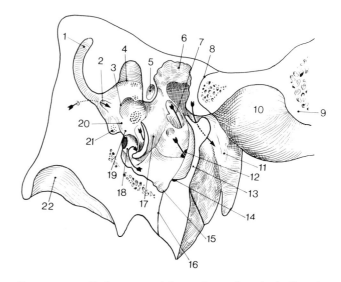

Figure 203. Right temporal bone (vertical cut). 1, Superior semicircular canal. 2, Orifice of the vestibular aqueduct. 3, Vestibular crest with the pyramid anteriorly. Beneath this crest is the hemispherical fossa and middle cribriform area. Above this crest is the semioval fossa. 4, Superior ampullary crest. Above it is the ampulla of the superior semicircular canal. Below it is the superior cribriform area. 5, Facial canal. 6, Attic. 7, Arrow in the canal for the tensor tympanic muscle. 8, Petrosquamosal suture ending above at the internal petrosquamosal fissure, and below at the anterior branch of the Glaserian fissure. 9, Temporal condyle. 10, Glenoid cavity. 11, Petrosal hernia (large)—the inferior prolongation of the tegmen tympani. In front is the anterior branch of the Glaserian fissure. Behind it is the posterior branch of this fissure. 12, Orifice of the eustachian tube. 13, Tympanic bone and external auditory canal. Note above, at the superior border of this bone, the section of the mallear groove (arrow) and the section of the mallear crest, which is outside this gutter. 14, Sulcus tympanicus. 15, Hypotympanic recess. 16, Posterior tympanopetrosal suture. 17, Promontory. Above lies the oval window. Behind it are two arrows. The superior arrow enters the scala vestibuli; the inferior enters the scala tympani. Between these two arrows is the osseous spiral lamina. 18, Posterior edge of the round window. 19, Part of the inferior wall of the vestibule situated between the origin of the spiral lamina and the inferior ampullary crest. 20, Inferior ampullary crest. 21, Ampulla of posterior semicircular canal and inferior cribriform area. In front is the inferior ampullary crest. Between this crest and the crest of the vestibule lies the cochlear fossa. 22, Jugular fossa.

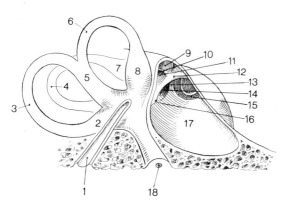

Figure 202. Bony labyrinth (internal aspect), internal auditory canal, cochlear and vestibular aqueducts. 1, Vestibular aqueduct. 2, Ampulla of the posterior canal. 3, Posterior semicircular canal. 4, Horizontal semicircular canal. 5, Common crus. 6, Superior semicircular canal. 7, Ampulla of the horizontal canal. 8, Ampulla of the superior canal. 9, Facial canal orifice. 10, Superior perpendicular crest. 11, Superior vestibular fossa. 12, Falciform crest. 13, Inferior perpendicular crest. 14, Inferior vestibular fossa. 15, Cochlear fossa with spiral cribriform area. 16, Foramen Morgagni. 17, Internal auditory canal. 18, Cochlear aqueduct.

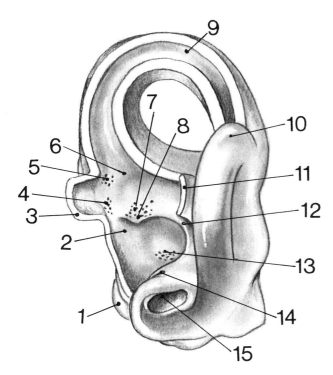

Figure 204. Interior view of the vestibule, showing the cribriform areas of the utricle, saccule, superior ampulla, and horizontal ampulla.[35] 1, Cochlea. 2, Interior wall of the vestibule. 3, Stump of the ampulla of the horizontal canal. 4, Cribriform area of the horizontal canal. 5, Cribriform area of the superior canal. 6, Superior ampullary crest. 7, Utricular cribriform area. 8, Pyramid of the vestibule. 9, Superior semicircular canal. 10, Posterior semicircular canal. 11, Stump of the nonampullary arm of the horizontal semicircular canal. 12, Vestibular crest. 13, Saccular fossa with its cribriform area. 14, Vestibulo-tympanic fissure. 15, Round window.

Vestibular Crest (crista vestibuli)

This is a slight, bony, linear ridge that is distinct in places and forms a semicircumference with inferior concavity on the vestibular wall (see Fig. 200). It circumscribes the spherical recess (hemispherical fossette). All of its midportion appears on the internal wall of the vestibule. However, its two extremities are prolonged—one onto the anterior wall, where it ends by a minute process called the *vestibular pyramid;* the other onto the floor, where it diminishes to lead to an almost imperceptible ridge on the free border of the osseous spiral lamina above the round window.

From the point where it curves to become vertical, the vestibular crest appears to be bifurcated at times. A second crest may detach and pass below the sulciform groove to join the inferior ampullary crest. Thus, it forms the superior limit of the cochlear fossette, whose anterior border is marked by the vertical portion of the vestibular crest and the posterior border by the inferior ampullary crest. The cochlear fossette extends externally onto the floor of the vestibule and will be discussed later.

The Vestibular Pyramid

This is a small bony process, triangular in shape with jagged borders that rises between the elliptical and spherical recess, forming a projection at the junction of the anterior and internal vestibular walls (see Fig. 200). At times, it projects as much as 2 mm. It marks the anterior extremity of the vestibular crest.

It is horizontal and contacts the superior and anterior angle of the oval window. It is a porous bone, with holes permitting passage for the terminal filaments of the utricular nerve. The interutriculosaccular membrane is strongly adherent to it (see Figs. 200, 204).

Utricular Cribriform Zone

The vestibular pyramid is included in the utricular cribriform zone. Ten to 15 foramina are present in the vestibular pyramid. The majority of these extend up into the elliptical recess to form the macula cribrosa superior. Others pass below into the spherical recess or onto the anterior wall of the vestibule. These tiny bony canals cross the labyrinthine capsule to enter the inferior aspect of the internal auditory canal (see Figs. 192, 194).

The cribriform plate of the ampullae of the external and superior semicircular canals occurs on the anterior wall of the vestibule, but it occasionally extends onto the internal wall to blend with the utricular zone in its inferior portion (see Figs. 200, 204).

Spherical Recess (hemispherical fossette, saccular fossette)

This is the deepest and most distinct of the vestibular recesses. It occupies the entire anteroinferior region of the internal wall. It is circumscribed above and behind by the vestibular crest, which separates it from the elliptical recess above and from the cochlear recess behind. Below, its inferior border marks the internal lip of the mouth of the scala vestibuli of the cochlea. In front, it makes a slight imprint on the anterior wall of the vestibule just inside the anterior commissure of the oval window (see Figs. 200, 204).

Saccular Cribriform Plate

In the center and inferior aspect of the cochlear recess is a porous elliptical zone, with a large anteroposterior axis. This is the saccular cribriform plate (macula cribrosa media), which contains numerous passages for transmission of the terminal filaments of the saccular nerve that reach the internal auditory meatus through the saccular recess. At this level, the spherical (saccular) recess is separated from the internal auditory canal by only a very thin and fragile bony lamella. It is located directly opposite the oval window, so that an instrument introduced through the oval window may penetrate through the spherical recess and into the internal auditory meatus.

There is danger of opening the meningeal spaces at this point.

Posterior Recess

This is located between the posterior wall of the vestibule and the inferior ampullary crest, which extends upward, forming the posterior wall of the sulciform gutter (see Fig. 200). A channel extends from the posterior ampullary orifice to the vestibular orifice of the common crus of the superior and posterior canals. It appears to become complete in the vestibule, with the outline of the circumference assumed by the posterior semicircular canal.

Sulciform Gutter (fossula sulciformis)

This is a small groove located above the posterosuperior region of the internal wall of the vestibule and a little below the anterior border of the vestibular orifice of the common crus of the superior and posterior canals (see Figs. 200, 205). It forms the boundary between the elliptical and posterior recesses. It is gently oblique from below upward, and from in front backwards. It goes deeper as it ascends, so that at the end, the groove becomes a canal ending at a minute orifice, which is the vestibular orifice of the vestibular aqueduct.

Floor of the Vestibule

It is 5 to 6 mm long and 2 to 2.5 mm wide. A large opening is found at either end. Posteriorly, it is the ampullary orifice of the posterior semicircular canal. Anteriorly, it is the opening of the scala vestibuli of the cochlea into the vestibule. Between these two openings, the floor extends from the internal to the external wall of the vestibule, and from the inferior ampullary crest to the point where the osseous spiral lamina curves inward toward the base to penetrate the cochlea. Thus, it forms a surface where one can distinguish:

1. The impression of the cochlear recess.
2. The origin of the osseous spiral lamina, of which the first 2 mm are apparent.
3. The vestibulo-tympanic fissure.

The inferior vestibular wall is irregular and uneven. It intersects the external wall of the vestibule horizontally at a point midway between the oval and round windows. It meets the internal vestibular wall below the spherical (saccular) recess, following the point of attachment of the origin of the osseous spiral lamina.

Ampullary Orifice of the Posterior Canal

It occupies the external and inferior angle of the posterior wall, but especially the latter; it is elliptical. Its great axis, 2 mm long, is in the plane of the canal. Its anterior border forms the inferior ampullary crest. This is a slightly roughened bony crest, which separates the posterior ampulla

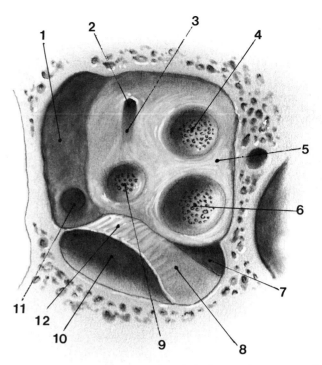

Figure 205. Internal wall of the vestibule showing the recesses and the cribriform plates. 1, Posterior wall of the vestibule. 2, Internal orifice of the endolymphatic canal. 3, Sulciform gutter. 4, Semioval (utricular) recess. 5, Vestibular crest. 6, Hemispherical (saccular) recess. 7, Origin scala vestibuli. 8, Osseous spiral lamina. 9, Cochlea recess. 10, Subvestibular cavity. Origin of the scala tympani. 11, Orifice of the posterior semicircular canal. 12, Floor of the vestibule. (From Poirier, P., and Charpy, A., *Traite d'Anatomie Humaine*, Vol. 5. Paris: Masson et Cie, 1904.)

from the cochlear recess. It extends from the external to the internal border of the floor of the vestibule. It passes over the internal wall, ascends it, and finally fades out in the region of the posterior lip of the sulciform gutter.

The posterior limit of the ampullary orifice is marked by a projecting edge, which is also the inferior limit of the posterior wall of the vestibule. The ampulla originates from this point, and overlaps this wall posteriorly. Also overlapping this wall posteriorly is the nonampullary orifice of the combined superior and posterior semicircular canal.

Posterior Recess

The deep wall of the posterior ampulla continues along the internal wall of the vestibule by a depression—the *posterior recess*. This extends vertically up to the orifice of the common crus of the superior and posterior canals, passing behind the sulciform recess.

The two vestibular orifices of the posterior canal face each other in a vertical plane at a distance of 3 to 4 mm. They are connected to each other by the posterior recess.

Cochlear Recess (cochlear fossette)

It is much smaller than the utricular and saccular recesses. It is limited in front by the vestibular crest and behind by the inferior ampullary crest. Above, it extends above the internal wall of the vestibule up to the level of the utricular recess, from which it is sometimes separated by a transversely oblique crest uniting the vestibular crest and the inferior ampullary crest (see Fig. 200); below, it extends up to the free edge of the osseous spiral lamina. It is the imprint of the vestibular extremity of the cochlear canal. It lodges the beginning of the ductus cochlearis.

Reichert's Spot

This refers to a cribriform area on the inferior portion of the cochlear recess. Tiny orifices may be seen, under magnification, that are situated on the superior surface of the ossseous spiral lamina near its origin and, indeed, near its free edge. Through these orifices, nerve filaments go to the initial part of the vestibular portion of the cochlea. They are in direct relation with the most external part of the spiral cribriform plate of the modiolus. They are not to be associated with the vestibular cribriform plate. The filaments passing through the vestibule are called the *nerve of Bechterew*. It has a small ganglion that is analogous to Scarpa's ganglion.

Vestibulo-tympanic Fissure

On the fresh bone, it is filled with soft tissue; but on the dry bone, it is an open, sickle-shaped fissure about 0.5 mm in size. It curves inward and is tapered at its extremity (see Fig. 200). Its internal convex lip is a portion of the free edge of the osseous spiral lamina. Its external concave lip is marked by a much less prominent lamina called the *secondary osseous spiral lamina,* which is inserted over the inferior edge of the external vestibular wall above the limits of the round window. The extremity of the vestibulo-tympanic fissure is closed at each end by the union of its two lips. The fissure is found 1 mm in front of the inferior ampullary crest, just above and behind the round window (see Fig. 200). On leaving this point, the spiral lamina and vestibulo-tympanic fissure run a horizontal course for about 2 mm, and then bend inferiorly to enter the cochlea. It is their short horizontal course that forms the floor of the vestibule. The vestibular cavity communicates with the scala tympani of the cochlea via the vestibulo-tympanic fissure (see Fig. 206).

Orifice of the Scala Vestibuli of the Cochlea

This is a large opening in the shape of a tunnel, which is flattened from outside to inside. It occupies the anterior third of the vestibular floor (see Fig. 193). Its inner edge is the inferior border of the spherical recess. Its posterior border is at the level of the inflection of the spiral lamina. Its external edge coincides with the inferior edge of the external wall of the vestibule (about 1 mm below the oval window).

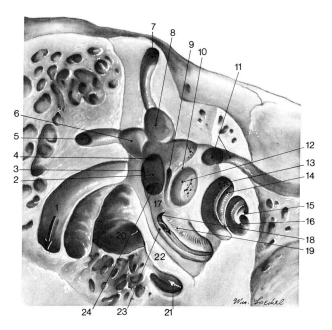

Figure 206.   Frontal section through the pars petrosa of the right temporal bone showing the medial wall of the vestibule. The basal winding of the cochlea has been opened to expose the scala vestbuli. 1, Facial canal. 2, Utricular recess. 3, Horizontal semicircular canal. 4, Common crus. 5, Horizontal semicircular canal. 6, Ampulla of the horizontal canal. 7, Superior semicircular canal. 8, Ampulla superior canal. 9, Aperture of the vestibular aqueduct. 10, Crista vestibuli and utriculoampullar cribriform area. 11, Facial canal. 12, Saccular recess and saccular cribriform area. 13, Scala tympani. 14, Scala vestibuli. 15, Lamina modioli. 16, Hamulus bony spiral lamina. 17, Floor of cochlear recess. 18, Hiatus semilunaris. 19, Bony spiral lamina. 20, Arrow through the round window membrane and into the scala tympani. 21, Arrow in the tympanic canaliculus. 22, Promontory. 23, Secondary spiral lamina. 24, Ampulla of the posterior canal.

Superior Wall of the Vestibule

The superior wall is not flat; in general, it is horizontal. It measures 6 to 7 mm long and 2 to 2.5 mm wide (see Fig. 200). Its greater anteroposterior axis forms an angle of 35° to 40° with the sagittal plane of the head. The ampullary orifice of the superior semicircular canal is at its anterior extremity, and the orifice of the common crus of the superior and posterior canals is at its posterior extremity. Its midportion between the two orifices is convex inferiorly, and follows the circular curve of the superior semicircular canal.

Ampullary Orifice of the Superior Semicircular Canal

The ampullary orifice of the superior canal is elliptical, with its long axis in the plane of the canal. Its external border is separated from the ampulla of the external semicircular canal by a distinct ridge (see Fig. 200). Its internal border is well marked by the crest, which clearly separates the superior ampulla from the elliptical recess. Its anterior border mingles with the superior edge of the anterior wall of the vestibule, with which it is prolonged to carry a few of the openings of the superior ampullary cribriform area. Its posterior border has a round graceful form where the posterior wall of the canal, in a vertical direction, turns gently to blend with the horizontal superior wall of the vestibule (see Fig. 200).

Orifice of the Common Crus of the Superior and Posterior Canals

The orifice is circular and measures 1.5 mm in diameter. Its external border is separated from the nonampullary orifice of the external semicircular canal by a distinct ridge (see Fig. 200). The posterior wall of the common crus is smooth, and forms part of the posterior and internal walls of the vestibule. In front, the anterior wall of the canal (in a vertical direction) is bound to the superior wall of the vestibule (in a horizontal direction) by a rounded angle. If a line is passed through the center of the vestibular orifices of the superior semicircular canal, it forms an angle of 37° with the sagittal plane of the head.

Anterior Wall of the Vestibule

The anterior wall of the vestibule is gently inclined from above below, and from front to back. It extends from the superior ampullary crest to the mouth of the scala vestibuli of the cochlea (see Figs. 200, 205). It is 1.5 mm wide and 5 mm high. It is divided into two levels by the anterior extremity of the crest of the vestibule, which thickens to form the pyramid of the vestibule. The inferior level, internally, blends with the spherical recess; and externally, it ends at the anterior end of the oval window. The superior level contains the anterior extremity of the elliptical (utricular) recess, with a few of the openings from the superior aspect of the vestibular pyramid and the utricular cribriform area. In the upper portion of this anterior vestibular wall, one finds the ampullary cribriform areas for the horizontal and superior semicircular canal ampullae.

External and Superior Ampullary Cribriform Areas

These cribriform areas are very close to each other and may even overlap. They spread out at the mouth of the ampullae into the vestibule (see Fig. 204). The superior cribriform area, with seven or eight openings, is at the anterior end of the bony crest separating the two ampullae. The external cribriform area, with a dozen smaller openings, is found a little lower, and may even extend towards the base to reach the utricular cribriform area above the anterior extremity of the pyramid of the vestibule. The openings of the cribriform area converge into canaliculi that lead to the superior cribriform area in the base of the internal auditory canal, terminating by one or two canals of considerable size (see Figs. 192, 194).

Posterior Wall of the Vestibule

The posterior wall of the vestibule extends from the common crus of the vertical canals to the inferior ampullary orifice. It is vertical and only measures 3 to 4 mm in height, although the height of the vestibule is about 5 mm. This is due to the common crus of the vertical canals and the ampulla of the posterior canal taking up a little of the space above and below. The posterior vestibular wall lies in a slightly more anterior plane than these two cavities.

Above its external border, the nonampullary arm of the horizontal semicircular canal will be seen. The peripheral walls of this nonampullary arm blend gently with the posterior vestibular wall without ridges or grooves (see Fig. 200).

From its internal edge, it joins the posterior recess described above.

Relations of the Vestibule

The vestibule presents as an intermediate piece situated between the tympanum and the internal auditory canal.

Placed openly at the bottom of the cavity of a petromastoidectomy, it appears to be found in the center of the petrosa. Its quadrangular form extends vertically and horizontally in the middle of the triangular form of the petrous pyramid. Its vertical anterior wall meets the anterior angle of the pyramid, its posterior vertical wall reaches the posterior surface of the pyramid, and its superior and inferior walls (both horizontal) are nearly equally distant, respectively, from the anterosuperior and anteroinferior surfaces of the pyramid, which forms an angle of about 90° between them. It follows that the ceiling and the floor of the vestibule form the one with the anterosuperior surface; while the other, with the anteroinferior surface of the petrosa, forms an angle of about 45° that is open posteriorly.

Having given the irregularities of the petrous pyramid, these relations should be discussed.

Relations of the Vestibule With the Cavities of the Middle Ear, or Relations of the External Wall of the Vestibule

The external wall of the vestibule corresponds to the superior and posterior region of the center of the tympanic cavity. This region is traversed from in front behind by the tympanic portion of the facial canal, whose projection against the vestibule divides the external wall into three levels (see Fig. 137):

1. An inferior or subfacial level, which includes the oval window in front and the space that separates the oval window from the inferior ampullary region behind.
2. A middle level covered by the aqueduct itself.
3. A superior level covered by the bow of the horizontal

semicircular canal, and containing the two vestibular orifices of this canal (see Fig. 137).

It is the oval window that reveals the presence of the vestibule. It opens in the center of the tympanum above the promontory. It faces externally and a little towards the base. It is at the base of a very revealing depression, which one designates the *oval window niche* and which one must recognize with confidence.

This niche is normally occupied by the stapes. Its superior or lintel edge carries an additional burden—The *facial canal,* which overhangs the oval window and often conceals the superior third (see Fig. 139). In order to see the window completely from the exterior, one is obliged to view it a little from below upward; besides, the arms and the head of the stapes are not placed horizontally, but are slightly inclined towards the base (Figs. 207, 208).

Anteriorly and posteriorly, the niche of the oval window is framed by two projecting structures. Anteriorly, it is the processus cochleariformis, which permits the tendon of the tensor tympani, in fresh state, to emerge. Posteriorly, it is the pyramid that bounds the box of the stapedius muscle (see Fig. 140); from its extremity emerges the tendon of this muscle.

Below, the window niche is united to the promontory by a round and smooth lip.

The oval window can be marked with the aid of the projection that the horizontal semicircular canal makes into the aditus. This projection is always clearly visible, and one finds the window below it (see Fig. 134).

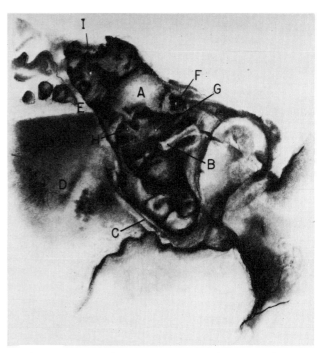

Figure 208.   View of posterior tympanum. A, Horizontal semicircular canal. B, Stapes. C, Sulcus tympanicus. D, External auditory canal. E, Scutum of Leidy. F, Processus cochleariformis. G, Pyramidal eminence. H, Posterior tympanic cells. I, Antrum mastoideum.

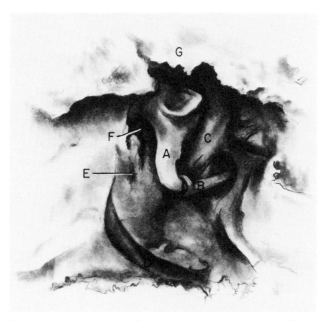

Figure 207.   Posterior wall of the tympanum with incus in place A, Incus. D, Sulcus tympanicus. C, Tympanic segment of facial canal. B, Stapes. F, Short crus of incus in fossa incudis. E, Iter chordae posterior. The posterior buttress or facial ridge lies below the fossa incudis, which contains the short process of the incus. The posterior buttress must be removed along with the necessary portion of the bone about the posterior part of the sulcus tympanicus before the drumhead is moved to the stapes head.

With the oval window and the projection of the horizontal canal, it is easy to trace the limits of the vestibule on the base of the tympanum and aditus. Actually, the anterior commissure of the oval window and the anterior extremity of the projection of the external canal mark the anterior limit of the vestibule. Its inferior limit passes 1 mm below the inferior edge of the oval window. Its posterior limit passes at 3 mm from the posterior commissure of the window, and its superior limit is on the projection of the horizontal canal.

Behind the oval window, the external wall of the vestibule glides towards the depth—it goes away from the tympanic cavity and corresponds to the sinus tympani, which is strongly overhung by the pyramid and the facial canal. This disposition makes access to the vestibule difficult from the tympanum in this spot.

Above the facial canal, the external wall of the vestibule is covered by the bow of the external semicircular canal, which forms a horizontal projection between the tympanum and the antrum. Anteriorly, in the aditus, the projection of the external canal, which corresponds to the anterior branch of the canal, constitutes an infallible landmark that is always visible (see Fig. 66) if it has not been eroded by osteitis or by a cholesteatoma. The vestibule is 3 mm deep at this point. Posteriorly, the external wall of the vestibule is deeply buried, and is covered by the bow of the horizontal canal (6 to 7 mm wide) and the bony mass separating the antrum from the external auditory canal. (see Fig. 209).

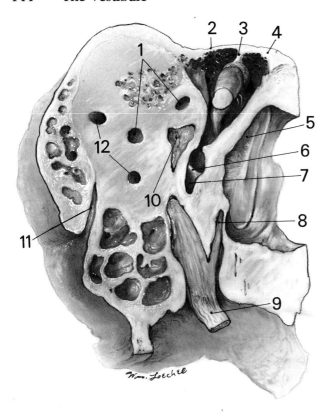

Figure 209.   Vertical cut through the petrosa just lateral to the descending facial canal. 1, Horizontal semicircular canal. 2, Tegmen tympani petrosa. 3, Superior mallear ligament. 4, Tegmen tympani squamosa. 5, Tympanic membrane. 6, Chordal ridge. 7, Facial sinus. 8, Chorda tympani nerve. 9, Stylomastoid foramen with emerging facial nerve. 10, Second turn of the facial canal. 11, Vestibular aqueduct. 12, Posterior semicircular canal.

Relations of the Vestibule With the Internal Auditory Canal

The vestibule is interposed between the tympanic bone and the internal auditory canal.

The floors of the vestibule and the internal auditory canal are on the same level. A wall separates the two cavities; its external surface is the internal wall of the vestibule, and its internal surface is the bottom of the auditory canal. Each of these two surfaces is divided into two levels by a bony crest—the vestibular crest on one side, and the falciform crest on the other. These two crests are of the same height on both sides of the party wall. At the inferior level, one finds on the tympanic side the hemispherical or saccular fossette; on the other side is the inferior vestibular fossette. The superior level is occupied by the elliptical or utricular fossette on the tympanic side, and by the superior vestibular fossette on the other side (see Figs. 192, 194).

The inferior level, which faces the oval window, is a surgical region used in the treatment of meningitis.

The wall of separation between the vestibule and auditory conduit is often thin and fragile at the level of the saccular cribriform spot, but it reaches more than 1 mm of thickness at the level of the falciform crest and at the periphery (see Figs. 192, 194).

Lateral Relations of the Vestibule

Posteriorly, the vestibule is separated from the cerebellar fossa by a bony mass whose thickness can vary from 2 to 12 mm. Compact in the majority of cases, this bony mass is sometimes cellular, so that the jugular fossa is absent. The group of sublabyrinthine cells can ascend behind the vestibule up to the height of the vestibular aqueduct (see Fig. 69).

Anteriorly, the distance separating the vestibular cavity from the middle cerebral fossa varies from 3 to 6 mm. This space is occupied above by the first turn of the facial canal, and below by the end of the basal coil of the cochlea, with its turning towards the tympanum (see Fig. 135). The front of the vestibule appears to engage the interior of the facial bend; between its two arms, it always remains removed less than 2 mm from what is called the *fold of the facial* (see Figs. 136, 138).

Vertical Relations of the Vestibule

Above, the vestibule is covered by the superior semicircular canal and the bony mass that encloses it and extends up to the arcuate eminence; that is, up to the anterosuperior wall of the petrosa. A distance of 6 to 10 mm separates, at this spot, the superior wall of the vestibule from the middle cerebral fossa.

Below, the vestibule is in relation with the subvestibular portion of the cochlea, which emerges from its floor anteriorly (see Fig. 200). Behind the cochlear exit, the vestibular substratum is made up more or less of compact bony materials, cellular materials; it can have a thickness of 10 to 12 mm if the jugular fossa is absent (see Figs 192, 194). This intervestibulo-jugular layer is reduced in proportion to the height of the jugular fossa; it can thus be reduced to the thickness of the labyrinthine capsule alone if it is 1 mm in certain cases, as already discussed.

In the majority of cases, the floor of the vestibule, like the floor of the internal auditory canal, does not have any limited relations with the intangible structures of the region. It corresponds to the sublabyrinthine space that is so well delimited on numerous petrosas by the carotid canal in front and the moderately developed jugular fossa behind (see Figs. 69, 123). Later, we will discuss the surgical approach to these two floors in order to reach the fundus of the internal auditory canal.

8 The Semicircular Canals

The semicircular canals have the form of an incomplete circle 7 to 8 mm in diameter; each end opens into the vestibule. The canals plus the vestibule house the vestibular apparatus or statokinetic labyrinth. When a patient is lying on the operating table, it may be considered as the posterior labyrinth. Embryologically, they arise from the walls of the labyrinth by evaginating and pleating. The labyrinth does not exist in invertebrates. It appears in the lowest vertebrates (Cyclostomes): The Myxine possess only a single canal and the Lamprey possesses only two canals.

Dimensions of the Semicircular Canals

The horizontal canal varies between 12 and 15 mm in length, the superior canal between 15 and 17 mm, and the posterior canal between 18 and 20 mm; the calibration varies. They are generally slightly flattened in the direction of the plane of the canal, giving it an ovoid form on sectioning. Their large diameter varies from 1 to 1.5 mm; their transverse diameter varies from 0.5 to 1 mm.

Orientation of the Semicircular Canals

The curvature of the semicircular canals varies with each person; indeed, from side to side in the same person. In order to trace the plane of a canal, one selects two fixed points, which are its vestibular orifices. The superior canal is vertical, and the external (lateral) is horizontal.

The plane of the horizontal canal is determined by passing a line straight through the center of its vestibular orifices, and building on this line a plane perpendicular to the sagittal plane of the head.

The plane of the superior canal is established in the same way. Its two orifices pierce the ceiling of the vestibule on a horizontal line. To obtain the plane of the canal, one raises a vertical plane on a line that passes through the center of the two vestibular orifices. This plane forms a right angle with the horizontal semicircular canal.

The plane of the posterior canal can also be found on the vestibular orifices (see Fig. 200). These two orifices—one on the ceiling, and the other on the floor of the vestibule—are found on a nearly vertical line. The plane that includes this line is also vertical; on the whole, the canal is nearly perpendicular to the plane of the superior canal.

The three orifices of the vertical canals are arranged in a right angle, with the common orifice rising to the summit of the angle. The three canals are therefore perpendicular to each other. There is a distance of 8 cm from one vestibule to the other.

The *horizontal canals* lie in the same plane. The two vestibular orifices of each canal are found on a line that forms an angle of 37° on the average, with the sagittal plane, and with the corresponding line of the opposite side an angle of 74°. The ampullae are both anterior and symmetrical. They both present their cribriform areas on their anterior border, and they are found placed face to face.

The *superior vertical canals* also function symmetrically. Each is found in a vertical plane, which forms with the sagittal plane an angle, open in front, of about 37°. Between them, it forms an angle of 74°. The superior canal is more sagittal than transverse, and it is not exactly diagonal. The ampullae are both anterior, with their cribriform area on the anterior border of their vestibular orifice. The superior canals are symmetrical without being parallel. They do not oppose one another like the horizontal ampullae.

The *posterior vertical canals* have a symmetry analogous to that of the superior canals. These two vertical canals of the same side form a right angle between them. Since the superior canal forms an angle of 37° with the sagittal plane, it follows that the posterior canal forms an angle of 53° (open behind) with the sagittal plane, and that the two posterior canals form an angle of 106° between them.

The superior semicircular canal is in a more sagittal direction than the posterior canals, which by contrast are more in the transverse direction. The superior canal of one side forms an angle of 16° with the posterior canal of the opposite side. These two canals are usually considered as parallel and coupled diagonally to simulate the coupling of the horizontal canals. Actually, each of the bony vertical canals deviates from the geometric diagonal by about 8°. If one subtracts this from the small divergence of 16°, the superior canal of one side and the posterior canal of the opposite side approach a true coupling effect. The ampullae are both anterior and appear to oppose their opposite canals with one ampulla downward and the other upward.

Termination of the Semicircular Canals

Each of the canals presents an ovoid dilation at one of its extremities (ampulla) that is flattened in the direction of the canal plane. They measure, on the average, 2 mm in lenth, 1.5 mm in width, and 1 mm in thickness. They correspond to a similar swelling of the membranous labyrinth.

The swelling of the bony ampulla is made at the expense of the central wall of the canal, whereas the distal wall has no special landmarks and is confined to the ampullary cribriform area of the vestibule.

The ampullary cribriform area is composed of 8 to 15 tiny openings located at the junction of the vestibule and the ampullary walls, with the exception of the posterior area, where they occur solely in the ampulla. They are centered on the distal edge of the ampullary orifice; that is, on the most elongated point from the center of the circumference described by the canal (see Figs. 200, 204). There are three ampullary orifices and only two nonampullary orifices; one is for the horizontal canal and the other is for the vertical canals, whose nonampullary arms unite to form a common crus as it approaches the vestibule.

The Horizontal Semicircular Canal (External, Lateral)

The horizontal semicircular canal is still called the *external canal*, because its two arms arise from the external wall of the vestibule and its curvature is where the labyrinth is brought closest to the external surface of the cranium.

It describes a semicircumference around a compact bony mass and present three regions: The *anterior arm,* which contains the ampulla, opens into the vestibule at the anterosuperior angle of its external wall. The *posterior arm,* which ends at the posterosuperior angle of the external wall of the vestibule by a crater-like widening that is sometimes wider than the ampulla (see Fig. 200). The *ring of the canal,* which connects the two arms. They form a curvature with a variable radius according to the length of the canal. It bends inferiorly in almost all temporal bones.

The horizontal semicircular canal is the shortest canal. It measures 12 to 15 mm in length. By contrast, it is wider, especially at the level of the arms. The transverse cut of the canal is elliptical and flattened in the plane of the canal. Its great axis may reach 2 mm, and the little axis may be 1 mm. The distance from the ringlet to the vestibular cavity varies

between 3 to 5 mm. The distance separating the two arms of the canal is 3 to 3.5 mm.

Orientation

The center of the vestibular orifices of the hoizontal canal are found on a horizontal plane. These two points are on a line that forms, with the sagittal plane of the head, an angle that is open in front and a little inferior of 45°. The canal expands external to and behind the vestibule, and its nonampullary or posterior orifice is more deeply situated than the ampullary or anterior orifice.

The ampullary arm runs from the anterior and superior angle of the external wall of the vestibule and is directed horizontally outward. Below, it overhangs the oval window. Above, by its extremity, it is contiguous to the ampulla of the superior canal (see Figs. 198, 199).

From the ampullary arm, the bow of the canal narrows and continues in a more or less regular arc. This arc does not always remain rigidly in the horizontal plane, but curves slightly towards the base, giving the canal on the whole a widening aspect.

The canal ends behind by its nonampullary arm, which reaches the posterosuperior angle of the external wall of the vestibule between the orifice of the common crus of the superior and posterior canals above, and the ampullary orifice of the posterior canal (see Fig. 200). The direction of the canal is lateral to medial and posterior to anterior, following a line that forms an angle 50° to 60° (open behind) with the sagittal plane. It is important to note these details, because the nonampullary arm of the horizontal canal is a guide when opening the vestibule.

The Superior Semicircular Canal

The two extremities of the superior canal terminate at each end of the superior wall of the vestibule—the ampullary end in front and the nonampullary behind. Three regions can be considered:

1. An anterior or ampullary arm, which rises above the vestibule and gently inclines outward (Fig. 210).
2. The bow, which is not inclined outward, but rises vertically or even takes an inverse inclination inward and then approaches the nonampullary end.
3. The nonampullary or posterior arm, which joins the nonampullary arm of the posterior canal.

Dimensions

The length of the superior canal is 15 to 17 mm. The distance separating the two arms varies between 4 to 5 mm. The most elevated point on the canal is between 5 to 6 mm from the roof of the vestibule. The lumen varies in shape from circular to oval. Its caliber is less than that of the other two canals (0.5 to 1 mm). The common crus is larger than

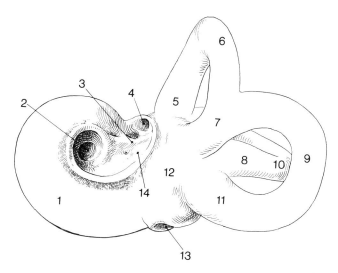

Figure 210. Right bony labyrinth seen from the inner side and from behind (× 7). 1, Cochlea. 2, Cochlear area in the internal auditory meatus. 3, Transverse crest. 4, Superior vestibular area. 5, Bony ampulla superior canal. 6, Superior semicircular canal. 7, Common crus. 8, Bony ampulla horizontal canal. 9, Posterior semicircular canal. 10, Horizontal semicircular canal. 11, Bony ampulla posterior canal. 12, Vestibule. 13, Round window. 14, Inferior vestibular area (internal auditory meatus).

each of the two arms that participate in its formation, and most often measures 1 to 1.5 mm.

Orientation

Most often, this canal is vertical. At times, it leans outward. This occurs when the common crus, in imitation of the ampullary arm, is also inclined outwards. The vertical plane of the superior canal is at right angles to the horizontal canal. It makes an angle of 37° (open in front) with the sagittal plane of the head. Its nonampullary or posterior arm is deeper than the ampullary or anterior arm in relation to the temporal surface of the cranium.

The Posterior Semicircular Canal

The posterior semicircular canal is in a plane that extends the posterior wall of the vestibule outward. It is outside the vestibule and behind the horizontal semicircular canal (see Figs. 198, 200).

Form and Course

It describes an almost complete circumference. Its ampullary orifice opens into the vestibule on the floor at the angle formed by the inferior, posterior, and external walls, and is directed upwards. Its nonampullary orifice, which is continuous with the common crus it forms with the supe-

rior canal, opens on the ceiling with its posterior extremity and looks downward (see Fig. 200). The two orifices face a nearly vertical line and are separated only by a space of 3 to 4 mm. The superior extremity is directed downward and the inferior is upward (see Fig. 200). The nonampullary arm is strongly curved on itself. Its last 2 to 3 mm contribute to the formation of the common crus. The ampullary arm is shorter and a little less curved. It terminates with an ampullary swelling. The bow of the canal describes an arc of a circle larger than that of the other two canals.

Dimensions

The posterior semicircular canal is the longest of the three canals (see Fig. 199). It measures 14 to 18 mm. The distance separating the bow of the canal from the posterior wall of the vestibule varies between 5 to 7 mm. The caliber of the posterior canal is slightly larger than that of the superior canal, but is less than that of the horizontal. Its greatest diameter barely surpasses 1 mm.

Labyrinthine Relations

The bow of the posterior semicircular canal is found about 2 mm from the posterior arm of the horizontal canal and crosses it at right angles. Nearer the vestibule, the relations of the two canals are different. The horizontal canal tends to lodge between the arms of the posterior canal without quite arriving there (see Fig. 198). From its opening in the vestibule, its posterior wall is included between the orifices of the posterior canal (see Fig. 200). The most sloped point of the posterior ampullary arm is found a little below the level of the vestibular floor and descends nearly to the level of the superior border of the round window (see Fig. 200). The ampulla is 1.5 mm behind and above the round window, and its vestibular orifice is at the level of the threshold of the oval window and 2.5 mm behind this opening (see Fig. 200).

Orientation

The two vestibular orifices of the posterior semicircular canal are lined up vertically; therefore, the canal is vertical (see Fig. 200). It is a little difficult to orient this vertical plane in relation to the plane of the superior canal, and also in relation to the sagittal plane. The ampulla and common crus are not in the same plane as the whole canal. These two extremities are gently curved in front, and thus leave the plane of the entire canal. This forms, with the superior canal, a right angle—and with the sagittal plane of the head, an angle of 53° (open behind). When establishing the plane of the posterior canal, one can take the vestibular orifices and the summit of the canal arc and find that the angle formed with the superior canal tends to exceed 90° and the incidence with the sagittal plane of the head approaches 45°

The posterior ampullary cribriform area is a small porous surface very near the zone where the ampulla unites with the internal wall of the vestibule. It is very near the inferior ampullary crest onto which it often encroaches (see Figs. 192, 194). The ampulla ascends as it approaches the floor of the vestibule. The cribriform area is found above this ascending portion on the internal or anterointernal wall of the ampulla and, at the same time, on the ampullary surface of the inferior ampullary crest, which limits the ampulla in front (see Fig. 200). The canaliculi of the porous area reunite rapidly to form a conduit 0.3 mm in diameter for passage of the inferior ampullary nerve through 3 to 4 mm of bone, opening into the internal auditory meatus by an orifice called the *foramen singulare of Morgagni* (see Figs. 127, 128).

Relations of the Horizontal Semicircular Canal

The cochlea appears in the tympanum through the medicum of the promontory and the round window. The vestibule is detected here across the oval window; the horizontal semicircular canal also indicates its presence by a characteristic projection that is always clearly visible in the aditus ad antrum.

Impossible to see through the external auditory canal, this projection is revealed if one performs a petromastoidectomy—or better yet—if in a simple mastoidectomy, one has care to push the procedure up to the immediate vicinity of the canal and of the tympanic framework (Fig. 211) with a length of 4 to 6 mm and a width of 3 mm rounded in all directions, and formed by a white compact tissue with a smooth surface, it appears on the internal border of the aditus between the antral cavity and the tympanum. By the gloss and whiteness of its surface, it contrasts with the (honey-combed) aspect of the bony environment.

It presents the following relations:

1. Superiorly, it is the petrous antrum, and its internal wall is all trabeculated cellular tissue. Below, it is the tympanic cavity; thus, it is interposed between these two cavities.

2. On the tympanic side, it enters in intimate relation with the facial canal, which insinuates under it (Fig. 134). And its smooth surface often enlarges inferiorly by the thickness of the canal unless there persists a very distinct line of demarcation between the two organs (see Fig 52).

3. Anteriorly, it is separated from the anterior wall of the petrosa by a distance that varies from 2 to 4 mm; it is the anterior part of the aditus, whose base is made up more often of a multitude of small cells.

4. Posteriorly, it is lost in the bony mass (more or less dense), which separates the antrum from the posterosuperior angle of the external auditory canal.

5. Externally, it corresponds to the posterior region of the attic, which lodges the horizontal apophysis of the

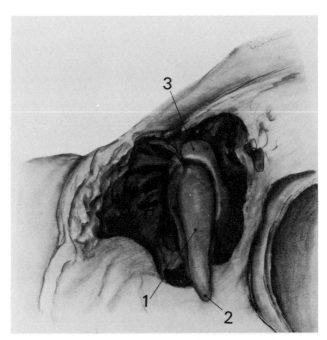

Figure 211.   Posterior tympanotomy. Aditus opened. 1, incus. 2, Short process of incus in fossa incudis. 3, Malleus head.

incus; it is the inferior edge that is found opposite the ossicular apophysis at 1.5 mm distant from the level of the incudo-petrosal articulation and 2 mm from the level of the incudo-mallear articulation. This relation is important from the surgical point of view—chiefly in a mastoidectomy and especially in the young infant, where the lesions and the bony friability often lead the curette onto the projection of the horizontal canal and very near to the ossicles, which it is important to respect. Of greater importance is incomplete removal or resection of the tympanic framework completely, while leaving the ossicles in place.

6.   Internally, the projection of the horizontal canal corresponds to the ampullary or anterior arm of the canal, and more profoundly to the external wall of the vestibule. It constitutes a surgical landmark of prime order. It covers the canal under a bony bed of 1 to 1.5 mm thickness. Its anterior extremity corresponds to the ampulla, which opens into the vestibule at the anterosuperior angle of its external wall. The vestibular cavity is found, at this spot, at only 2 or 3 mm from the aditus in the depth.

The anterior extremity of the projection is found above the anterior commissure of the oval window, it is separated from it by the thickness of the facial canal (see Figs. 134, 140).

Its posterior part corresponds to the bow of the horizontal canal. It overhangs the fundus of the tympanum by 4 to 5 mm above the round window. Below it overhangs the facial canal.

Considered in its entirety, the horizontal semicircular canal is found in the center of the petrous pyramid—and at a certain distance from all the walls of the petrosa with which it never enters into contact.

We have seen that its ampullary arm, which projects into the aditus, is always separated from the anterior cortex by a space that varies from 2 to 4 mm; its posterior arm, covered in a compact bony mass, is placed almost between the two branches of the posterior vertical canal, and is separated from the cerebellar fossa by a distance varying from 3 to 13 mm.

On its superior surface, the horizontal canal forms with its two congerers a trihedral right angle whose opening corresponds to the base of the petrous antrum, and is usually filled with a compact bony tissue—the name *solid angle* is given to this region. At times, air cells are developed there.

The distance separating the external semicircular canal from the anterior wall of the petrous pyramid in the vertical direction is measured by the height of the superior semicircular canal augmented by the thickness of the cortex; it is from 6 to 10 mm. The distance that separates it from the petrous ridge is slightly greater.

By its inferior surface, the horizontal canal acquires some relations with the tympanum which was mentioned earlier. The ampulla arrives at the vestibule 1 mm above the lintel of the oval window and overhangs the tympanum (see Fig. 134). The middle of the bow dominates and overhangs the tympanum above the oval window. The nonampullary branch of the canal is in relation inferiorly with the bony mass, which on the inside of the facial canal separates the tympanum from the deep subantral mastoid cells. Occasionally, the sinus tympani pushes a prolongation up to its contact. To this inferior surface of the canal is hung the facial canal, which passes under the ampulla and makes its second turn under the nonampullary branch.

Relations of the Posterior Semicircular Canal

When one follows the posterior arm of the horizontal canal with a gouge in order to thrust towards the vestibule above and behind the second turn of the facial canal, one soon encounters the midregion of the bow of the posterior canal. This is found deeper than the horizontal canal by about 2 mm. It is placed behind its congerer and the right angle crossing by a distance of 2 mm.

The posterior canal is always deeply buried in the petrous bone. Nothing reveals its presence in the cavity during a petromastoidectomy.

From its vestibular emergence, it extends towards the exterior nearly parallel to the posterior border of the petrosa, and thus tends to approach the lateral sinus—sometimes up to 6 mm, but more often 8 or 10 mm from the sinus, Bellocq[11] indicates an extreme distance of 15 mm.

Its superior vestibular origin has been discerned. It is the common branch, with its 2 or 3 mm length and ascending direction above the ceiling of the vestibule. The portion following it attracts the circular movement of the canal. It is the superior branch, which acquires with the petrosal

ridge and the superior petrosal sinus relations that at times, are very narrow (1 mm) or more distant. To surgically seek the superior branch of the posterior canal results in excavating the petrosal ridge.

In general, the posterior semicircular canal has very variable relations with the cerebellar fossa. Its superior arm sometimes projects. Mouret[86] has seen dehiscence. More often, it is separated by 3 to 4 mm; in the large petrosas, which are very full of cells, the retrolabyrinthine space can have up to 12 mm. This space is always 2 to 4 mm larger below than towards the crest, because the petrous pyramid enlarges toward its base. It is divided into two levels by the vestibular aqueduct (see Figs 131, 202): (1) the superior level, which mingles with the superior retrolabyrinthine space belonging to the system of superior perilabyrinthine spaces; and (2) the inferior level, which is the inferior retrolabyrinthine space and is compressed between the vestibular aqueduct above and the jugular dome below if it reascends high enough (see Fig. 69)—and the posterior sublabyrinthine space in the contrary case.

We have previously summarized the relations of the posterior canal with the vestibular aqueduct.

We must now consider the special relations of the ampullary branch. Its curve descends a little below the level of the vestibular floor. It enters in relation with the sublabyrinthine space (see Fig 57) or with the jugular dome (see Fig. 131). It is more removed from the cerebellar fossa than the superior branch because of the enlargement of the petrous pyramid at its base.

Anteriorly, the ampulla of the canal approaches the posterosuperior angle of the tympanum by the intermediary of the sinus tympani. One knows that this diverticular cavity, situated above and behind the round window, is insinuated behind the facial mass, entering in relation with the ampullary region of the posterior canal almost with the extremity of the nonampullary branch of the horizontal canal and the region below and posterior to the external wall of the vestibule.

The sinus tympani varies in development, but it is a point at which the labyrinth can enter in immediate relation with the tympanum. Also, independent of the sinus tympani, the ampulla of the posterior canal is not more than 2 mm behind and a little above the opening of the round window (see Fig. 57).

Externally, the inferior branch of the posterior canal acquires some important relations with the facial canal (see Fig. 57).

By its general orientation, from its loop to its vestibular orifices, the posterior canal is directed anteriorly and medially like the petrosa itself; its two extremities—common branch and ampulla—have an anterior inclination a little more accentuated than the loop. This inclination causes the ampullary arm to be concealed externally by the facial canal, and it appears to glide behind it when one considers the region from the mastoid route (see Fig. 57). If one reaches the ampulla of the posterior canal surgically, one is obliged to outline the aqueduct from behind in order to come to the region below it or behind it.

The distance separating the second turn of the facial

canal from the posterior ampulla is usaully 3 to 4 mm. This distance can be reduced to 2 mm in certain contracted petrosa.

The loop of the posterior canal, a little below its crossing with the horizontal canal, is found behind the facial turn at a distance of 2 or 3 mm. On narrow petrosas, the two structures touch each other, with 1 mm or less separating them. This is a surgical region; hence, the importance of these relations.

Relations of the Superior Semicircular Canal

The superior canal, which forms with the sagittal plane of the cranium an angle open in front of 37° (on the average), is placed vertically across the petrous pyramid where it occupies the superior level (see Fig. 194).

It is not visible at the bottom of a simple petromastoidectomy; yet its ampulla is adjacent to the aditus, where it has an excellent landmark in the projection of the external canal. One knows that the anterior extremity of this projection conceals the ampulla of this canal, and that by the superior edge of its vestibular orifice, it is contiguous to the corresponding edge of the ampulla of the superior semicircular canal. It suffices to excavate the internal wall of the petrous antrum to a depth of 2 or 3 mm, just above the projection of the external canal near the aditus, in order to find this ampulla (see Fig. 203). It is this point where the superior canal is nearest the antrum. It progressively withdraws up to its nonampullary termination, where one finds it 8 or 10 mm deeper, when measured from the antral wall.

The bony mass that separates the canal from the antrum is the solid angle which was defined earlier. It is generally compact; yet one often encounters below the anterior cortex of the petrosa a cellular tissue that, parting from the antrum, insinuates up to the region of the canal following the petrous wall in a puffiness situated a little outside of the canal—the *eminentia arcuata fossa.* In this case, the solid mass is reduced and occupies only the bottom of the angle of the three canals.

The solid angle is sometimes crossed by cells passing under the arc of the superior canal along with the antrocerebellar canal.

The internal surface of the superior canal looks toward the petrous apex. In the newborn, it is free and rises on the side of the petrosa at the entrace of the subarcuate fossa like the vault that forms the entrance of a tunnel (see Fig. 18). In the adult, the tunnel is filled, its entrance is leveled, and the slope of the petrosa no longer presents any uneveness at this level (see Fig. 184). Therefore, this is not an eminent arch of feeble relief, which reveals the presence of the subjacent canal during the three first years, but disappears most often in the adult. When the arcuate eminence is visible, it appears on the anterior slope of the petrosa in front of the petrous ridge. More often, it is dominated 2 to 3 mm externally by a blowing up or puffiness of the petrosal wall, which certain authors designate as the arcuate eminence. This puffiness, due to the presence of subcortical cells, contributes to erasing the true arcuate eminence, but would not be a substitute for it.

By its internal surface, in the adult, the superior semicircular canal is in relation with the bony material overloading the roof of the internal auditory canal. There, one encounters the endocranial orifice of the petromastoid canal, which opens 5 mm from the semicircular canal into the cerebellar fossa. One may also find air cells there. Here lies the crossroads of the superior perlabyrinthine cell tracts (Fig. 182). Even more distinctly in the cerebellar fossa, the internal auditory meatus opens 10 or 15 mm from the canal.

At its periphery, the superior semicircular canal is in relation by its ampulla with the superior antelabyrinthine space, which marks its posterior limit, and (beyond this space) with the anterior wall of the petrosa. Below, the ampullary branch and petrosal wall are about 3 mm from each other; they are brought nearer, while rising and ending, by entering in intimate contact after a distance varying from 2 to 4 mm.

The entire loop of the canal, at times up to its reunion with the posterior canal, is in relation with the middle cerebral cortex, which it raises (or not) into an arcuate eminence. The bony plate separating the canal from the cerebral fossa is more often minimal (0.5 to 1 mm); it is sometimes thicker, going up to 2.5 mm according to Bellocq[11]. At times, the canal is dehiscent.

The petrous ridge acquires some variable relations with the nonampullary branch of the superior semicircular canal. It is generally 3 mm behind and above the canal; but it can deviate for 6 to 7 mm posteriorly in large petrosa—like it can, at other times, adhere to the canal when flattened.

Finally, the superior semicircular canal redescends towards the vestibule not far from the cerebellar fossa. Sometimes it is very near and even raises the cerebellar cortex of the petrosa (which is rare) and sometimes it is separated by 6 or 7 mm of bony tissue (which is generally rare); most often it is separated by 3 mm.

The portion that is common with the posterior canal deviates slightly more to the cerebellar fossa, because it is a little oblique from behind forward and from above downward, and because the cerebellar fossa also deviates in an inverse direction.

Air cells sometimes occupy the interior of the petrous ridge and the space separating the superior semicircular canal from the cerebellar fossa.

Inferiorly, we know that the superior semicircular canal is in relation with the vestibule by the intermediary of the bony mass circumscribed by its bow. A cut carried in the plane of the canal causes the regular appearance of a circle 5 to 6 mm in diameter. One can note the petromastoid canal in the region of the nonampullary arm (see Figs. 183, 187) and, sometimes, some air cells.

9 Anatomy of the Cochlea

The cochlea is a bony tube that is rolled up on itself into a decreasing spiral of two-and-a-half turns ending in a cul-de-sac. This spiral form is found only in mammals. In birds, it is short and straight. In reptiles, it is even more rudimentary. In amphibians and fishes, there is only the *expanded saccula,* called the *lagena.* It does not exist in lower forms such as the lamprey.

In the human embryo, and in other vertebrates, the cochlear duct is formed by expansion of the inferior wall of the saccule. The canalis reunions persists between the saccule and the cochlear duct, and the cochlear duct epithelium originates in the interior of the vestibule.

The connection between the cochlea and the vestibule is formed by a wide orifice (Figs. 193, 212). It occupies the anterior third of the vestibular floor. Its inner edge is the inferior border of the hemispherical recess in the vestibule (Figs. 205, 213). Its posterior border is marked by the spiral lamina at the level of its inflection (see Figs. 193, 205). Its external edge coincides with the inferior edge of the external wall of the vestibule, stopping 1 mm below the oval window (see Fig. 212). Its anterior border is at the base of the anterior wall of the vestibule. The bony cochlea leaves the vestibule as it extends to become the basal coil.

Orientation

The cochlea lies under the vestibule for 3 to 4 mm, and then extends toward the petrous apex. In relation to the vestibule, it is found partly below—but in greater part medially and anteriorly—at a level slightly inferior.

The first turn of the cochlear spiral is open to the vestibule. It immediately takes the form of a tubular, spirally wound cylinder whose caliber continually decreases. It begins below the vestibule and extends medially and anteriorly, withdrawing from the tympanum to pass under the internal auditory meatus; it then extends forward until it is found below the cochlear recess.

The distance from the vestibule to the cochlear recess (the noncoiled part of the cochlea) is 5 to 6 mm. It includes

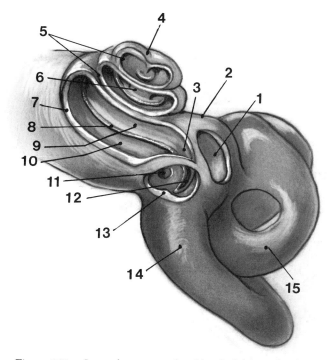

Figure 212. Internal structure of cochlea. Left labyrinth of newborn, viewed from below and a bit anterior. The inferior region of the otic capsule has been resected on the three turns of the cochlear spiral ($\times$ 5).[35] 1, Oval window. 2, Anterior wall of the vestibule. 3, Orifice of the scala vestibuli. 4, Apex. 5, Spiral partition. 6, Modiolus. 7, Otic capsule. 8, Osseous spiral lamina. 9, Scala vestibuli. 10, Scala tympani. 11, Orifice of the cochlear aqueduct. 12, Vestibulotympanic fissure. 13, Round window. 14, Posterior semicircular canal. 15, Horizontal semicircular canal.

the round window, and lies medial to the posterior half of the promontory. It is of great surgical importance.

Apart from the point where it becomes tangential to the inferior border of the cochlear recess, the first turn of the spiral coils more closely. It passes in front of the anterior wall of the meatus in a vertical circular movement, with the

151

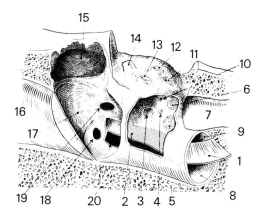

Figure 213. A general schema of the ear, particularly the bony labyrinth. 1, Spiral lamina. 2, Floor of the vestibule. 3, Orifice of the ampullary end of posterior semicircular canal. 4, Cochlear recess. 5, Hemispherical (saccular) recess. 6, Utricular recess. 7, Internal auditory meatus. 8, Scala tympani. 9, Scala vestibuli. 10, Endolymphatic canal. 11, Nonampullary orifice of the superior and posterior semicircular canals. 12, Nonampullary orifice of the horizontal canal. 13, Ampullary orifice of the superior canal. 14, Ampullary orifice of the horizontal canal. 15, Antrum. 16, External auditory canal. 17, Tympanum. 18, Round window. 19, Oval window. 20, Subvestibular cavity. From Poirier, P., and Charpy, A., *Traite d'Anatomie Humaine,* Vol. 5. Paris: Masson et Cie, 1904.

center opposite the cochlear recess. It rises to the height of the meatal roof, redescending while nearing the anterior wall of the vestibule, and terminating its revolution 1.5 mm in front of and medial to the anterior margin of the oval window.

The second turn of the spiral is located in front of the first. It is smaller and more compact. The third turn is even smaller. It is located in front of the second turn and terminates in the apex. It is incomplete, forming a half turn more or less (see Fig. 212).

Form

The cochlea has a conical form with a slightly bulging surface, a rounded summit, and an opening—the *round window*—set in a lightly flaring niche that is gracefully contoured. The axis of the spiral is made up of very porous bone, forming a core called the *modiolus.* The base of the modiolus is made up of the cochlear cribriform area, which is call the *spiral foraminous tract.* Its holes give passage for the terminal branches of the cochlear nerve.

Dimensions

The cochlear tube has a total length of about 30 mm. The diameter of the basal coil is 9 to 10 mm. The tubular cavity, which has a diameter more than 2 mm at the level of the

round window, has less than 1 mm at the apex of the cochlea.

Orientation

The cochlear cone lies on its side, with the apex of the cochlea directed forward and the base posteriorly. The modiolus, which is equally conical, has the same recumbent position. A line joining the middle of the base to the apex is the axis of the cochlea. This axis is oriented from behind forward, and from within outward, in the same plane as the superior semicircular canal. It is inclined outwards and downwards. The coiling of the cochlear tube is so well done that each turn of the spiral is in a general vertical plane, but is still a little inclined from above downward and nearly parallel to the longitudinal axis of the petrous bone.

Labyrinthine Relations of the Cochlea

The first 3 to 4 mm of the basal turn of the spiral are found under the vestibule, topographically, below the oval window. This is called the *subvestibular portion of the cochlea.* Here it is separated from the vestibule by a cleft whose inner wall is formed by the last quarter of the first turn of the cochlea, and the external wall by the anterointernal angle of the vestibule. This *vestibulo-cochlear cleft* is opposed to that portion of the facial canal passing over the labyrinthine block at this level.

The next portion of the basal coil is carried anteriorly by the helicoid form of the cochlea. It closely approximates the floor of the internal auditory meatus, passes in front of the anterior meatal wall, and completes its first turn in front of the vestibule.

The base of the cochlea is in intimate relation with the internal meatus via the *tractus spiralis foraminosus.* This cribriform area, in the form of a ribbon rolled into a spiral, begins at the union of the base and the floor of the internal auditory meatus, and has a length of 3 to 4 mm. At this level, the cavities of the cochlea and the meatus are superimposed and separated from each other by 1 mm thickness of bone.

Leaving the floor of the internal meatus, the tractus spiralis foraminosus passes onto the anterior wall of the meatus, where it makes a spiral and a half in the cochlear recess. The cochlear tube follows the same course, passing in front of the internal meatus and completing its first spiral turn at the end of the cochlear recess. The cochlear bed curves from the floor to the anterior wall in the depth of the internal auditory meatus.

These relations are of great surgical importance. They indicate the pathway of the spread of infection in otitic meningitis, and they underscore the potential risks incurred in the insertion of cochlear implants for hearing improvement.

Constitution

The labyrinthine capsule is easily dissected in a five-month old (or older) fetus. It is formed by a thin plate of compact bone that is very distinct from the normal bone making up the mass of the petrosa. It is very thin in the fetus, thicker in the newborn (0.3 mm), and reaches 1 mm in the adult. The capsule encloses the cochlear cavity except for four openings:

1. The oval window opening into the vestibule and occluded by the footplate of the stapes.
2. The round window opening into the scala tympani at the beginning of the basal turn and occluded by the round window membrane.
3. The foramina for the cochlear nerve filaments and the vessels accompanying them.
4. The orifice of the cochlear aqueduct.

Internal Structures

All of the internal bony structure of the cochlea can be considered as part of the otic capsule. The osseous spiral lamina is also a portion of the otic capsule. The term *otic capsule,* however, usually refers to the peripheral circumferential lamina housing the entire inner ear. The capsule at the periphery and the modiolus in the center form the lateral walls (external and internal) of the cochlea tube. The dorsal and ventral walls of this tube are made up by the two surfaces of a bony partition call the *spiral partition.*

The internal or axial wall of the bony cochlea is the external cortex of the modiolus. It is made up of compact bone overlaying the porous inner portion. It is divided along its entire length, in the cochlear tube, into two parts by the spiral lamina (Fig. 214). Its anterior part is the *scala vestibuli* of the cochlea and its posterior part is the *scala tympani.*

Along the entire length of the first spiral turn, orifices are seen on the anterior part of the axial wall of the scala tympani. These are irregularly arranged and extend onto the posterior aspect of the osseous spiral lamina. These orifices (*habenula perforata*) are separated by a type of column—*columns of the scala tympani of Cotugno* (Domenico Cotugno, Neapolitan anatomist, 1736–1822). These begin, like the osseous spiral lamina, on the floor of the vestibule and end at the extremity of the modiolus (see Fig. 212).

The peripheral wall of the otic capsule is connected to the free edge of the osseous spiral lamina by the basilar membrane. Along the line of insertion of the basilar membrane, it carries a little bony crest call the *secondary spiral lamina,* which is clearly visible only at the origin of the cochlear tube—where it constitutes the external lip of the *vestibulo-tympanic fissure* (see Figs. 212, 214) and on a part of the first spiral turn.

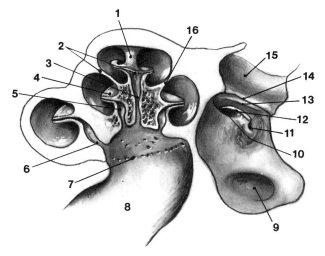

Figure 214.   Section of cochlea through the axis of the modiolus and floor of the vestibule. 1, Terminal end of the spiral septum (modiolar lamina). 2, Spiral wall or partition. 3, Central canal of the modiolus. 4, Osseous spiral lamina. 5, Spiral canal of Rosenthal. 6, Cochlear canaliculus. 7, Spiroid cribrosa (spiral foraminous tract—Sobotta). 8, Internal auditory meatus. 9, Ampullar end posterior semicircular canal. 10, Beginning of scala vestibuli. 11, Internal orifice cochlear aqueduct. 12, Intervestibulo-tympanic fissure. 13, Secondary osseous spiral lamina. 14, Oval window. 15, Promontory. 16, Spiral partition.

The Spiral Partition (Fig. 215)

The anterior wall of a spiral turn and the posterior wall of the following turn form a bony partition between the two spiral cavities. It extends from the origin of the second spiral turn to the extremity of the third. It presents as a bony ribbon that describes a declining spiral, or a turn and a half. Its external edge corresponds externally to a groove outlined by the juxtaposition of two turns of the cochlear tube (see Fig. 212). Its axial edge, with its spiral insertion on the circumference of the modiolus, ends at the summit; that is, at the point where the spiral lamina becomes free in order to form its terminal hook (Figs. 216, 217).

The second spiral turn, smaller than the first, partially dovetails into the first. The third spiral turn, smaller than the second, does the same.

The modiolus ends at a point where the osseous spiral lamina becomes free to form its terminal hook. It does not extend to the cochlear apex. Arriving at the summit of the modiolus, the spiral partition ends by a free edge that goes from the summit of the modiolus to the dome of the apex (Fig. 216). This terminal free edge of the spiral partition measures 1 mm in length. It appears as the column of the apex (see Fig. 216).

In the apex, the spiral partition appears as a spiral and funnel-like incline or scala. The external edge of the tunnel, which is thus realized, would be the foundation of the apex. In the anterior, widened part (in front of the hook of

POST.   ANT.
←   →

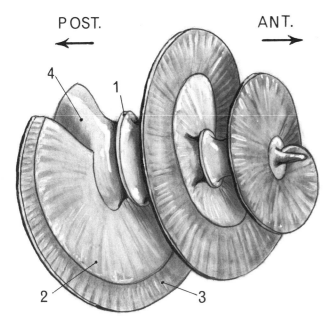

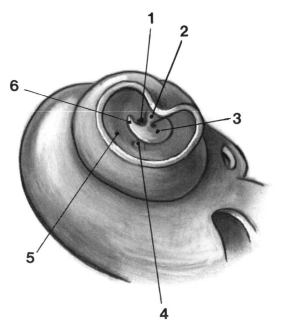

Figure 215. Modiolus showing the osseous spiral lamina and the membranous spiral lamina (basilar membrane). The right ear is viewed laterally and slightly anteriorly. The bony spiral lamina is broad in the basal turn and narrow in the apical turn (bony spiral partition, which separates the cochlear turns is deleted; only its anchorage to the modiolus is shown). The scala vestibuli is situated anterior to the osseous spiral lamina, and the scala tympani is posterior. 1, Bony spiral partition. 2, Osseous spiral lamina. 3, Membranous spiral lamina. 4, Modiolus. Note that the osseous spiral lamina is much larger at the base, and that the basilar membrane is much larger at the apex.[10]

Figure 216. Apex of cochlea and termination of the modiolus (× 6).[35] 1, Helicotrema. 2, Terminal edge of the spiral partition. 3, Scala tympani. 4, Summit of modiolus. 5, Scala vestibuli. 6, Hamulus.

the spiral partition) ends the scala vestibuli. In the narrow part (behind the hamulus) ends the scala tympani. The two scalae communicate with each other through a narrow orifice at the apex—the *helicotrema* (Greek: helix, a spiral + trema, a hole).

Modiolus

The modiolus is a small, irregular mass of porous bone in the shape of a cone. In the center of the cochlea, it occupies the space enclosed by the first two turns of the spiral. Its base in the first turn of the cochlear spiral is 4 mm in diameter. At its summit, it is less that 0.5 mm in thickness, and corresponds to the terminal part of the second spiral turn. Its axis from base to apex measures no more than 3 mm (see Fig. 212).

The modiolus has nothing to do with the framework of the cochlear apex. Its summit is marked by the point where the osseous spiral lamina becomes free of all adherent bone in order to form its terminal hook (Fig. 216). However, a bony edge seems to continue the modiolus axis and extend up to the dome of the apex. This structure, however, does not belong to the modiolus; rather, it is the free and terminal edge of the spiral partition.

The outer surface of the modiolus is covered by a thin layer of compact bone that belongs to the otic capsule. The otic capsule contains two spiral bony laminas that are inserted on the modiolar cone like the thread of a screw adherent to its metallic hub. One is the osseous spiral lamina, which in two turns of the screw goes through the modiolar surface from base to summit. The other is the spiral partition whose peripheral edge inserts on the otic capsule (see Fig. 212).

The base of the modiolus, which is made up entirely of porous bone, forms a part of the anterior wall of the internal auditory meatus. A lesser area is found in the inferior wall of the meatus. This is the beginning of the spiral foraminous tract. It is formed from a ribbon of bone, with channels 1 mm wide, which rises at the junction of the floor and the terminal (or vestibular) wall of the internal auditory meatus. It extends on the floor in a forward direction for 3 to 4 mm. From where it reaches the anterior border of the meatus, it rolls up into a rapidly decreasing spiral, making a turn and a half, to end at its center at an orifice much larger than the others called the *central canal of the modiolus.* The tightly spiraled part of the spiral foraminous tract terminates on the anterior wall of the meatus at the cochlear recess.

Each hole of the spiral foraminous tract is the origin of a canaliculus that, after a variable course for each of them, proceeds to the *spiral canal of Rosenthal* (Fig. 218). The central canal of the modiolus (*cup of Vieussens*—French anatomist Raymond Vieussens, 1641–1716) is visible with the naked eye. It proceeds in a straight line to the summit of the modiolus (see Fig. 212), where it stops with the

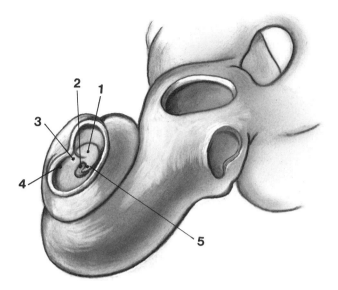

spiral canal of Rosenthal, which also ends at this point. All of these little canals conduct axons of the cochlear nerve, which they deliver to the spiral ganglion (see Fig. 212, 218).

The spiral canal of Rosenthal (see Fig. 218) is an oval-shaped conduit located at the periphery of the modiolus, opposite the zone of adherence of the osseous spiral lamina. It is 0.1 to 0.2 mm in diameter. Its origin corresponds to the origin of the osseous spiral lamina. It makes two turns paralleling the edge of the osseous spiral lamina, and ends at the top of the modiolus.

On its entire course, it receives on its inferior aspect the canaliculi of the modiolus. From its superior aspect emerge the canaliculi of the spiral lamina. It ends at the top of the modiolus, where it occupies most of the thickness of the bone. Here it also meets the large central canal of the modiolus. It is from here that all of the canaliculi leave to proceed onto the hook of the spiral lamina (see Fig. 212).

In humans, the spiral canal of Rosenthal is occupied by bipolar ganglion cells that together constitute the *spiral ganglion* or *ganglion of Corti.* The canaliculi that emerge carry nerve fibers from the organ of Corti via the osseous spiral lamina, and then carry them towards the internal auditory meatus via the modiolus.

Figure 217. The apex of the cochlea and its internal structure viewed from its inferior and anterior aspect—left side (× 6).[35] 1, Osseous spiral lamina. 2, Helicotrema. 3, Terminal edge of the spiral wall. 4, Spiral wall. 5, Hamulus (termination of osseous spiral lamina).

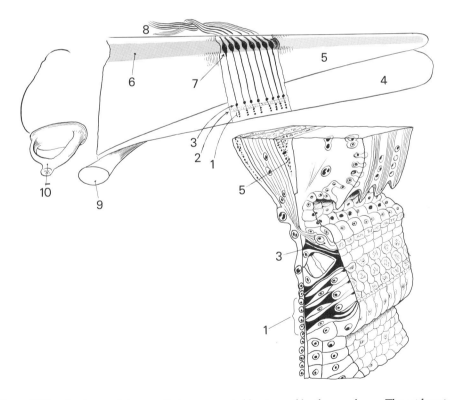

Figure 218. A schema of the uncoiled osseous spiral lamina and basilar membrane. The midportion of the spiral lamina has been dissected to show the neural anatomy. 1, Outer hair cells (three rows). 2, Supporting cells (pillar). 3, Inner hair cell (one row). 4, Basilar membrane. 5, Osseous spiral lamina. 6, Rosenthal's canal. 7, Spiral ganglion cells (bipolar). 8, Cochlear nerve in the internal auditory meatus. 9, Round window. 10, Stapes.

The Spiral Lamina

An osteomembranous partition (see Fig. 215) divides the cochlear duct into two semicylindrical compartments called the scala vestibuli and the scala tympani. It begins on the floor of the vestibule, and ends in the apex at the helicotrema. By its external membranous portion (basilar membrane plus spiral ligament), it adheres to the otic capsule; by its internal bony portion, to the modiolus (the osseous spiral lamina).

In the dry bone, the basilar membrane has disappeared, and the osseous spiral lamina appears like a very accentuated thread of a screw. It has a width of 1 mm at the vestibular exit and 0.5 mm at the top of the modiolus. Its free edge extends nearly up to the middle of the cochlear duct. Its adherent edge is fixed to the modiolus, following a spiral line that leaves the vestibular floor and travels from the base to the top of the modiolar surface (see Fig. 212).

The osseous spiral lamina makes two and one quarter turns. It has the same orientation as the cochlear spiral; that is, it is vertical in a plane vaguely parallel to that of the posterior semicircular canal, or to the longitudinal axis of the petrosa. It presents an anterior and a posterior surface. The anterior surface faces the scala vestibuli, and the posterior faces the scala tympani.

The osseous spiral lamina is composed of two distinct lamellae—dorsal and ventral—united to each other by bony spicules (see Fig. 212). Between these two lamellae is found a system of small canals directed transversely from the adherent to the free edge. These canals originate, medially, on the superoexternal edge of the oval canal of Rosenthal (see Fig. 212), and give passage for the myelinated nerve fibers that go from the spiral ganglion to the organ of Corti (Alfonso Corti, Italian anatomist, 1822–1888) (see Fig. 218).

Origin of the Osseous Spiral Lamina

The osseous spiral lamina arises on the vestibular floor, near the external edge of the cochlear recess (see Fig. 205)—from 1 mm in front of the inferior ampullary crest to above the superior edge of the round window. At first, it has a horizontal course from posterior to anterior and contributes to the formation of the floor of the vestibule (see Figs. 193, 205, 212, 213), then it gradually bends inward toward the base, leaving the vestibular floor in its midportion (nearly so) in order to penetrate the cochlear duct (Fig. 205).

Opposite the free border of the osseous spiral lamina, on the external wall of the otic capsule above the round window, there is a little crest called the *secondary spiral lamina* (Figs. 193, 212, 219). The sickle-shaped fissue that, on the dry bone, separates the osseous spiral lamina from the secondary spiral lamina is called the *vestibulo-tympanic fissure*. In humans, it is filled by the basilar membrane.

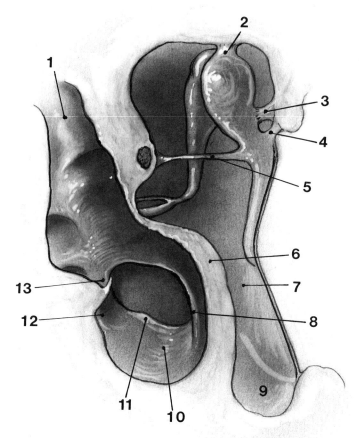

Figure 219.   The osseous spiral lamina has been removed in order to expose the floor of the scala tympani and the round window looking forward in the vestibule. 1, Superior semicircular canal. 2, Superior mallear ligament. 3, Lateral mallear ligament. 4, Membrane flaccida. 5, Tensor tympani tendon. 6, Promontory. 7, Middle ear. 8, Secondary osseous spiral lamina. 9, Hypotympanum. 10, Floor of the scala tympani. 11, Crista semilunaris. 12, Inner orifice of the cochlear aqueduct. 13, Attachment of primary osseous spiral lamina. (From Siebenmann, F., Sinnesorgane: Mittelohrn und Labyrinth. Jena: Gustave Fischer, 1897.)

Above and in front of the osseous spiral lamina, at a point where it bends back towards the base, one finds the origin of the scala vestibuli (see Figs. 193, 205). Below and behind its first millimeter, the scala tympani originates in a cul-de-sac whose base is made up chiefly by the round window membrane (see Fig. 212).

Termination of the Osseous Spiral Lamina

The osseous spiral lamina makes two complete turns around the modiolus, arriving at the helicotrema or at the anterior extremity of it. It leaves there and ends in a type of hook, in the form of a very curved sickle, which free of all bony attachments still makes a quarter turn (see Fig. 212). This hook (hamulus, bec, rostrum, crochet) is found in the cochlear apex.

By its absolutely free edge, even on the fresh bone, the hamulus faces the terminal funnel-shaped part of the spiral partition, and with it forms a tunnel-shaped passage (see Fig. 216). On the fresh bone, the basilar membrane, after having filled the spiral fissure along the entire cochlear duct, ends by a free concave border that goes from the point of the hamulus to the wall of this tunnel. The concave border of the hamulus, the free terminal concave edge of the basilar membrane, and the terminal infundibuliform part of the spiral partition form a pinhole-sized orifice called the *helicotrema*. It is across the helicotrema that the scala vestibuli and the scala tympani communicate with each other.

The free border of the osseous spiral lamina forms the axial edge of the spiral fissure (see Figs. 212, 214, 219). At the floor of the vestibule, it constitutes the internal lip of the vestibulo-tympanic fissure. Along its course, it is pierced by a multitude of little holes (*habenula perforata, foramina nervosa*) that transmit the terminal fibers of the cochlear nerve. It ends in the apex at the hamulus.

The attachment of the osseous spiral lamina in its first 2 mm forms a portion of the floor of the vestibule (the region of the hook) (see Figs. 193, 205, 212, 214). The rest is inserted on the modiolus following a spiral line that makes two complete turns that progressively decrease in size, running from the base to the summit of the modiolar canal. The attached edge is thicker that the free border. The two lamellae of the osseous spiral lamina diverge and bend back—one in front and the other behind—on the cortical modiolus to blend with it. The cortical layer of the modiolus is considered the axial portion of the otic capsule (see Fig. 214).

The Cochlear Scalae

The cochlear scalae are formed by the division of the cochlear duct into two semicylinders by a vertical partition composed of the spiral lamina and basilar membrane (see Fig. 212).

The scala vestibuli is separated from the basilar membrane by Reisner's membrane, thus forming the *scala media,* which closes up the cochlear canal with the organ of Corti. The scala vestibuli arises in the anterior and external region of the floor of the vestibule by an elliptical orifice that measures 1 mm by 2 mm. This orifice is situated 1 cm below the inferior edge of the oval window (see Fig. 212).

The scala vestibuli follows the same spiral course as the otic capsule and ends in the apex, where it occupies the anterior or terminal part situated between the hook of the spiral lamina and the vault (see Fig. 212).

The scala tympani arises from a cul-de-sac at the round window below that portion of the vestibular floor formed by the origin of the osseous spiral lamina. The round window from where the scala tympani leaves is a nearly circular orifice measuring a little more that 1 mm in diameter. It is situated 2 mm below the posterior edge of the oval window. It is directed posteriorly, while the oval window is directed externally.

The superior edge of the round window corresponds to the initial and horizontal part of the vestibulo-tympanic fissure; that is, the superior border of the window is found slightly below the level of the floor of the vestibule (see Fig. 212).

From the external edge of the round window rises a spiral crest (see Fig. 219) directed toward the interior of the scala tympani, passing over the floor and going on the posterior wall, where it ends under the spiral lamina—supporting it like the support of a bracket (see Fig. 212).

Immediately in front of this crest on the posterior wall of the scala tympani is the orifice of the cochlear aqueduct (see Fig. 212).

The round window in humans is closed by a membrane called the *secondary tympanic membrane,* whose external surface is in contact with air in the tympanum and internal surface is in contact with the perilymph of the scala tympani.

A drawing is included of the membranous labyrinth enclosed within the bony labyrinth, for study purposes (Fig. 220).

Relations of the Cochlea

When one views the cochlea during a classic radical mastoidectomy, it appears on the medial tympanic wall from the rear of the carotid canal (on which it appear to rest) to the first turn of the facial canal, which meanders on its superior side (see Fig. 141). The tympanum externally, the carotid canal below, and the facial canal above are its prin-

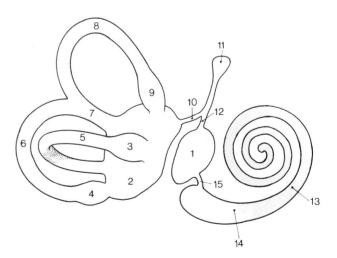

Figure 220. Membranous labyrinth (right side). 1, Saccule. 2, Utricle. 3, Ampulla horizontal canal. 4, Ampulla posterior canal. 5, Horizontal semicircular canal. 6, Posterior semicircular canal. 7, Common crus. 8, Superior semicircular canal. 9, Ampulla superior canal. 10, Utricular duct. 11, Endolymphatic sac. 12, Saccular duct. 13, Cochlear (coiled) duct. 14, Cochlear duct (non-coiled) or vestibular portion. 15, Ductus reunions.

cipal relations. Externally, the cochlea is in relation not only with the tympanum—at the base of which it indicates its presence by a rounded curve called the *promontory*—but also with the eustachian tube and the canal for the tensor tympani.

Relations With the Promontory

The promontory is limited above by the threshold of the oval window, in front and above by the canal for the tensor tympani, below and in front by the internal lip of the tubal orifice that spreads out on its surface without demarcation, below by the cells of the base of the tympanum or by the carotid canal when it is highly situated, and posteriorly by a prominence of 2 to 3 mm that forms the recess of the round window (see Fig. 140).

Under a compact bony layer 1 mm thick, the promontory covers:

1. The subvestibular portion of the cochlea or external side of the first helical turn, whose width equals the length of the oval window.
2. The external side of the second helical turn below the processus cochleariformis.

The promontory is seen at the bottom of the tympanum on otoscopic examination when the drumhead is absent.

Relations With the Eustachian Tube

The internal lip of the tubal orifice adheres to the anteroinferior region of the promontory (see Fig. 140). It is very close to the two basal spirals of the cochlea at the point where they turn in order to sink into the depth.

Relations With the Canal for the Tensor Tympani

The canal for the tensor tympani muscle is applied on the anterosuperior surface of the eustachian tube (see Fig. 140). At the level of its inferior border and anterior to the promontory, the tympanic end of the eustachian tube ends; but the muscular canal continues and extends on the external surface of the promontory up to the facial canal in the immediate neighborhood of the anterior commissure of the oval window, where it terminates at the processus cochleariformis. It is this tympanic portion, 6 to 7 mm long, which enters in relation with the cochlea. The processus cochleariformis is opposite the end of the first spiral or the beginning of the second (see Fig. 140). The external side of the cochlear apex is opposite the body of the muscular canal.

The Inferior Relations

Inferiorly, the cochlea rests on the carotid canal at its curve. In small petrosas, the three spirals apply their inferior side upon the carotid canal and may indent it; on large petrosas, the contact is less pronounced. Variations occur in the depth of the carotid. If the carotid is recessed several millimeters, the space left free is often occupied by a group of air cells (intercarotico-tubal-cochlear cells) that may form the inferior antelabyrinthine cell tracts (see Figs. 57, 118).

Behind the ascending arm and the turn of the carotid canal, the posteroinferior side of the subvestibular portion of the cochlea is found above a space called sublabyrinthine, which is occupied by bone (either compact or pneumatic), or even by the jugular fossa whose dome may rise until it hides the opening of the round window (see Fig. 24). Nevertheless, there is always found between the carotid canal and the dome of the jugular fossa a triangular sublabyrinthine space that contacts the subvestibular portion of the cochlea.

The Superior Relations

Superiorly, the cochlea is in relation with the first turn of the facial canal and its two arms, as well as with the site of the geniculate ganglion.

The highest part of the basal turn of the cochlea is found in front of and within the vestibule (see Fig. 197), and is separated from it by a groove where the first part of the facial canal passes while encircling in its curve the top of the first spiral turn (see Figs. 131, 136). The second spiral turn and the apex, which are less deviated and more anterior in position, are found directly under the geniculate ganglion. From the tympanic aspect, the external flank of the second spiral turn and the apex are surmounted and overhung by the tympanic segment of the facial canal from the site of the geniculate ganglion up to the anterior commissure of the oval window (see Figs. 134, 135).

Medial to the site of the geniculate ganglion and immediately behind the hiatus facialis, the apex adheres by its superior flank to the cortex of the anterior wall of the petrosa. At this point, one almost never encounters air cells (see Figs. 69, 134, 136).

Medial to the intervestibulo-cochlear groove and the facial canal (see Figs. 135, 136), the top of the cochlea is seen in relation with the anterior wall of the petrosa. Here the cells of the crossroads of the superior perilabyrinthine spaces can be interposed; or, in the same way, diploic tissue may be present.

The Anterior Relations

The small apex is in relation with the portion of the anterior petrosal wall included between the hiatus facialis above and the carotid canal below (see Fig. 134). Here there is a precochlear space measuring, on the average, 3 mm in height and 3 mm in width. This space is usually filled with compact bone, but it may contain precochlear cell tracts or diploic tissue.

The Posterior Relations

The initial portion of the first turn, which is found beneath the vestibule and the internal auditory canal, is in relation with the large sublabyrinthine and retrolabyrinthine space, which the jugular fossa may fill in certain cases. The rest of the cochlear base reaches the anterior wall of the internal auditory canal at the cochlear recess.

The Medial Relations

The internal side of the cochlea is in relation with the petrous apex in the region included between the internal auditory canal superiorly and posteriorly, the carotid canal inferiorly and anteriorly, and the anterior wall of the petrosa superiorly and anteriorly.

It is difficult to surgically approach the internal auditory meatus or the petrous apex via the intercarotico-cochlear route, because one must pass between the carotid canal inferiorly and the facial nerve superiorly. The average space is 3 mm at the level of the apex and 6 mm at the level of the oval window.

The Niche of the Round Window

Bela Bollobas, M.D.[95]

On the posterior surface of the promontory facing the sinus tympani is a well-defined cavity of variable size and shape (Fig. 221). This is the chamber of the *round window,* containing in its cranioventral part the bean-shaped round window, with its secondary tympanic membrane. It is found between the sustentaculum promontorii and the subiculum. Its opening into the tympanic cavity is oblique, in most cases, as it follows the posterolateral edge of the promontory. Keratinous adhesions may fill the niche and obscure the round window membrane. Folds of mucous membrane may obstruct the entrance of the niche, and may be misjudged as the secondary tympanic membrane. Rarely, the round window may be missing when the cartilage ring, preventing the osseous obliteration of the window, does not develop or is obliterated by an otosclerotic focus.

Inframicroscopic Anatomy

This study was made with the surgical microscope. A large number of temporal bones were examined. Observations were also recorded during surgery on the ear, especially when the round window niche could be seen from the aditus.

Certain structures, such as fustis, postes, and sinus concamerati, proved to have an ontogenic and phylogenetic

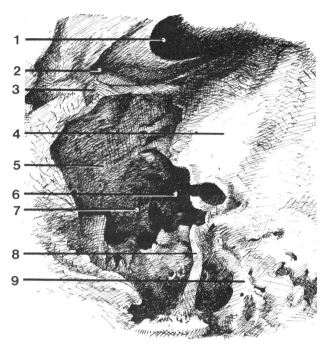

Figure 221. The round window niche area. 1, Oval window. 2, Posterior tympanic sinus (subfacial sinus). 3, Pyramidal eminence. 4, Promontory. 5, Sinus tympani. 6, Round window. 7, Area concamerata. 8, Trabecular sustentaculum of the promontory. 9, Hypotympanum. The area concamerata is found between the hypotympanum and sinus tympani dorsomedially to the sustentaculum of the promontory. It is an antechamber to the round window niche.

importance, and their appearance was indicative even of extratympanic anatomic situations. For example, deep concamerate sinuses are indicative of the topography of the jugular fossa. Incongruence in the area of the fustis suggests a developmental retardation of other tympanic cavity structures. Broad niche entrance is suspicious of a narrow hypotympanum and vice versa.

The following details can be distinguished in the round window niche.

Fundus

This is the upper process of the concamerate area of the hypotympanum. Posteriorly, it forms the floor of the sinus tympani. This is the cranial part of the jugular wall. The bone plate of the fundus varies in thickness. The bony wall of the jugular fossa bends laterally at the middle of the fundus, and leaves the tympanic cavity. Cranially, the fundus plate is always full; but caudally, it gradually thins out, and it is often dehiscent around the sustentaculum.

Craniocaudally, on the fundus, three areas can be distinguished:

1. The medial or superior part found near the upper wall (*postis posterior*). This is an uneven compact bone surface.

2. The lateral or inferior part found near the lower wall (*postis anterior*). For the most part, it is smooth, forming the thinnest area in the floor of the niche.

3. The pars media in between the above. Horizontal and perpendicular to the plane of the entrance, a solid bone column extends into the niche. It varies in shape, but is always present as a typical structure of the fundus. This bony column resembles a stick thickening towards the niche; therefore it is called the *fustis*. The fundus is composed of trabecular, lamellar, or cellular bone. The jugular fossa is more distant; therefore, the space between the floor of the tympanic sinus and jugular fossa is filled with bone.

The above-mentioned three areas of the fundus differ ontogenetically. The upper part is a process of the periosteal layer of the periotic capsule. This process grows on top of the bone plate of the fundus; therefore, it is more uneven and compact than the lower part of the fundus formed by the thin plate of the jugular fossa. The tympanic surface of the jugular fossa constitutes the floor of the tympanic cavity (jugular wall) formed in the second half of embryonic life as the *pavimentum pyramidis* to close the tympanic cavity.

The pavimentum pyramidis is an independent covering part of the tympanic cavity developing in the peritympanal embryonic-connective tissue. It contacts the otic capsule with a thin process. Below and ventrally, it forms the tympanic floor, the carotid canal, and the ventral segment of the canalis musculotubarius.

The relatively smooth, thin bone plate covering the jugular vein is separated from the upper part of the fundus of the round window niche where the jugular fossa bulges into the tympanic cavity. Its contact with the labyrinthine capsule is well visualized with the surgical microscope.

The fustis develops between the periosteal layer of the labyrinthine capsule and the thin, smooth plate of pavimentum pyramidis. Up to a certain maturational stage, the fustis protects and then narrows the entrance of the round window niche.

Tegmen of the Round Window Niche

This is formed by the oblique dorsolateral edge of the promontory, which forms a convex edge over the round window niche. The tegmen is narrowest on its free edge. It widens as it approaches the floor of the niche. The free edge of the tegmen can have various forms. It can be sharp, straight, spiny, undulated, or doubled. Occasionally, an isolated arciform trabecule connects it with the fundus.

The tegmen consists of the periosteal bone of the labyrinthine capsule. At the separation of the tympanic cavity, peritympanic embryonic-connective tissue cords bridge the space between the promontory and posterior tympanic wall. These are surrounded by the tubotympanic epithelium forming the tympanic cavity. Some of them degenerate, but others survive and give rise to precartilage and cartilage. The cartilage does not transform to bone until after the complete development of the inner ear.

The first ossification center appears in the 16th week around the cochlea. By the 22nd week, four ossification centers are seen. The full ossification of the labyrinthine capsule takes one week, with the exception of a ring around the oval and round windows, the fissure ante fenestram, and above the horizontal semicircular canal.

The periosteal layer of the labyrinthine capsule is initially very thin, but it slowly thickens until early adulthood. The tegmen of the round window niche is only the thinned periosteal process on the posterior tympanic wall of the labyrinthine capsule.

Anterior Postis of the Round Window Niche

The postis anterior is usually the thinner column of the fenestra entrance running parallel to the sustentaculum. It connects the basal helix of the cochlea with the jugular wall of the tympanic cavity. It is usually thinner, less developed, and more variable than the postis posterior. It is also derived from the periosteal layer of the labyrinthine capsule, and is thinner than the postis posterior due to the following reasons:

1. Its base will later participate in the broadening of the tympanic cavity, the elongation of which includes the base of the postis anterior.

2. The neighboring bone to which it joins by synostosis does not reach its full maturation with development of the labyrinthine capsule. The structure next to the postis anterior is the sustentaculum, connecting caudally the labyrinthine capsule and jugular wall.

3. Pneumatization goes on in its surroundings and makes the postis anterior thinner.

Posterior Postis of the Round Window Niche

This is the upper rear edge of the niche entrance forming an acute angle with the tegmen. Posteriorly and superiorly, it fuses with the subiculum. It is consistently thicker than the postis anterior. Its insertion toward the sinus tympani may vary. It can reach the fundus perpendicularly, and may bend outwards to the floor of the sinus tympani; but, in most cases, it turns inwards through the entrance of the fenestra.

Behind the round window, the postis posterior joins the middle avascular periosteal protective layer of the labyrinth to the jugular wall, which is capable of osteogenesis after trauma or infection.

The subiculum and postis posterior are made of thick periosteal bone to protect the origins of the scala tympani and vestibuli and the area of the round window. The postis posterior is always thicker than the postis anterior due to the following reasons:

1. Its base is stable and does not change during maturation.

2. The neighboring periosteal bone to which it adheres cranially is also stable. The subiculum, due to the constant size of the underlying cochlear helix, is altered during the second half of fetal life only by periosteal thickening without any change of its internal dimensions.

3. It is not—or is hardly—pneumatized. Even in the latter case, pneumatization is restricted to the base and its vicinity.

The walls forming the entrance of the niche may be of different lengths; however, in most cases, the tegmen and fundus are longer than the postis. This relation changes to its opposite under pathologic conditions, or when the whole tympanic cavity is compressed in the craniocaudal direction. Square or rhomboid entrances are not infrequent. According to the position, direction, shape, and size of the walls and the fustis, the entrance and constituent structures of the fenestra show a number of variations as follows.

Embryology

It is well established that during ossification of the otic capsule, a cartilage located in the round window niche prevents ossification of the opening. In the three-month-old embryo, the round window niche is completely filled with embryonic mesenchyme (Fig. 222). This cartilage ring is differentiated in the third month, transforming desmally to give rise to the secondary tympanic membrane.

The tympanic cavity is not yet formed. The round window niche is filled with embryonic mesenchyme. If, in the four-month-old embryo, the mesenchyme is removed at a stage when the stapes is still cartilaginous and the oval window is not yet formed, the large round window chamber can be seen craniolaterally on the inferoposterior part of the promontory (Figs. 223-225). The edges of the chamber are rounded off, having a sulcus only at the angle between the subiculum and promontory.

In this stage of maturation, the subiculum extends up to the tympanic frame because the tympanic sinus has not developed and the tympanic cavity has not yet opened. However, from the subiculum, a thick semicylinder bends into the round window chamber, which ensures the bean shape of the later secondary tympanic membrane. On the lower part of the fundus of the round window niche, a layer of bone and a smaller excavation develops below and above the recurrent bone cylinder, respectively. They are

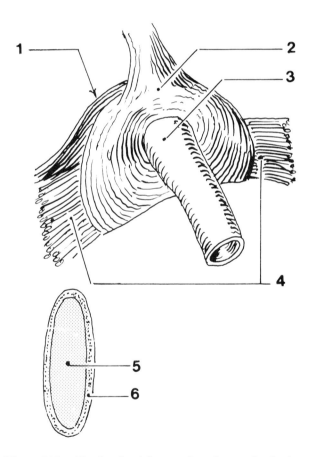

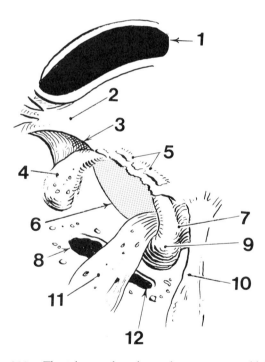

Figure 222. The right round window niche in a one-year old child. As a result of further covering bone formation the tegmen of the round window niche becomes stratified. 1, Oval window. 2, Subiculum promontorii. 3, Joining part of subiculum promonorii with the postis posterior. 4, Postis posterior. 5, Layer of covering bone on top of the niche. 6, Secondary tympanic membrane. 7, Tunnel of promontory. 8, Sinus concameratus medialis. 9, Postis anterior. 10, Sustentaculum promontorii. 11, Fustis. 12, Sinus concameratus lateralis.

Figure 223. The fossula of the round window in the third embryonic month (from the external auditory meatus). In the third embryonic month, the fossula of the round window is completely filled with embryonic mesenchyme. Between the desmalcartilaginous stapes arches the stapedial artery, which disappears after this period. 1, Desmally preformed stapedius muscle. 2, Stapes. 3, Stapedial artery. 4, Facial nerve appearing in the tympanic cavity of a two-month-old fetus and running uncovered without a canal. 5, Fossula of the round window from the direction of the sound conductor. 6, Cartilage ring preventing ossification of the round window.

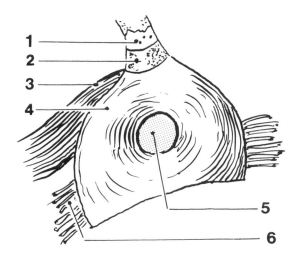

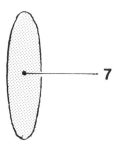

Figure 224. The fossula of the round window in a four- month-old fetus seen from the acoustic meatus. In the fourth month of in-trauterine life, the chamber of the round window is unaltered. The stapedial artery has disappeared and the fibers of the stapedius muscle are separated from the facial nerve. 1, Long process of the incus. 2, Head of the stapes. 3, Developing stapedius muscle and tendon. 4, Posterior crus of the stapes during desmalcartilaginous transformation. 5, Intercrural space after regression of the stapedial artery. 6, Fibers of the facial nerve. 7, Fossula of the round window from the direction of the sound conductor.

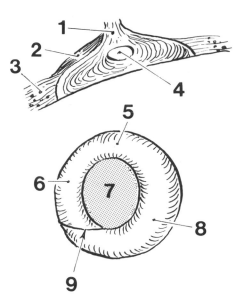

Figure 225. The right round window fossula in a four- month-old fetus seen from the posterior wall of the tympanic cavity. In the otic capsule, ossification has started and surrounds the round window chamber with a thickened ring. Caudally, the arms of the ring cross over each other. 1, Stapes. 2, Tendon of the stapedius muscle. 3, Facial nerve. 4, Intercrural space. 5, Anlage of the tegmen of the round window niche. 6, Anlage of the postis posterior. 7, Fossula (niche) of the round window. 8, Anlage of the postis anterior. 9, Crossing over of the arms of the ring.

caudally bordered by the embryonic mesenchyme and tubotympanic epithelium. The ventrocaudal wall of the chamber is constituted by well-developed mucous membrane folds. The secondary tympanic membrane closing the scala tympani develops by the gradual dedifferentiation from the cranial aspect of the cartilage ring.

Between the semicylinder bending into the chamber and the secondary tympanic membrane, the cartilage persists on a fan-like area, which instead of dedifferentiating ossifies to form the inferior wall of the round window. Ossification starting in the cartilage establishes a connection with the semicylinder constituting the floor the the chamber (Fig. 226).

In the five-month-old fetus, ossification between the semicylinder and secondary tympanic membrane is complete; then a gradual regression of the semicylinder takes place. Its medial part will be the process of the postis posterior in the chamber that is fixed to the osseous capsule of

the scala tympani under the secondary tympanic membrane. Its lateral part gives rise in one or two months to the fustis (Fig. 227).

In the seventh fetal month, the periosteal layer of the promontory grows further, the tegmen of the chamber elongates dorsally, the process of the sinus tympani digs a large pneumatic cavity behind the postis posterior, and the part of the postis bending into the chamber gradually regresses near the window frame. The postis anterior forms either a thin plate or a sharp protrusion at the lateral edge of the chamber. The fustis developing and penetrating into the chamber occupies mostly the ventrolateral edge of the round window chamber, so that the secondary tympanic membrance becomes more craniodorsal in its position (Figs. 228, 229). Somewhat later on the lateral part of the chamber, a tunnel appears in the covering osseous substance.

In the eight-month-old fetus, the edges of the chamber entrance get thicker, and small cells develop on the fundus. The postis anterior fuses partially or totally with the sustentaculum formed around the inferior tympanic artery, and the tunnel becomes deeper under the basal helix and toward the tubal funnel (Figs. 229, 230).

In the last fetal month, the periosteal layer of the promontory thickens further, its edge above the round window chamber becomes either elongated or rounded off. The secondary tympanic membrane changes its position from

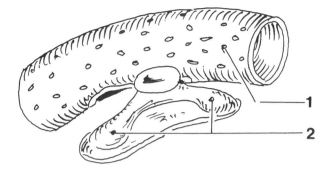

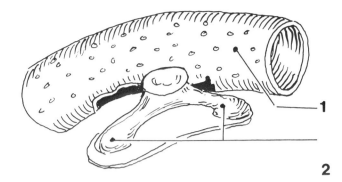

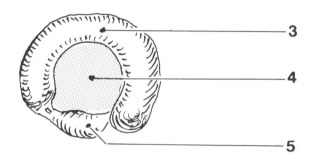

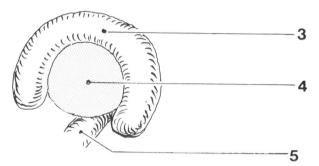

Figure 226. The right fossula of the round window in a 4.5-month-old fetus. The two caudal ends of the ring regress, but a part of the postis posterior remains in the chamber. This gives rise to the fustis. 1, The osseous facial canal. 2, Cylindrical arms of the osseous stapes. 3, Anlage of the tegmen of the round window niche. 4, The front of the round window niche viewed from the posterior tympanic wall. 5, Part of the postis posterior remaining in the chamber.

Figure 227. Fossula of the round window in a five-month- old fetus. Part of the postis posterior remaining in the round window chamber becomes isolated from its surroundings and starts to grow dorsolaterally. 1, Facial canal. 2, Arms of the stapes. 3, Tegmen of the round window niche. 4, Round window membrane. 5, The growing fustis isolated on the floor of the round window chamber.

nearly horizontal to almost vertical as its ventrocaudal edge is transposed towards the posterior wall of the tympanic cavity. On the fundus, the formation of pneumatic cellules is invariably seen. Below and above the fustis, deep sinus concamerati develop (Fig. 230).

In the newborn, the round window chamber is nearly vertical—only its lower part declines ventrally. It resembles a lyre in shape with its rounded angles. The tegmen does not extend too deeply over the chamber entrance. It has an uneven edge, with a protrusion at its dorsal third that turns inside the chamber towards the tube and is inserted on the labyrinth block. The lateral angle of the chamber, formed by thin plates, is always open. These plates extend toward the tympanic frame, forming a continuous osseous plate with excavations, small protrusions, and trabecules.

The medial part of the fundus has a variable appearance. The postis posterior may fuse with the fustis. In other cases, the fustis and postis posterior may be connected with a trabecule in the plane of the chamber entrance. More ventrally in the chamber and dorsally in the arched area, structures are separated by cellules of various size.

The lateral part of the fundus is wide, trabecular, or cellular, with a number of dehiscences. Dehiscences seen in the adult indicate an incomplete neonatal development of the hypotympanum. The network of trabecules extend dorsally to contact the styloid complex. Networks around the time of birth contain cellules in the jugular wall that occasionally open caudally into the jugular fossa.

In intrauterine life, the relative size of the round window niche is larger than in the adult. In the last intrauterine months, the chamber forms together with the hypotympanum a joint cavity reaching to the tubal funnel. Its ventral border is determined by the inferior tympanic artery, which initially has a bony cover ventrally and partly toward the promontory and the tympanic ring, while dorsally it is completely open. The artery enters the tympanic cavity at its floor through a sharply edged irregular or roundish opening. Until the lateral part of the tympanic cavity develops, the area of the hypotympanum—through which the inferior tympanic artery enters the tympanic cavity—is steep ventrocranially in the direction of the tympanic ring. Above the entry, a perforated cavity is found sending a pro-

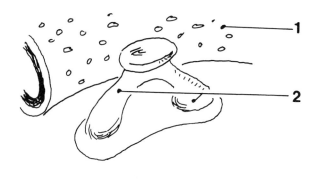

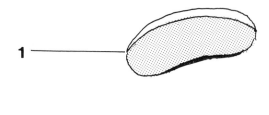

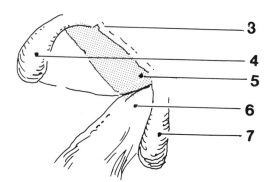

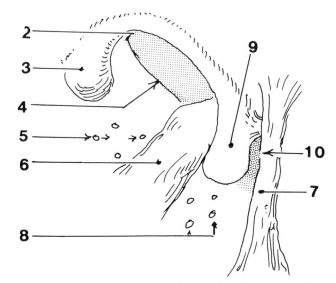

Figure 228. Niche of the round window in a seven-month-old fetus. The fustis is markedly elongated, and the round window chamber resembles its mature appearance. 1, Facial canal. 2, Crura stapedis. 3, Tegmen of the round window niche. 4, Postis posterior. 5, Secondary tympanic membrane. 6, Fustis. 7, Postis anterior.

Figure 229. The right niche of the round window in an eight-month-old fetus. Pneumatic cellules are formed on the fundus of the round window chamber. 1, Oval window. 2, Tegmen of the round window niche. 3, Postis posterior. 4, Secondary tympanic membrane. 5, Pneumatic cellules medial to the fustis. 6, Fustis. 7, Sustentaculum promontorii. 8, Pneumatic cellules lateral to the fustis. 9, Postis anterior. 10, Tunnel of promontory.

cess above the tube. This process is the anlage of the medial infundibular sinus that is present in the adult. Above, the sinus develops an open ring corresponding to the later channel of the sustentaculum. The open ring is closed about the end of intrauterine life. On the promontory, a slightly ventrally directed sulcus is formed for the vessel; dorsally, the bone plate completing the channel extends with a spinous edge into the area concamerata. Around the vessel, the channel gradually grows longer; after birth, a vascular channel is found at the dorsolateral edge of the hypotympanum (sustentaculum). However, the chamber entrance is open in this direction.

In infants, the tegmen of the round window shows stratification. Duplicatures occur between the protrusions of the postis anterior mucosa. In the covering osseous substance of the postis posterior, the bottom of the cellules is deepened by secondary cellules. The sinus concamerati also becomes deeper due to the cranial elongation of the osseous substance forming their walls. The fustis is usually a wider semicylinder than in the adult, and is fixed by low bone plates to both postes. The brachium pyramidale can be well developed, so that the underlying medial sinus concameratus may reach a size equal to that of the sinus tympani.

Variation in the infant is as frequent as in the adult. Longitudinally or transversely elongated chamber entrances are readily observed. The fundus of the infant chamber is not always dehiscent. Fine cellular trabecules may occur in the pars interior, and are separated from the jugular fossa by a thin bone plate. Occasionally, the dehiscences of the hypotympanum are situated near the tympanic ring, and not in the vicinity of the chamber or on the fundus of the chamber. However, these are rather infrequent situations. Connections between the tympanic cavity and jugular fossa are mostly found in the medial part of the fundus—less frequently laterally from this site and sporadically near the tympanic ring.

In the infant, when the inferior tympanic artery is covered with bone and the thick sustentaculum develops around it, the lateral part of the chamber floor continues between the labyrinthine capsule and sustentaculum

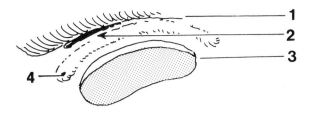

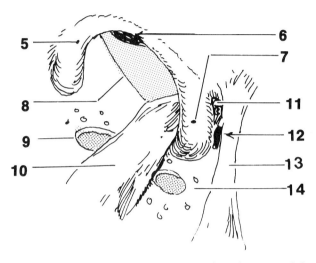

Figure 230. The right fossula of the round window around the time of birth. On the floor of the round window chamber, two large cavities appear—the sinus concamerata medialis and lateralis. 1, Facial canal. 2, Subfacial sinus. 3, Oval window. 4, Subfacial disc. 5, Postis posterior. 6, Tegmen of the round window niche. 7, Postis anterior. 8, Secondary tympanic membrane. 9, Sinus concameratus. 10, Fustis. 11, Lamina sustentaculopostica. 12, Tunnel of the promontory. 13, Sustentaculum. 14, Sinus concameratus lateralis.

towards the tube in the immature tunnel. The lateral part of the chamber floor and the fundus of the tunnel show an identical structure. It is usually composed of a fine meshwork of bone trabecules, with cellules and shallow excavations between them.

During childhood and adolescence, the tunnel becomes deeper between the fustis and sustentaculum, cellules of the lateral part of the chamber floor grow larger, and trabecules occupy a vertical postion due to cranial growth—narrowing the lateral part of the chamber. In adulthood, trabecules become thicker and fuse with each other. The cellules are filled with bone tissue, and the lateral part of the fundus is narrower forming a single bone surface.

It must be noted that in the jugular fossa, round, elliptical or irregular holes correspond to the dehiscences of the hypotympanum. During the last intrauterine month, flattened thin lamellas with tiny cellules developing between them are found on the wall of the jugular fossa. In extrauterine life, these lamellas coalesce and form an initally folded and later smoothed osseous surface. Cellules grad-

ually narrow and disappear; however, dehiscences persist for the penetrating vessels.

Inframicroscopic Variants

According to Postion

According to position, the variants of the round window niche can be classified into three groups as described in the following paragraphs.

Horizontal Aperature of the Round Window Niche (68%). In this position, the lateral entrance to the niche is nearly in a horizontal position (Fig. 231). This is usually coupled with a wide entrance; the promontory is laterally acute, the postis posterior is poorly developed, and the edge of the tegmen is sharp, spinous, and has a ventral slope so that the postis anterior is considerably lower than the postis posterior. The fustis is on the fundus of the chamber, and is well demarcated from its surrounding. It is always located closer to the postis posterior. It often bifurcates towards the posterior wall of the tympanic cavity. The absence of a postis anterior is a rather frequent variant. In these cases, the edge of the fenestra entrance is constitued by the sustentaculum promontorii.

Behind the sustentaculum promontorii, towards the infundibulum, a well-developed promontory tunnel is consistently found. The tunnel narrows ventrally. If the postis anterior is missing, a trabecule, spine, or lamella is present in place of the missing postis. In this variant, the subiculum is usually narrow, the sinus tympani is well developed, the area concamerata is broad, and the regions of the posterior

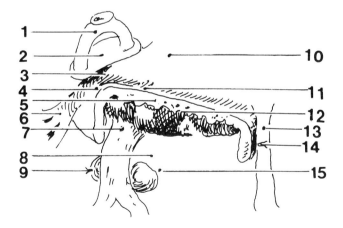

Figure 231. Fossula fenestrae rotundae horizontalis (horizontal round window niche). 1, Stapes. 2, Stapes foot plate. 3, Subiculum promontorii. 4, Covering bone connecting the subiculum to the postis posterior. 5, Dentated plate of the tegmen of the round window niche. 6, Arms of the subiculum promontorii. 7, Insertion of the fustis on the window frame. 8, Pneumatic cellules on the chamber floor. 9, Sinus concameratus medialis. 10, Promontory. 11, Backward slope of the promontory. 12, Secondary tympanic membrane. 13, Sustentaculum promontorii. 14, Tunnel of the promontory. 15, Sinus concameratus lateralis.

part of the tympanic cavity are (except for the styloid prominence) poor in structure.

The horizontal development of the round window niche is determined by the development of surrounding structures:

1. The subiculum is lengthy; therefore it is far from the apex of the promontory and extends towards the posterior tympanic wall.
2. The basal helix of the cochlea also has a horizontal course, which widens the tympanic cavity horizontally.
3. When the tympanic cavity gets its lumen, only a small amount of peritympanic embryonic tissue remains at the posteroinferior part of the promontory. This does not substantially thicken the promontory caudally.
4. The subepithelial-connective tissue participating in the pneumatization and the tubotympanic epithelium surrounding the structures of the tympanic cavity may destroy more of the posteroinferior than other promontory surfaces.
5. The inferior tympanic artery enters the tympanic cavity more ventrally than usual, and reaches the promontory close to the tubal funnel—as a result, the sustentaculum develops ventrally.

In the development of oblique round window chambers, the same developmental factors occur as in the case of horizontal or vertical chambers, but their proportion is different.

Dorsal Aperture of the Round Window Niche (23%).   Similar to the horizontal entrances, the dorsal entrances can be of two types (Figs. 232, 233). One has a straight tegmen, while in the other, the lower and upper parts of the tegmen meet in an obtuse angle. The tegmen is straight when the upper posterior angle of the promontory is almost a right angle, and when the promontory has a straight edge to the sustentaculum either because of a retropositioned sustentaculum or a postis anterior localized near the posterior tympanic wall. When the postis anterior is missing and the sustentaculum develops in front near the tubal funnel, the edge of the tegmen is broken in an angle. This angle is the promontorial remnant of the missing postis anterior, opposite of which a protrusion is always seen in the area concamerata. This is the lower remnant of the postis anterior. Together, with an angular tegmen, we find the fustis always running under the upper part of the tegmen. In these cases, it might be developed to such an extent that it fills the entire upper part of the entrance. An oblique tegmen narrows the tympanic sinus, which is occasionally abridged in front of the brachium pyramidale by a trabecule or spine. The hypotympanum is the broadest between the niche entrance and the outer aperture of the chorda channel.

Vertical Aperture of the Round Window Niche (9%).   In this case, the lateral entrance is in the sagittal or nearly sagittal plane. The promontory is rectangular, the tegmen is thick with a rounded edge, the postis posterior is fused with the brachium pyramidale of the subiculum, and the postis an-

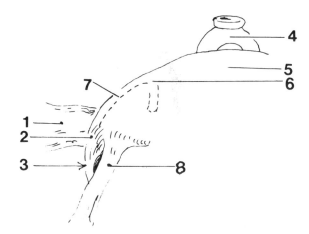

Figure 232.   Fossula fenestrae rotundae posterior dorsalis. From the direction of the sound conductor, there is no insight into the round window chamber as it opens towards the posterior tympanic wall. The tegmen is cranially convex. 1, Fustis. 2, Postis anterior. 3, Tunnel of the promontory. 4, Stapes in situ. 5, Promontory. 6, Postis posterior. 7, Tegmen of the round window niche. 8, Sustentaculum promontorii.

terior is (as usual) thinner, lamellated, and spinous. The entrance is wide; hence, the sinus tympani is less developed. The area concamerata is trabecular, uneven, or cellular. The hypotympanum is deep, and the promontorial area is wider than the area concamerata—the latter being narrowed by the styloid prominence (Fig. 234).

A vertical round window niche develops when:

1. The basal helix of the cochlea runs caudally and widens the promontory in this direction.
2. At the formation of the tympanic lumen, a substantial amount of peritympanic-connective tissue is left back on the pars sacculocochlearis of the inner ear.

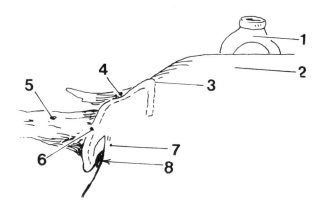

Figure 233.   Fossula fenestrae rotundae dorsalis. The tegmen is broken in an angle. 1, Stapes in situ. 2, Promontory. 3, Angle between the tegmen and postis posterior. 4, Dentated plate extending backwards from the tegmen. 5, Fustis. 6, The laterally declining part of the tegmen broken in an angle. 7, Sustentaculum promontorii. 8, Tunnel of promontory.

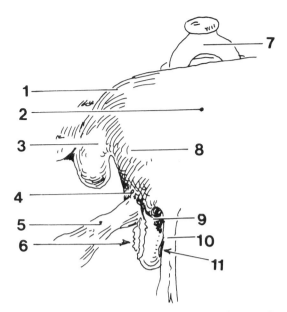

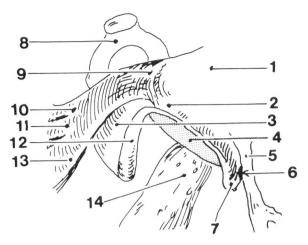

Figure 234. Fossula fenestrae rotundae verticalis. 1, Subiculum promontorii. 2, Promontory. 3, Postis posterior. 4, Secondary tympanic membrane. 5, Fustis. 6, Dentated plates on the postis anterior. 7, Stapes in situ. 8, Tegmen of the round window niche. 9, Postis anterior. 10, Sustentaculum promontorii. 11, Tunnel of the promontory.

Figure 235. Fossula fenestrae rotundae lata (wide). 1, Promontory. 2, Tegmen of the round window niche. 3, Covering bone between the postis posterior and subiculum. 4, Secondary tympanic membrane. 5, Sustentaculum promontorii. 6, Tunnel of the promontory. 7, Postis anterior. 8, Stapes in situ. 9, Subiculum promontorii. 10, Facial arm of the subiculum promontorii. 11, Pyramidal arm of the subiculum promontorii. 12, Postis posterior. 13, Styloid arm of the subiculum promontorii. 14, Fustis.

3. The tubotympanic epithelium leaves intact large areas on the promontory.
4. The tympanic branch of the ascending pharyngeal artery—the *inferior tympanic artery*—reaches the promontory near the posterior tympanic wall; as a result, the sustentaculum develops in a more posterior position. The subiculum is short and does not extend back towards the posterior tympanic wall.

According to Size

According to the size of its aperture, the round window niche has variants, as described in the following paragraphs.

Fossula Fenestrae Rotunda Lata (Wide) (22%). This is encountered in deep, wide tympanic cavities. Its position is never sagittal; it is oblique or nearly horizontal. The tegmen is not thick. The postis posterior is high, running perpendicularly from the promontory down to the floor of the niche, and is well separated from the brachium pyramidale of the subiculum. The postis anterior is often missing, or is just indicated by two spines of its insertion points. The sustentaculum, as a rule, is lower than the postis posterior. The fustis located at the upper part of the round window entrance is usually wide and thick, and can readily be distinguished from its surroundings. All three areas of the hypotympanum are wide; the sinus tympani is cranially narrower, and caudally wider. The promontorial tunnel is a broad, short, ventrally narrowing cavity (Fig. 235).

Occasionally, the lower, more horizontal part of the aperture extends towards the infundibular area, thus being an extremely large size. In contrast to the tegmen of the lower part, the promontorial area of the hypotympanum contains a cranially convex trabecule running parallel to the tegmen. The trabecule is well separated from the jugular wall. Between its lower ventral insertion and the tegmen, long spines extend from the sustentaculum into the aperture.

The extremely large apertures of the round window niche are accompanied by a number of developmental variations. The sustentaculum is low, shortened, and displaced ventrally. The postis anterior is missing—both of its insertions are marked with spines. The promontory tunnel is wide, usually extending deep and laterally, and can be readily seen. The cavity of the tunnel is divided by spines and septa between which deep excavations extend towards the jugular fossa. In a poorly structured tympanic cavity, the large tunnel forms a common, undivided cavity due to the scarcity of structures. Here also the fustis lies near the postis posterior and occasionally under the promontory. More often, it branches towards the sinus tympani. The fustis is generally broader in all directions than usual.

The long tegmen is undulated or dentated. A single protrusion is often found around the middle of the roof of the aperture. The postis posterior is well separated from the subiculum, and a wide fundus is observed between the fustis and postis posterior. In some cases, the fustis bifurcates towards the sinus tympani. The upper branch fuses with the postis posterior. This bifurcated fustis usually does not extend perpendicularly into the window frame, but its promontorial end deviates caudally. Thus, it is in a horizontal position even if the window frame is oblique. In such cases, the jugular wall is formed by a poorly structured smooth bone surface that follows the convexity of the jugular fossa. The fustis is located at the corner where the jugular wall meets the scala tympani of the cochlea.

An extremely large aperture of the round window niche is accompanied by developmental anomalies:

1.   The archiform horizontal trabecule of the hypotympanum develops as a result of special maturational conditions. The broad postis anterior and the backward-extended protrusion of the tegmen are, respectively, the cranial and caudal remnants of trabecules.

2.   A wide and large tunnel develops because the osseous cover of the cochlea extends far down. A large cavity is formed between the cover and the capsule of the scala tympani by the penetrating subepithelial-connective tissue.

3.   Usually, between the fustis and postis posterior, a wider fundus region is found than under normal circumstances, as there is ample room for the fustis to diverge caudally from the postis posterior.

The divergence of the two structures also occurs when the fustis bifurcates towards the posterior tympanic wall and its upper process is fused with the postis posterior. In these cases, the larger area available is not occupied by a divergence of the fustis from the postis posterior, but the closely adhering part remains in contact with the postis while the lower branch of the fork bends caudally.

The horizontal development of the fustis is generally determined by the postion of the encounter of the jugular wall and labyrinthine block.

Fossula Fenestrae Rotunda Alta (10%).   Between the jugular wall and the posterior promontorial edge, the aperture of the round window niche is located in such a fashion that the nearly rectangular aperture is formed at its longer sides by the two postes—whereas at the shorter sides, it is formed by the fundus and tegmen of the round window niche. The compressed, high cleft-like chamber entrance produces peculiar situations. The postis posterior cannot be distinguished from the styloid brachium of the subiculum. Both structures are smooth surfaced and well developed, forming tall columns. Ventrally, under the window frame proper, the remnants of the fustis can be seen. A typical fustis does not develop on the fundus. It is only indicated in the cranial part of the chamber by a smooth-surfaced process emerging from the postis posterior. The tegmen is wide, and convex, but rather short and poor in structures. In its continuation, the short, bulky medial ponticulus is found. Under the ponticulus, the short distance between the rear edge of the subiculum and the osseous capsule of the pyramidal eminence is often bridged by one or more isolated bone trabecules (Fig. 236).

The postis anterior is the continuation of the tegmen towards the jugular wall. Its course is parallel to that of the postis posterior. It resembles the tegmen in structure; that is, it is smooth surfaced and convex. Its posterior inferior part forms a downward-directed protrusion. The distance between the postis anterior and the sustentaculum is con-

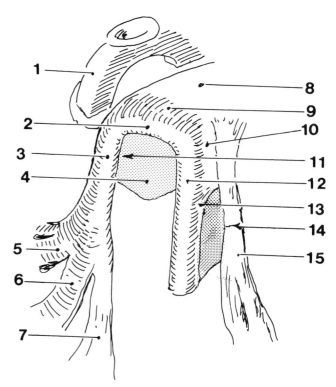

Figure 236.   Fossula fenestrae rotundae alta (high). 1, Stapes. 2, Tegmen of the round window niche. 3, Postis posterior fused with the subiculum promontorii. 4, Secondary tympanic membrane. 5, Arms of the subiculum promontorii. 6, Styloid arms of the subiculum promontorii. 7, Fustis fused with the postis posterior. 8, Promontory. 9, Surface of the promontory curving posteriorly and laterally. 10, Lamina sustentaculopostica. 11, Intrachamber surface of the postis posterior. 12, Postis anterior. 13, Bone plate between the tunnel and postis anterior. 14, Tunnel of the promontory. 15, Sustentaculum promontorii.

siderable. Between them, a parallel excavation occurs. The fundus is a smooth, poorly structured portion of the jugular wall penetrating into the round window chamber. It is fixed on the postis posterior, and forms an acute angle with the fustis. On the fundus, towards the postis anterior, the above-mentioned protrusion is found.

A high, cleft-like chamber entrance is also encountered when the postis anterior fuses with the well-developed, horizontally located fustis. In these cases, a well-developed tunnel leads between the postis anterior and sustentaculum towards the tubal funnel. The entrance of the tunnel is found between the high bone trabecule connecting the fustis with the styloid prominence, the postis posterior, and the sustentaculum. This is a hypotympanum area of uneven walls. The entrance proper is a deep cavity, with the spinous plate elevating craniodorsally from the promontorial area of the hypotympanum. The dorsal process of the tunnel is almost as large as the sinus tympani. From its posterior wall, curved trabecules and irregular plates stand out.

This variant belongs to those rare chamber entrance

situations in which the fustis is near to the postis anterior, and not the postis posterior. Embryologically, it is explained by the development of the jugular fossa caudally to the tympanic cavity. In this way, a deep tunnel is formed in front of the fustis, along with an equally deep and voluminous tunnel entrance. An unusually high, well-developed fustis is necessary for development of this variant. The periosteal layer of the promontory grows toward the fustis when forming the chamber.

Coupled to the high, narrow round window chamber are found:

1. A very deep hypotympanum.
2. A deep tympanic sinus.
3. A styloid prominence bulging into the area concamerate.
4. A tall, well-developed pyramidal eminence.

Fossula fenestrae rotundae alta develops when the jugular fossa is located medial to the otic capsule; that is, far from the promontory. In these instances, the chamber fills the space between the covering bone of the otic capsule and the jugular fossa. This region is elongated craniocaudally, causing a similar elongation of the chamber as well. The resulting narrow cleft allows no room for the formation of an isolated fustis on the chamber floor; therefore, in these situations, the fustis is connected to or fused with the postis posterior.

Horizontal elongation brings about a separation on the postis anterior and a spine formation towards the fundus. Because of the high chamber entrance, the distance between the postis anterior and sustentaculum is longer. The medial dislocation of the jugular wall causes the unusual depth of all three hypotympanic areas. An additonal consequence is that in this variant, a deep, steep-walled tube funnel and an infundibular sinus extending deeply beneath the inferior infundibular septum are found.

Transitional Forms

Between the large and wide chambers and the narrow and high chambers are found a number of transitional forms. These are classified according to their shape as described in the following paragraphs.

Fossula Fenestrae Rotundae Lateritia (15.2%). The rectangular chamber entrance is nearly vertical, medium sized, and usually smaller than the oval window niche (Fig. 237). The chamber entrance is thus a rectangle directed dorsally towards the sinus tympani, and standing parallel to the posterior wall of the tympanic cavity. The postis posterior is missing, and is replaced by the lower lateral wall of the subiculum. The postis anterior is an isolated perpendicular trabecule between the floor of the tympanic cavity and the promontory. Its lower insertion is widened and continues behind the tunnel in a bulky column composing its dorsal wall. The tegmen has an undulating course that is moderately developed. The fundus is typical. At its midportion, a broad fustis is present, with wide excavations on its sides. The fustis flattens under the promontory, but dorsal-

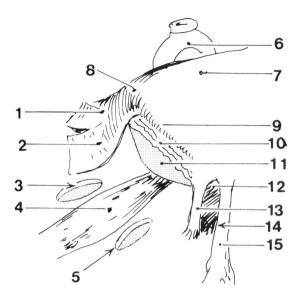

Figure 237. Fossula fenestrae rotundae lateritia. 1, Facial arm of the subiculum promontorii. 2, Pyramidal arm of the subiculum promontorii. 3, Sinus concameratus medialis. 4, Fustis. 5, Sinus concameratus lateralis. 6, Stapes in situ. 7, Promontory. 8, Subiculum promontorii. 9, Backward slope of the promontory. 10, Stratified, lamellar tegmen of the round window niche. 11, Secondary tympanic membrane. 12, Lamina sustentaculopostica. 13, Postis anterior. 14, Tunnel of the promontory. 15, Sustenaculum promontorii.

ly towards the styloid prominence, it gradually becomes more marked. Its angles are nearly right angles.

Accompanying this variant, the promontory is smooth surfaced; the nearly square subiculum is high and bound by trabecules to the body of the pyramidal eminence. The brachium pyramidale is well developed, and the retrofenestral sinus above it has uneven walls. The sinus tympani is divided by the fustis into an upper, smaller part and a lower, larger part; the latter extends to below the styloid prominence. The sustentaculum is low, wide, and canalized, and forms with the postis anterior a medially open acute angle. The jugular fossa is far below the tympanic cavity. Thus, the jugular wall of the tympanic cavity is thick, and the area concamerate is narrow. Under the trabeculolamellar structure of the promontorial and infundibular areas, well-developed cellules can be seen. The infundibular sinus is medially located and wide, and reaches far to the area between the labyrinth capsule and the carotid canal. The carotid canal deviates laterally. Its wall is thin. The infundibular septum is found on the territory of the infundibulum of the tube and uneven-surfaced transverse bone plate.

The development of this variant can be explained by the developmental parameters of its surroundings. The labyrinth capsule is covered by a thick periosteal bone layer extending dorsally far over the chamber entrance. The pavimentum pyramidis inserted to the labyrinth block under the subiculum runs steeply towards the jugular fossa. Between the pavimentum and the promontory, the area is bridged by an isolated trabecule—the *postis anterior*. Its isolation is due to the fact that the thick jugular wall is composed not of solid bone, but partly of well-developed cellules, and partly of plates and trabecules narrowing towards the promontory. Similarly isolated bone trabecules develop in front of the narrow tympanic sinus, and between the pyramidal eminence and upper posterior tip of the promontory. These delicate structures were mostly observed in female labyrinths.

Fossula Fenestrae Rotundae Quadrata (10.2%)   These are medium sized or small chambers. Their shape is square as the two postes, and the tegmen and fundus are parallel and of equal length (Fig. 238). The postis posterior is usually fused with the subiculum, and has a straight course with a smooth surface convex towards the chamber. The postis anterior is thinner, and almost consistently forms a protrusion towards the fundus. This protrusion is formed by the interruption of the postis short of its lower insertion. An incisure develops that continues at the insertion in a prominent spine. The edge of the tegmen meets the postes at right angles. The surface of the promontory is convex dorsally; that is, towards the tegmen. Between the upper edge of the chamber and the most curved surface of the promontory, a nearly sagittal, convex bone surface is observed. The fustis contributes substantially to the formation of the fundus. This fustis, in all instances of this variant, has a wide and smooth surface, almost entirely filling the fundus and bifurcating inside the chamber. It may fill only the upper posterior part of the fundus, and closes various angles with the postis posterior. Occasionally, the lower

front region of the fustis is made up of a bone surface lower and flatter than the fustis.

In the tympanic cavity, the following anatomic situations can be observed. The oval window is usually larger than the round window chamber. The surface of the promontory is convex. The sustentaculum is thick and canalized. Between the postis anterior and sustentaculum, a full or partial plate is present. In these cases, the tunnel begins between the postis anterior and sustentaculum, goes under the above plate, and penetrates deep under the basal helix of the cochlea below the tube funnel. Its lateral wall is wide open. In front of it, the promontory area is filled by plates, trabecules, and cellules of different sizes. The area concamerata is usually cellular as well, because there is a considerable distance between the chamber floor and the jugular fossa filled by spinous plates, slender trabecules, and well-developed cellules. The tympanic sinus is small, because the subiculum reaches far posteriorly. The pyramidal eminence is connected to the promontory by a full or partial plate called the *ponticulus medialis lamellosus*. Above it, a retrofenestral sinus is found extending behind the pyramidal eminence. The tympanic cavity can thus be considered enriched in structures.

A square chamber entrance develops when the tympanic cavity has an excess amount of covering bone and the perosteal layer covering the labyrinthine capsule is also thicker than usual. These factors result in the demarcation of the postis posterior, the isolated development of the postis anterior and sustentaculum, the deep impression of the tegmen into the entrance, and the well-developed fustis and tegmental part of pavimentum pyramidis. Angles between the postes, tegmen, and fundus are right angles that—in addition to the well-demarcated, slender, densely packed structures of the tympanic cavity—are a sign of enhanced subepithelial-connective tissue activity. This is also indicated by the separation of structures and the size of various recesses and sinuses.

Fossula Fenestrae Rotundae Ovalis (8.2%).   The postis posterior is well developed and smooth surfaced. The postis anterior is missing (Fig. 239). Its cranial remnant is indicated by a spinous bone plate within the area concamerata. The plate is fixed towards the chamber entrance on the fustis. Towards the hypotympanum, the plate is fixed to a bulky archiform bone eminence running from the styloid prominence to the tunnel. The tunnel is so wide that, on its central eminence, a row of thin plates is located. The tegmen of the chamber entrance is sharp edged and extends ventrally. The postis posterior bends over to the tegmen. On the tegmen, the remnant of the postis anterior is marked by a spine that continues medially into the sustentaculum. The fustis is situated close to the postis posterior, and has no continuation towards the tympanic sinus, but divides inside the chamber into cranial and caudal branches inserted to the scala tympani of the cochlear basal helix (Fig. 239).

The wide oval round window chamber occurs in pyramid bones, where the fossula of the oval window is small and almost rectangular, the promontory has an uneven sur-

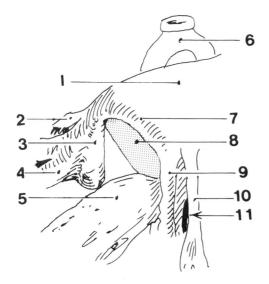

Figure 238.   Fossula fenestrae rotundae quadrata. The round window chamber is square. 1, Promontory. 2, Facial arm of the subiculum promontorii. 3, Postis posterior. 4, Styloid arm of the subiculum promontorii. 5, Fustis. 6, Stapes in situ. 7, Tegmen of the round window niche. 8, Secondary tympanic membrane. 9, Postis anterior. 10, Sustentaculum promontorii. 11, Tunnel of the promontory.

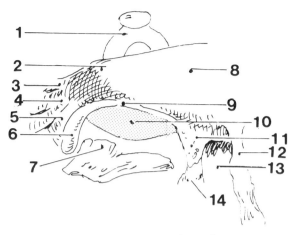

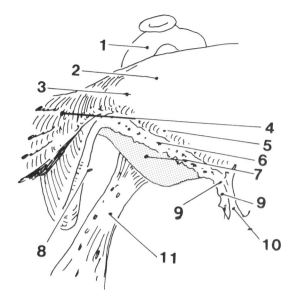

Figure 239. Fossula fenestrae rotundae ovalis. 1, Stapes in situ. 2, Subiculum promontorii. 3 and 4, Arms of subiculum promontorii. 5, Covering bone plate connecting the subiculum to the postis posterior. 6, Postis posterior. 7, Bifurcating fustis. 8, Promontory. 9, Tegmen of the round window niche. 10, Secondary tympanic membrane. 11, Postis anterior. 12, Sustentaculum promontorii. 13, Lamina sustentaculopostica. 14, Protrusions underneath the postis anterior.

Figure 240. Fossula fenestrae rotundae trapezoides. 1, Stapes. 2, Promontory. 3, Subiculum promontorii. 4, Arms of the subiculum. 5, Backward slope of the promontory. 6, Tegmen of the round window niche. 7, Secondary tympanic membrane. 8, Postis posterior. 9, Protrusions of the sustentaculum promontorii penetrating into the chamber. 10, Short sustentaculum promontorii. 11, Fustis.

face, and the hypotympanum is deep, lamellar, and cellular. The sinus tympani is of similar character; the styloid prominence is thick and spinous-lamellar, and the retrofenestal sinus is open laterally and fuses with the sinus tympani. The pyramidal eminence is fixed to the facial canal, but has a thick wall. Behind it, a deep (rather than wide) retropyramidal sinus is found.

Accordingly, wide and oval round window chambers develop when the periosteal part of the labyrinth capsule is thick, and the hypotympanum is deep. The sinus tympani is similarly wide due to insertion of the pyramidal eminence to the wall of the facial canal. In addition to the thick periosteal layer of the promontory, the whole tympanic cavity has a well-developed osseous cover in which the subepithelial-connective tissue and the tubotympanic epithelium cause deep excavations with wide lamellae and deep cellules. This subepithelial mesenchymal activity seen in the hypotympanum and sinus tympani widens the entrance of the window chamber by separating the postis anterior from the periosteal layer of the promontory.

Fossula Fenestrae Rotundae Trapezoides (8%). The round window chamber is mostly horizontal and larger than usual (Fig. 240). The postis posterior is fused with the subiculum, but fusion sutures cannot be seen. Its lower insertion is on the fustis, while toward the tegmen, it continues in a sharp angle. At the lower insertion, either a bone protrusion, tuberosity, or a tubercle is found. Opposite to it on the tegmen, dorsally or laterally or at both sites, a spine emerges. Thus, the postis anterior of the chamber corresponds to the sustentaculum. The sustentaculum is short, wide, and longitudinally permeated by several blood vessel and nerve canaliculi. The tegmen connects obliquely the

cranioventral end of the postis posterior with the sustentaculum. It has an undulated edge, and extends deeply over the chamber entrance. The sustentaculum-substituting postis anterior is much shorter (generally half) compared to the postis posterior, and deviates in its craniocaudal course to ventral. The fundus consists usually of four or five parts:

1. The upper medial part, which is a narrow area between the insertion of the postis posterior and the cranial edge of the fustis.
2. The fustis caudolaterally.
3. The excavation between the fustis and the posterior spine of the postis anterior.
4. The spine.
5. The narrow bone surface between the spine and sustentaculum.

The postis posterior stands in a nearly right angle to the fundus; whereas with the tegmen, it forms an acute angle. Similarly, an acute angle is found between the sustentaculum and fundus, and an obtuse one between the sustentaculum and tegmen. These angles—together with the difference in length between the postis posterior and sustentaculum and the oblique course of the tegmen—make the chamber trapezoid.

The promontory is uneven, aerolated, and richly canaliculized. The subiculum is wide, the promontorial wall of the stapes chamber is steep, and the arms of the subiculum are well developed. Between the facial and pyramidal arms, a deep retrofenestral sinus is encountered, communicating with the tympanic sinus. The sinus tympani is medium sized with an uneven surface. The styloid prominence, with its uneven lamellary and trabecular remnants and deep cells, bulges conspicuously into the tympanic sinus and the area concarmerata of the hypotympanum.

The promontory tunnel is doubled. Its upper part is situated behind the sustentaculum, and its surface is uneven, while the lower part is united ventrally to the sustentaculum by a thick spinous bone plate. Some trapezoid chamber entrances were seen to possess an equally destroyed postis anterior and sustentaculum, with the latter being represented by a spine directed downward from the promontory and an uneven plate from the hypotympanum. The promontorial upper part of the lateral plate of the tunnel is irregularly perforated. Behind it, the large cavity of the tunnel extends far below the promontory and behind the fustis. The cavity narrows towards the tube funnel. Here the tunnel wall is uneven and macerated, suggesting pathologic alterations. A trapezoid round window chamber is seldom found without pathologic alterations at other sites of the tympanic cavity.

A necessary prerequisite for the development of a trapezoid niche of the round window is the lack of a jugular fossa and the presence of a low sustentaculum. The postis anterior is usually destroyed by some pathologic process. This is suggested by several pathologic bone surfaces throughout the tympanic cavity. In rare cases, when no pathologic bone surfaces were seen along with a trapezoid round window chamber, the lack of a postis anterior is most likely due to developmental factors. The upper oblique side of the trapezoid is provided by the thick periosteal layer of the promontory, which is so developed that it extends deeper than usual above the chamber entrance.

Fossula Fenestrae Rotundae Rhomboidea (6%). This is a medium-sized type of round window chamber roughly equal to the ovoid chamber. The postis anterior and postis posterior meet the tegmen in obtuse and acute angles, respectively (Fig. 241). Postes are either of equal length to the tegmen and fundus or somewhat shorter. In addition to the rhomboid shape, this variant is also characterized by its straight walls.

The postis posterior is fused with the subiculum and continues under the promontory in a wide bone cylinder parallel to the fustis. It is demarcated from the fustis by a narrow sulcus. The tegmen is dorsally convex, straight, or slightly undulated. Above it on the promontory, a conical bone surface is found directed from the apex towards the tegmen. Occasionally, the promontory apex has spines. The postis anterior is a thin, straight bone plate. Behind it, under the basal helix of the cochlea, runs the long promontory tunnel communicating with the tympanic cavity through a lateral opening. The partition of the fundus is easily recognized. The upper part is smooth; the lower part contains spines of various size. In the middle part, the fustis bulges moderately into the chamber. If the floor and roof of the chamber entrance are longer than the postes, the promontorial apex and the anterior-inferior part of the

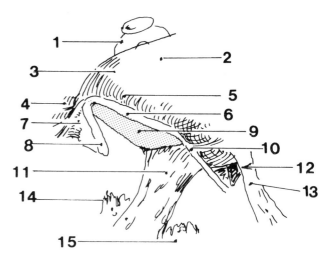

Figure 241.   Fossula fenestrae rotundae rhomboides. 1, Stapes. 2, Promontory. 3, Subiculum promontorii. 4, Arms of the subiculum. 5, Backward slope of the promontory. 6, Tegmen of the round window niche. 7, Secondary tympanic membrane. 8, Postis posterior. 9, Secondary tympanic membrane. 10, Postis anterior. 11, Fustis. 12, Tunnel of the promontory. 13, Sustentaculum promontorii. 14 and 15, Protrusions and cellules around the fustis.

fundus contain antagonizing bone spines. These are developmental remnants. It appears that the postis anterior proper has been resorbed during maturation; only spines have been left behind at its upper and lower insertions. The thin plate in place of the postis anterior is thus the remaining edge of the plate connecting the original postis with the sustentaculum. The fustis is usually the lowest at the chamber entrance, and thickens ventrally under the promontory and posteriorly to the styloid prominence.

The rhomboid round window niche develops in pyramid bones in which the promontory is covered by a thick periosteal layer, the jugular fossa penetrates high into the tympanic cavity, and the pavimentum pyramidis dislocates laterally the floor of the chamber with the inserted postes. Perhaps if the jugular fossa would not bulge so highly into the tympanic cavity, growth of the pavimentum pyramidale could not have a pulling effect on the postes. In such cases, the hypotympanum is abundantly structured with plates and trabecules. The partial lack of a postis anterior, marked angles between the postes, tegmen, and fustis, and the depth of the sinus tympani and smooth infundibular sinus are all indicative of enhanced subepithelial mesenchymal activity. In the development of this variant, enhanced osteoclast and decreased osteoblast activity may also be of importance.

Fossula Fenestrae Rotundae Semilunaris (5.8%)   The chamber entrance is almost horizontal. The postis posterior is low and wide. It branches off from the pyramidal arm of the subiculum; in the chamber, it diverges cranially from the fustis (Fig. 242). The angle between the postis posterior and tegmen is part of a circle line. The tegmen is con-

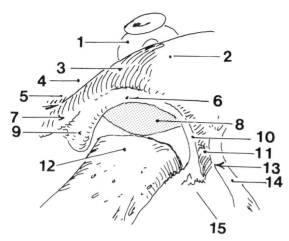

Figure 242. Fossula fenestrae rotundae semilunaris. 1, Stapes in situ. 2, Promontory. 3, Subiculum promontorii. 4, Fenestral arm of the subiculum promontorii. 5, Facial arm of the subiculum promontorii. 6, Tegmen of the round window niche. 7, Pyramidal arm of the subiculum promontorii. 8, Secondary tympanic membrane. 9, Postis posterior. 10, Postis anterior. 11, Lamina sustentaculopostica. 12, Fustis. 13, Tunnel promontorii. 14, Sustentaculum promontorii. 15, Protrusions at the lower insertion of the postis anterior.

vex, moderately thick, and smooth surfaced. The postis anterior is separated from the sustentaculum by a shallow sulcus. At its lower insertion, the signs of separation are seen with a spine on the fundus. The same applies for the sustentaculum. The fustis occupying almost the entire fundus inserts thinly to the styloid prominence. Ventrally, in the chamber, it flattens and widens. Despite that, the fustis fills almost the whole fundus; its cranial edge runs still closer to the postis posterior. The semilunar shape of the chamber is a result of the flat, wide fustis, low postes, and slightly archiform course of the tegmen.

A semilunar round window chamber with rudimentary promontory develops because the periosteal layer of the promontory is thin, the jugular fossa penetrates deep into the tympanic cavity, and the wide, flat, and low fustis further narrows the sagittal diameter of the chamber. Thus, the periosteal layer of the promontory is underdeveloped, and is the covering bone structure of the tympanic cavity. Nonpathologic impoverishment in structures may be a consequence of alimentary, metabolic, hormonal, or vitamin supply disturbances, and may be indicative of increased subepithelial mesenchymal activity.. This is suggested by the spine found on the subiculum as the remnant of the ponticulus, the nonprotruding variant of pyramidal eminence, and (rarely) the poorly developed osseous structures in the infundibular area of the hypotympanum.

A subvariant of this situation is the lyre-shaped round window chamber, which differs from the semilunar by the longitudinal ventral opening of the thin, wide plate between the postis anterior and sustentaculum. The postis posterior is broad and smooth surfaced. In its upper part, it

fuses with the brachium pyramidale, while it is separated at the caudal insertion. Here the postis posterior fuses with the fustis. The fustis has a horizontal course within the chamber. However, at the edge of the chamber, it bends ventrally in a right angle and is inserted on the lower spine remnant of the postis anterior. The two stems of the fustis surround, between the branching plates of the postis anterior, an extremely deep cavity that continues into the tunnel. The tegmen of the chamber is thin and undulated. The sustentaculum deviates downward in the direction of the infundibulum.

Lyre-shaped round window chambers occur in aerolated tympanic cavitites possessing a deep hypotympanum. The tympanic sinus develops behind the lower posterior portion of the fustis. It is very deep and narrows upward because the distance between the pyramidal eminence and subiculum is short. From the meeting point of the fustis and lower plate of the postis anterior, a septum constituting the lower posterior wall of the tympanic sinus runs to the uneven styloid prominence. Below this, the hypotympanum, at the corner between the area concamerata and the promontory, is formed by a cavity matching the sinus tympani in size. This cavity is the *hypotympanic sinus.* The inferior tympanic artery runs obliquely ventrally to the promontory. This results in the oblique postion of the sustentaculum. The acute angular encounter of the deep hypotympanum and the separated lamelles of the postis anterior constitutes towards the sustentaculum the long, gradually thinning part of the lyre-shaped entrance.

Fossula Fenestrae Rotunda Rotundae (5%). This type belongs to the smaller class of chambers. Both postes are well developed, smooth surfaced, and thick, the tegmen is arched, and the fustis is the closure of a circle (Fig. 243).

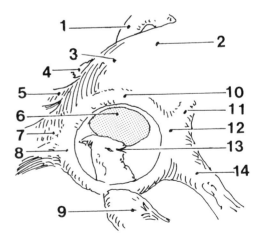

Figure 243. Fossula rotunda fenestrae rotundae. 1, Posterior crus of the stapes. 2, Promontory. 3, Subiculum promontorii. 4, Fenestral arm of the subiculum promontorii. 5, Facial arm of the subiculum. 6, Secondary tympanic membrane. 7, Pyramidal arm of the subiculum promontorii. 8, Postis posterior. 9, Fustis. 10, Tegmen of the round window niche. 11, Canal of Jacobson. 12, Postis anterior. 13, Intrachamber part of the fustis. 14, Sustentaculum promontorii.

The fustis consists of two parts. The inner part runs below the promontory between the concavity of the fundus and the postis posterior. The outer part connects the fusion point of the two postes with the styloid prominence. The postis posterior is fused with the brachium pyramidale of the subiculum. Its narrowest part is in the corner formed with the tegmen. From there, it broadens gradually until it bifurcates near its lower insertion. One branch runs to the inner part and the other to the outer part of the fustis. In such cases, the postis anterior is wider and thicker than the postis posterior. The postis anterior—although limiting a narrow round window—is fused with the sustentaculum; together the two form a thick, smooth-surfaced column. The postis anterior is also thinner at the tegmen and thicker at the fundus. At its lower insertion, it gives rise to a lateral process to the lateral edge of the fustis.

We find in this type of round window configuration: (1) a wide, flat subiculum; (2) a markedly convex, poorly structured promontory; (3) a moderately developed, well-demarcated tympanic sinus; and (4) a thick jugular wall. Thus, the edges of the small, round-shaped round window chamber are thick and similar to other tympanic cavity structures. Also, the hypotympanum has a thick wall with deep recesses. In the tube funnel, extremely deep infundibular sinuses and complicated lamelles and cellules can be observed.

The round-shaped round window chamber with a wide opening develops when the labyrinth block is covered by thick periosteal bone. This constitutes the edges of the window chamber and rounds off corners. In general, this variant is characterized by the abundance of bone tissue.

Fossula Fenestrae Rotundae Triangularis (3.4%). The chamber is smaller than the average. It is triangular because it practically has no tegmen. What can serve as a tegmen is the apex of the triangle. The two postes are the sides of the triangle, whereas the fundus is its base. (Fig. 244).

The postis posterior is a well-defined bone column fused medially with the subiculum. Its course is oblique, and its cranial part leans laterally. This cranial part continues without transition into the tegmen, and it is thinner than the caudal insertion that bifurcates. The dorsolateral process fuses with the fustis whereas the ventromedial process joins the bone frame of the secondary tympanic membrane and follows its lower edge to the sinus tympani. The tegmen has, caudally, a sharp edge towards the inside of the chamber that ends far from the most prominent edge of the promontory. The tegmen has no prominent edge towards the tympanic sinus, since the chamber roof forms at the cranial end of the fustis, part of a circle and turns downward in a roughly 60° angle to continue in the postis anterior.

Despite the usually joint occurence of triangular round window chamber with a moderately sized tunnel entrance, this proportion is occasionally altered; and the back entrance of the tunnel may be equal in size to the window chamber. This variant is seen in tympanic cavities with poorly developed covering bone. The edges of the round window niche and tunnel entrance are formed by mod-

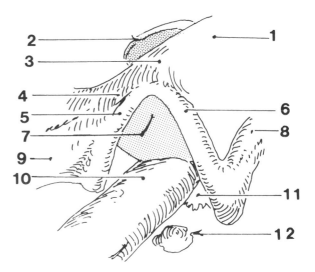

Figure 244. Fossula fenestrae rotundae triangularis. 1, Promontory. 2, Oval window. 3, Subiculum promontorii. 4, Facial arm of the subiculum promontorii. 5, Postis posterior. 6, Postis anterior. 7, Secondary tympanic membrane. 8, Sustentaculum promontorii. 9, Pyramidal arm of the subiculum promontorii. 10, Fustis. 11, Dentated plate on the fustis. 12, Sinus concameratus lateralis.

erately spinous, sharp-edged bone plates. Even the postis anterior separating the two openings is sending only a thin plate between the two cavities.

The postis anterior is hardly isolated from its surroundings. It is a convex bone plate that thickens caudally. Its edges are dentated or undulated. The hypotympanum meets the sustentaculum in a corner as the postis leans backwards, while the sustentaculum deviates towards the tube funnel. These two form a caudally open acute angle. The periosteal layer of the promontory between the postis anterior and sustentaculum may smooth or uneven. The corner formation between the postis anterior and sustentaculum is typical in young persons. In adults, these structures are usually parallel. In these cases, the sustentaculum is canaliculized, but the caudally opening vascular canal does not bend immediately towards the tube funnel; it runs in the periosteal layer of the promontory to appear at the apex of the promontory. Then it runs in the Jacobson's sulcus directly to the lower plate of the semicanal of the tensor tympani, pierces it in the subcanalicular area, and merges with the muscular canal.

The medial part of the fundus of the round window niche is always formed by the fustis. Its lateral part is rather variable. In some instances, a flat bone plate is found between the lateral edge of the fustis and the caudal insertion of the postis anterior, forming a 60° angle with the postis anterior. In other cases, an isolated bone plate extends from the lower insertion of the postis anterior to above the fustis, also forming a 60° angle with it. The thin lamella does not reach the fustis; behind it, the chamber entrance continues in a deep, richly structured excavation. This excavation turns medially towards the tubal funnel; hence, it forms the floor of the promontory tunnel. In the chamber, the fustis runs near the postis posterior. In front of the chamber towards the tympanic sinus, it either merges with the flat bone surface of the area concamerata of the hypotympanum or crosses the tympanic sinus and continues parallel to the brachium styloideale into the styloid prominence.

Although the sides of the triangle meet at 60° angles, we find different situations at each angle. The smoothest and widest of all is the cranial meeting point of the postes—the tegmen. Here the transition is a smooth arch, and the bone edge is convex and structureless. More acute is the corner between the postis posterior and fundus because, just underneath, the fustis bulges into the chamber. The sharpest angle is found between the postis anterior and fundus due to a caudal excavation of the chamber floor.

The promontory is generally square or rhomboid. The apex of the promontory occurs far from the chamber edge, at about the middle of the promontory. The subiculum is broad, with well-developed arms that diverge dorsally. A sinus retrofenestralia is often present, because the ponticulus continues caudally in a plate. Under this plate, there may be a communication with the sinus tympani. The sinus tympani is, at some places, bridged towards the styloid prominence not only by the arms of the subiculum, but also by long trabecules. The hypotympanum is usually deep. The jugular fossa is located far from the tympanic cavity. In a child's pyramid bones, the spine formation lateral to the postis posterior is not infrequent, and spines may be found occasionally in the corner between the postis anterior and sustentaculum.

From the developmental point of view, the formation of the triangular round window chamber is explained by an unusually thick periosteal layer that posteriorly does not form a horizontal edge, but extends dorsally towards the postes. The backward deviation of the chamber roof bone narrows the chamber entrance to such a degree that the two postes meet in an angle, and practically no tegmen is formed. The course of chamber formation also depends on the shape, size, and position of the mesenchymal ring remaining in the fenestra after ossification of the cartilaginous otic capsule. The great distance between the jugular fossa and labyrinth block, together with isolated development of the postis anterior and sustentaculum, favor deep tunnel formation. For similar reasons, all three hypotympanic areas show a lamellar-cellular structure.

Fossula Fenestrae Rotundae Semicirularis (2.6%). This is a subvariant of the semilunar type. The chamber entrance is deepened dorsally between the postis posterior and brachium pyramidale, and between the postis anterior and the caudal edge of the fustis. Thus, postes are elongated so that the chamber entrance extends over the fundus, forming a semicircle. Its characteristics are a wide, well-developed fustis, an excavation above and under the fustis, and an arciform tegmen-postis encounter. In these cases, the postis posterior bends in the chamber entrance under the promontory and fuses with the fundus in the chamber. The tegmen has an undulating course; dorsally, it reaches

to above the entrance. The postis anterior is short and hardly separable from the sustentaculum. The round window chamber is obliquely positioned and smaller than the oval window niche. The promontory is rhomboid, the apex of the promontory is uneven and aerolated, and sustentaculum is canaliculized, and the subiculum is fixed to the tympanic cavity wall by well-developed facial and pyramidal arms. Between the arms, a deep sinus tympani is found penetrating below the pyramidal eminence. There is no separate retrofenestral sinus. The pyramidal eminence is attached to the facial canal, and is connected to the subiculum by a narrow medial ponticulus. The styloid prominence is particularly marked. It borders caudally the tympanic sinus, and its ventral, well-developed process continues into the fustis. The styloid prominence and its process extend into the corner between the area concamerata and promontory. Towards the annulus tympanicus, a dorsally hemispheric hypotympanic sinus makes the tympanic cavity deeper. The floor of the sinus is bumpy and spinous. The promontory area has an uneven surface. The infundibular area is packed with trabecules and lamelles. The jugular fossa reaches high; its cranial edge extends up to the lower third of the tympanic sinus. The jugular wall is moderately developed. In some cases, the sulcus between the postis anterior and fustis continues under the fustis; thus the fustis has a sharp edge caudally towards the hypotympanum.

This variant develops when the promontory is covered by thick periosteal bone that rounds off the angles of the window edges. The jugular fossa is separated from the tympanic cavity by a bone plate of medium thickness. The floor of the tympanic cavity is not deep enough to accommodate cellules and lamellas, but there is still ample room for the formation of excavations under and above the fustis. These excavations elongate the chamber entrance dorsally, yielding a semicircular shape to it. The strong styloid prominence extends a well-developed fustis into the chamber entrance, accentuating the semicircular shape on the fundus.

Fossula Fenestrae Rotundae Inversa (0.4%). Its description will be given later when considering the pseudofustis dentatus.

Structure

According to structure, three variants of the round window chamber can be distinguished as described in the following paragraphs.

Fossula Fenestrae Rotundae Dentata (18.8%). The chamber entrance is vertical or oblique, and usually is smaller than the oval window niche. At the edges of square, lyre-shaped, or trapezoid chamber entrances on the lower or upper segment of the tegmen, one or more protrusions extend dorsally into the tympanic cavity or the chamber entrance narrowing their diameter. Protrusions occur most often where the postis anterior and tegmen meet. On the opposite area of the fundus, no antagonizing protrusion or spine is visible (Fig. 245).

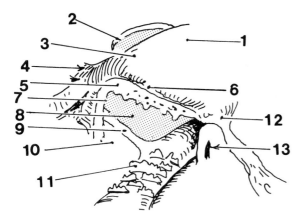

Figure 245. Fossula rotundae dentata. 1, Promontory. 2, Oval window. 3, Subiculum promontorii. 4, Facial arm of the subiculum promontorii. 5, Dentated plates extending from the tegmen into the chamber. 6, Tegmen of the round window niche. 7, Postis posterior. 8, Secondary tympanic membrane. 9, Medial branch of the fustis inside the chamber. 10, Covering bone protrusions on the fundus of the round window chamber. 11, Dentated plates on the fustis. 12, Sustentaculum promontory. 13, Tunnel of the promontory.

The postis posterior is fused with the brachium pyramidale to such an extent that they cannot be distinguished from each other. The postis posterior forms an acute angle with the tegmen. The tegmen has an undulated course, and its edge is sharp where it is spinous, while it is thick at other sites. The fundus is a flat bone surface. The fustis is present only ventrally in the form of a spinous trabecule connecting the styloid prominence with the jugular wall deep inside the chamber. The two structures are in line; but on the fundus, their connection is interrupted.

Another form of appearance of the dentate chamber entrance is when the fundus contains a well-developed fustis beginning from the upper corner of the chamber entrance. However, from the corner between the postis posterior and tegmen, the promontory edge forms a protrusion opposite of which a similar structure emerges from the upper edge of the styloid prominence. The postis posterior bifurcates on the fundus beginning from the pyramidal arm, and runs in the chamber entrance to the frame of the round window. The tegmen is thick at its upper part, while sharp-edged at the lower part. The postis anterior is missing. The tegmen continues downwards into the sustentaculum. The fundus is divided into three areas. Its ventrocaudal part is usually dentated or lamellated and contains remnants of a postis anterior.

The promontory has an uneven surface, and the sustentaculum is low with a channel in its axis. The oval window niche is smaller than that of the round window. The subiculum is narrow and short. The retrofenestral sinus is absent. The upper back part of the tympanic cavity is constituted behind the pyramidal eminence by a cranially smooth, laterally uneven tympanic sinus. The margins of the pyramidal eminence and the subiculum are connected by a short, bulky medial ponticulus. The styloid promi-

nence is caudally dislocated, occupying the posteroinferior angle of the hypotympanum. The jugular wall is thin and, at some parts dehiscent.

The dentate round window chamber is found when the jugular fossa strongly protrudes into the tympanic cavity, the jugular wall is thin, and the lower back region of the hypotympanum is occupied by a well-developed, aerolated styloid prominence. In these cases, the area concamerata is horizontally short and narrow. The edge of the chamber, the styloid prominence, and the high fundus are bridged by mucosa duplicatures. At their insertion, a bone protrusion develops by primary angiogenic ossification. This protrusion may be the remnant of the postis anterior, or it may be directed from the chamber edge towards the styloid prominence. The spine remnant of the postis anterior is indicative of its covering bone origin, rather than of bone destructive processes. Osteoblasts only partly build up the postis anterior. In late fetal and neonatal temporal bones, the chamber of the round window is wide open ventrally. The fissure also extends to the sustentaculum.

Fossula Fenestrae Rotundae Spinosa (12.2%). The chamber is oblique, small, and usually smaller than the oval window niche. It may be rectangular or low triangular. In the latter case, ventrally from the brachium pyramidale, a wide structure bulges into the chamber lumen, which develops in place of the postis posterior (Fig. 246). This is a rare variant, because the postis posterior is one of the most stable structures of the chamber. The tegmen is a thick, smooth convex bone surface. The postis anterior is low, thinning towards the fundus where it does not insert fully. The sustentaculum is low, oblique, and found not at the lower back, but at the front back part of the promontory. The postis anterior is connected with the sustentaculum by a slender, unevenly surfaced covering bone. The distance between the two is extremely long.

The three fundus regions are well expressed. The fustis is a wide, high, smooth-surfaced semicylinder, preserving this character in the chamber also. It is inserted on the beginning of the scala tympani of the cochlear basal helix. It bifurcates dorsally. The cranial branch disappears in the floor of the tympanic sinus, while the caudal branch continues into the styloid prominence. At the meeting point of the fustis and fundus, a small cellular structure is seen. A notable feature of this variant is a long spine forming an upward convex arch from the corner of the postis anterior in the direction of the styloid eminence without reaching it. The styloid eminence has a rough, uneven surface. It is low and extends far into the area concamerata on the cranioventral area, from which it continues to the postis anterior by an undulated lamelle. The tubal variant of the pyramidal eminence is present. The retropyramidal sinus is well developed and continues far under the basal lamina of the aditus. It replaces the lower angle cellules. The ventral apex of the styloid prominence is located near the spine directed backwards from the chamber frame. On the cranial surface of the styloid prominence, a ventrally narrowing bone trabecule is found inserting with a plate

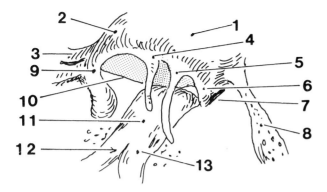

Figure 246. Fossula fenestrae rotundae spinosa. 1, Promontory. 2, Subiculum promontorii. 3, Facial arm of the subiculum promontorii. 4 and 5, Protrusions on the tegmen of the round window niche. 6, Short postis anterior. 7, Tunnel of the promontory. 8, Sustentaculum promontorii. 9, Postis posterior. 10, Secondary tympanic membrane. 12 and 13, Part of the fustis bifurcating in the area concamerata.

on the pyramidal eminence. Neither the front end nor the caudal edge of this trabecule area fuse with the styloid prominence. Both the trabecule extending from the chamber frame into the tympanic cavity and the trabecule of the pyramidal eminence resting on the styloid prominence and directed toward the promontory can be regarded as identical structures. It seems that in the mucosa duplicature between the pyramidal eminence and promontory, ossification has started. The osseous bridge formed this way might have been complete had it not been dislocated cranially by the cranioventral growth of the styloid prominence and separated by mechanical forces. It is also possible that within the mucosa duplicature, *a priori* incomplete trabecules have developed. When the styloid prominence was dislocated cranially, the trabecule fixed on the pyramidal eminence—the promontorial spine—deviated to dorsolateral.

The most common and simple form of this variant is the occurrence of a few spines at the rear edge of the promontory inside the chamber. Spines may be different sizes, but their consistent feature is a wide base and narrow free end. They are directed either towards the styloid prominence or the area concamerata of the hypotympanum. These vis-a-vis structures are, however, always lower and less developed than their promontorial continuations, since the bloody supply of the promontory is better than that of the posterior tympanic wall.

If the chamber entrance is square, spines generally occur at the promontorial insertion of the postis anterior. Frequently, not a single well-developed spine is found here; rather, a number of spines of different size are situated closely parallel to each other. In the area concamerata, slightly distant from the chamber entrance, similar but more pronounced structures appear directed towards the promontorial spines. The differences in size are also explained by the different blood supplies of these structures.

The development of the spinous round window cham-

ber is relatively simple, and can be explained mostly by the lack of a postis anterior and the remaining rudimentary postis portions of the upper and lower insertion sites. Such spines occur in square or rectangular chamber entrances. Low triangular- or heart-shaped chamber entrances are usually coupled to horizontally smaller sinus tympani and hypotympanum in the tympanic cavity; whereas the promontory is covered by a thick periosteal bone layer. The abundant vasculature of the periosteal layer produces bone to fill the tympanic cavity, to thicken edges, and even to bridge the posterior space of the tympanic cavity. As a result of enhanced osteogenesis between the promontory and posterior tympanic wall or styloid prominence, the development of an osseous bridge is guided by the mucosa duplicatures, which may be either partial—producing a long spine on both walls—or complete. It cannot resist the cranial growth of the styloid prominence; therefore, its central, poorly vascularized portion degenerates. The infolding on the cranial plate of the styloid prominence argues for its later growth. Thus, the variant develops when the periosteal layer of the promontory shows a higher developmental activity than the covering bone of the posterior tympanic wall. As mentioned above, developmental differences are explained on the basis of local blood supply.

Fossula Fenestrae Rotundae Trabecularis (1.6%). This variant was mostly present in rhomboid or rectangular chambers. Fine trabecules extend into the chamber from one or both postes (Fig. 247). Usually, the postis itself is also a trabecular structure. This structure, however, does not end at the lower insertion of the postis, but spreads in a fan-like fashion over the chamber floor and even on the fustis. It is mostly found perinatally because the trabecular chamber entrance occurs in adults only if the formation of covering bone is slowed down or stopped. In adults suffering

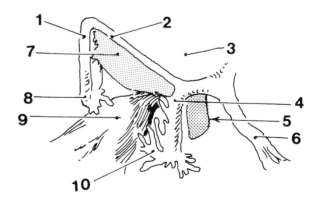

Figure 247. Fossula fenestrae rotundae trabecularis. 1, Postis posterior. 2, Tegmen of the round window niche. 3, Promontorial apex. 4, Postis anterior. 5, Tunnel of the promontory. 6, Sustentaculum promontorii. 7, Secondary tympanic membrane. 8, Caudally divergent trabecules of the postis posterior. 9, Fundus of the round window niche with the fustis. 10, Trabecules diverging on the base of the postis anterior.

from malnutrition (e.g., Australian aborigines), it is more frequent.

Of the constituting elements of the round window niche, we shall consider in detail the postes and fustis because these structures can be readily distinguished embryologically, functionally and inframicroscopically anatomically, surgically, and pathologically. In addition to their inframicroscopic description, their variants will be dealt with in the following chapters.

Variants of the Postis Posterior

The variants of the postis posterior are a result of its own development and relation to its surroundings. The lower insertion of the postis posterior is located on the fundus, so that one or two cristae continue ventrally in the chamber. There may be no isolated cristae present, but the fusion of the two may form a ventrally widening bone cylinder whose cranial end adheres where the osseous spiral lamina emerges cranially. This, in fact, is the angle between the scala tympani and scala vestibuli. The postis posterior is limited medially from the round window by a semilunar excavation, and laterally by a sulcus between the chamber entrance and fustis. Ventrally, it is usually isolated from its surroundings by a triangular excavation. This is called the triangular fossa of the round window and is bordered:

1. Ventrally by the upper posterior edge of the scala tympani on the basal helix of the cochlea.
2. Caudally by the fustis.
3. Dorsolaterally by the ventral end of the postis posterior.

The triangular fossa of the round window is mostly deep and smooth surfaced, with well-demarcated walls and pronounced angles between them. The deepest point of the fossa is found at the ventromedial part of the round window chamber.

Postis Posterior Promontorialis (34.4%).   This occurs mainly in triangular chambers. The postis posterior is not isolated from the periosteal layer of the promontory and subiculum, but remains connected to it. The periosteal layer of the promontory accumulates at the medial superior angle, filling in the angle and extending to the fundus of the chamber. In this variant, other tympanic cavity structures also have a thick covering of bone.

Postis Posterior Cellularis (21.6%).   The completely separated postis posterior inserts only caudally onto the subiculum. From the subiculum, a pronounced crest—the *styloid brachium*—runs to the styloid prominence. In the angle between this crista and the postis posterior, cellules are found on the fundus, also making cellular the dorsal aspect of the postis. Between the crista and fustis, a narrow, deep sulcus develops, continuing into the chamber where it is found between the cellular postis posterior and the intrachamber segment of fustis (Fig. 248).

It seems that the cellular structure of the postis posterior develops because subepithelial mesenchymal activity between the well-developed brachium styloidale and the

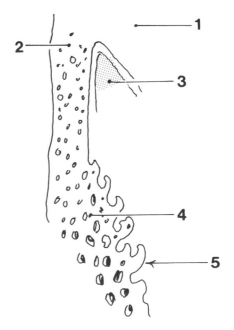

Figure 248.   Postis posterior cellularis. 1, Promontory. 2, Postis posterior. 3, Secondary tympanic membrane. 4, Large pneumatic cavities at the caudally widened insertion of the postis posterior. 5, Cranially elongated spines.

similarly well-developed fustis produces not only a deep fissure, but also cellules in the brachium postis angle and the postis.

Postis Posterior Lamellosus (17.4%).   The postis posterior fused with the subiculum forms a thin plate parallel to the chamber entrance. The plate has caudoventrally a sharp edge; upwards and backwards, it is slightly thicker. The subiculum has no pyramidal arm, and towards the scala tympani either the fustis alone penetrates into the chamber or a rudimentary process of the postis posterior separates from the postis inside the chamber, behind the edge of the plate. The fustis is low, wide, and fused on the fundus with the lamellar postis posterior. Laterally, at the level of the plate, it ends abruptly, and only its caudal edge bridges the tympanic cavity ending on the styloid prominence with a thin plate. The promontory is convex and smooth surfaced. The subiculum is broad and bound, with a thick lamellar ponticulus to the pyramidal eminence. The retrofenestral sinus is narrow, but it reaches deeply below the pyramidal eminence. The tympanic sinus is also a narrow, deep excavation with smooth walls. Caudally, it is bordered by the persisting lower plate of the fustis. The sinus does not extend below the pyramidal eminence, and its floor is concave. (Fig. 249).

The lamellar postis posterior occurs in the tympanic cavity when the distance between the pyramidal eminence and promontory is short and this space is occupied by a uniform, smooth-walled tympanic sinus. The ventral wall of the sinus is constituted by the common plate of the sub-

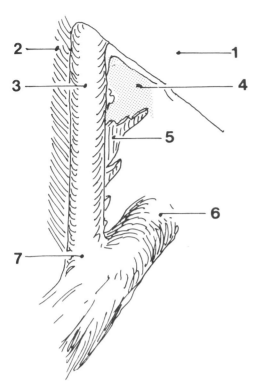

Figure 249. Postis posterior lamellosus. 1, Promontory. 2, Subiculum promontorii. 3, Postis posterior. 4, Secondary tympanic membrane. 5, Plates on the postis posterior extending into the chamber. 6, Fustis. 7, Joint of the postis posterior and fustis.

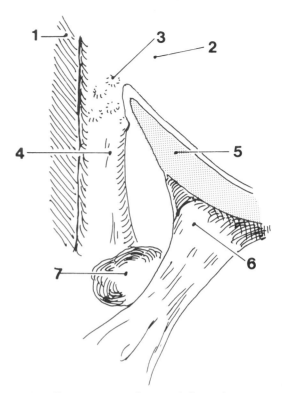

Figure 250. Postis posterior tuberosus. 1, Bony plate connecting the subiculum promontorii with the postis posterior. 2, Promontory. 3, Bony tubercles on the postis posterior. 4, Postis posterior. 5, Secondary tympanic membrane. 6, Fustis. 7, Sinus concameratus medialis.

iculum and postis posterior; and in its continuation is located the cut edge of the cranial two thirds of the fustis. It appears as if subepithelial mesenchymal activity starting from the tympanic sinus would have cut off the subiculum, postis posterior, and a substantial part of the fustis dorsally in a straight line. The caudal plate of the fustis, adhering in an upward convex arch to the styloid prominence, has remained because subepithelial-connective tissue did not affect the caudal part of the postis, nor was this structure later rebuilt by osteoblasts.

Postis Posterior Tuberosus (12.8%). On the wide lateral surface of the postis, fused with the subiculum, some tubercles occur near the tegmen (Fig. 250). Behind the lower bone tubercle, the postis is interrupted towards the fundus. Its insertion is seen only ventrally on the posterior wall of the scala tympani. The fustis is often caudally dislocated, and a cavity is formed between the place of the missing postis insertion and fustis. The deepest point of this cavity is found between the tubercle and ventrally deviating process. Backwards, this cavity merges with the tympanic sinus; thus, it can be interpreted as an extension of the sinus into the chamber (Fig. 250).

The tuberous postis posterior with an underlying cavity develops when the tympanic sinus extends towards the chamber. In such cases, a larger cavity is formed on the

fundus, between the fustis and postis posterior, but the subepithelial mesenchyme also invades the postis, which becomes tuberous.

Postis Posterior Dentatus (8.8%). From the angle of the promontory and subiculum, an isolated semicylinder extends to the fundus of the round window chamber. On its surface, at various levels of the postis posterior, bone protrusions develop (Fig. 251). The tip of these protrusions are most frequently directed towards the manubrium. The dentate postis posterior is quite common in the last months of embryonic life. Protrusions, as at other sites of the tympanic cavity, develop along arterioles. It seems that due to trophic disturbances valleys between protrusions are not filled up either embryonically or postnatally. Dentation remains for the rest of life.

Postis Posterior Duplex (5%). The postis posterior is doubled along its entire course. In fact, it consists of two fused cylinders. The two cylinders do not separate towards the tegmen, but this occurs usually near the fundus. One arm of the postis runs in the chamber, while the other runs dorsally towards the tympanic sinus and adheres to the posterior tympanic wall. The dorsal arm has no continuation on the floor of the sinus tympani (Fig. 252).

Embryologically, duplication of the postis posterior can

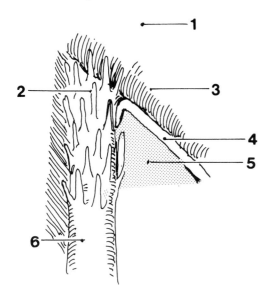

Figure 251.   Postis posterior dentatus. 1, Promontory. 2, Spines on the postis posterior. 3, Tegmen of the round window niche. 4, Ridge of the tegmen. 5, Secondary tympanic membrane. 6, Postis posterior.

be explained by a partition at its wide base by enhanced osteoclastic activity. It is also possible that the pyramidal arm of the subiculum adheres to the postis, but its dorsal growth towards the pyramidal eminence is arrested by enhanced osteoclastic activity.

Variants of the Postis Anterior

Postis Anterior Apertus (Disjunctus) (69.6%).   If the anterior window frame is not made of a solid bone cylinder, but the cylinder is incomplete, and ventrolaterally open a variant of

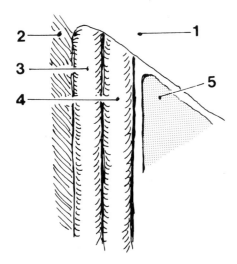

Figure 252.   Postis posterior duplex. 1, Promontory. 2, Subiculum promontorii. 3 and 4, The double column of the postis posterior. 5, Secondary tympanic membrane.

the open postis anterior develops. The sustentaculum is isolated from the postis anterior; the chamber entrance is usually not square, but lyre-shaped, semilunar, or semicircular. The fustis on the chamber floor may be different in size. The promontory is thick and rounded off on the territory of the tegmen. Some places on the apex of the promontory are covered with protrusions and hooks. The opening of the postis anterior can be of various extent. The opening occurs consistently caudally on the postis, being wider towards the chamber entrance. The angle of the opening is directed mostly towards the angle between the sustentaculum and hypotympanum (Fig. 253).

The smallest opening is caused by a minimal ventral interruption at the lower insertion of the postis anterior. The postis may also be open by the lack of its lower third, when the postis anterior is fixed not to the jugular wall, but to the sustentaculum. Thus, ventrolaterally on the fundus, the chamber entrance is constituted by a smooth-surfaced, usually canaliculized, circumscribed vertical trabecule of the sustentaculum. The larger upper part of the postis is made of arciform bone covering the promontory, and connecting the chamber entrance with the sustentaculum. This bony covering, although adhering to the sustentaculum, still has well-recognized contours on the sustentaculum. Occasionally, the caudal opening of postis anterior is diminished or bridged by a bone protrusion emerging from the fundus. In these cases, cellules are observed between the sustentaculum and postis anterior in

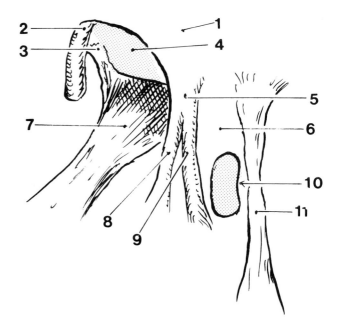

Figure 253.   Postis anterior apertus (disjunctus). 1, Promontory. 2, Postis posterior. 3, Osseous frame of the round window in the medial part of the chamber. 4, Secondary tympanic membrane. 5, Postis anterior with a common stem. 6, Lamella sustentaculopostica. 7, Fustis. 8, Medial branch of the open postis anterior. 9, Lateral branch of the open postis anterior. 10, Tunnel of the promontory. 11, Sustentaculum promontorii.

the periosteal bone layer of the promontory. Cellules may be present on the apex of the promontory, lifting the periosteal layer towards the chamber.

An open postis may result when it curves towards the promontorial area of the hypotympanum, and is inserted with a thin plate on the jugular wall. Between the postis and sustentaculum, the plate forms an area containing small indentations or cellules. Opposite to the open plate, a cranially emerging bone plate occurs in the area concamerata, forming an acute angle with the oblique lower segment of the postis. This antagonizing plate of the postis anterior may be situated either in the chamber entrance parallel to the promontorial edge, or may continue towards the styloid prominence in the form of a dentated crista in the area concamerata.

The plate forming the lower segment of the postis anterior may reach ventrally far into the promontorial area. It may even bridge it by adhering to the lower tympanic wall. In such instances, the plate continues under the sustentaculum, taking part in the formation of the vascular channel and the tunnel. Dorsally from this transverse plate of the postis anterior, the edge of the styloid prominence has a lamellocellular structure protected on the inferior promontorial wall by a wide shallow sulcus. This sulcus is covered from the tube funnel by a bony process originating ventrally and laterally on the periosteal layer of the promontory. This rises by widening in the craniocaudal direction to the bony plate of the sustentaculum that protects vessels.

In this stage of development, the fustis is more distant, running ventrally to the postis posterior and joining the chamber by a smooth-surfaced wide bone emerging dorsally from the promontory. This dorsal process of the promontory is derived from the periosteal layer of the promontory, and corresponds to the upper segment of the postis anterior. Simultaneously, on the floor of the hypotympanum, a bone protrusion is formed that emerges from the pavimentum pyramidis and approaches the edge of the promontory; that is, the upper process of the postis anterior. Postnatally, the process of the hypotympanum reaches the promontory, and closes the sustentaculum. The tegmen becomes thinner towards the fustis, separating from the periosteal layer of the promontory. Under the process, the tunnel appears. However, from the jugular wall, a bony plate adheres to the fustis, closing an acute angle with the covering bone of the sustentaculum. The plate connecting the hypotympanum and fustis is later separated from the fustis. This separation takes place when the jugular fossa widens, and the base of the tympanic cavity enlarges ventrally. Nevertheless, the remnant of the plate still forms an acute angle with the covering bone plate of the sustentaculum. Under the guiding effect of mucosa duplicature connecting the plates with each other and with the chamber roof, the two bone plates meet to form the postis anterior. In this process, an increased osteoblastic activity is instrumental. If osteoclastic activity predominates, the plates degenerate. The interaction of these factors determine the development of various postis anterior forms, and it may also bring about different openings at the lower segment of the postis anterior.

Postis Anterior Lamellosus (8.4%). This is a frequent variant of the window frame. It accompanies square- or lyre-shaped chamber entrances. The plate seldom connects the roof and floor of the chamber in a vertical plane. The downward and ventrolaterally directed plate runs to the sustentaculum, and is inserted on its dorsal surface. The tegmen of the chamber has a dentated edge; on the fundus, vis-a-vis structures, sharp lamelles are found. Similar structures occur on the cranial surface of the fustis. The fustis is poorly developed and hardly stands out of the fundus. The vis-a-vis structures of the fundus continue dorsally into the lamellocellular structure of the styloid prominence. This variant was observed mostly in young individuals. Occasionally, the sustentaculum also displays a similar structure. The lamellar and slender types of the postis anterior are both due to increased vascularization. This is supported by the richly structured area concamerata.

An additional role is played by the mucosa duplicatures partially covering the window frame, and by the developmental dynamics of the pavimentum pyramidis. In the soft tissue surrounding the arteriole, the slender trabecule of the postis anterior develops first. Then, in the membrana sustentaculopostica connecting this trabecule with the sustentaculum, covering bone develops that results in a plate connecting the two structures (Fig. 254).

The guiding role of mucosa duplicatures is indicated by vis-a-vis structures between the tegmen and fundus, while the effect of developmental dynamics of the pavimentum pyramidis is underlined by the gradually more distant position of the lower insertion of the plate and the transposi-

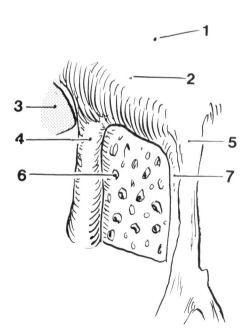

Figure 254.   Postis anterior lamellosus. 1, Promontory. 2, Tegmen of the round window niche. 3, Secondary tympanic membrane. 4, Postis anterior. 5, Sustentaculum promontorii. 6, Plate linking the postis anterior and sustentaculum. 7, Covering bone process of the promontory behind the sustentaculum.

tion towards the dorsal tympanic wall of vis-a-vis structures, whereby their free edges approach each other. The unusual thickness of the jugular wall may also be held responsible for the development of this variant. Parallel to the transverse plate, the area promontorialis and infundibularis are filled with plates continuing towards the hypotympanum in well-developed cellules.

In other cases, the postis anterior is incomplete due to an oblique course of the thick undulated tegmental edge to the sustentaculum. In such instances, the postis anterior may also be incomplete on its upper part. However, the lower insertion is marked by a protrusion, plate, or slender trabecule emerging from the jugular wall. This represents the lower part of the postis anterior.

The incomplete postis anterior occurs mostly in a wide chamber entrance. In fact, the chamber entrance is widened because of the incompleteness of the postis anterior, the openings of which add to the chamber entrance. However, a sporadically open postis anterior is coupled to a narrow, high chamber. The chamber entrance is vertically elongated, the promontory is square, the subiculum is well developed and smooth surfaced, and the postis anterior is conspicuously thick.

The fustis adheres to the postis posterior, and is fused inside the chamber with the bone process, which extends to the fustis from the definitive postis anterior. The fustis with the fused postis anterior fills the entire chamber, narrows cranially the window frame, and gives room caudally for a narrow tunnel. Here the fundus consists of two parts: (1) medially, the territory of the fustis; and (2) laterally, that of an uneven bony surface from which a well-demarcated, trabecular upwards-narrowing spine emerges towards the tegmen running parallel to the sustentaculum. The spine represents the lower part, while the bone trabecule directed from the tegmen to the fustis is the upper part of the postis anterior.

The hypotympanum is short and narrow. On its deep floor, trabecules are lying surrounded by bulky plates and minor cellules. The tube funnel is also narrow and poor in structures. The sacellus is shallow, and its edge is marked by slender trabecules. The protectum is present only towards the sacellus. It is indicated on the inferior promontorial wall by small spines. The styloid prominence is a well-developed, smooth bone surface that extends trabecule and plates into the area concamerata from its central edge. The tympanic sinus is narrow, deep, and has smooth walls.

The opening of the postis anterior also occurs in the form of a narrow cleft directed towards the lower insertion of the sustentaculum. This cleft forms ventrolaterally an acute angle, and interrupts the thin dehiscent bone plate that developed between the postis and sustentaculum in the membranae sustentaculo-portica. At the upper and lower edges of the postis anterior, thin spines stand opposite to each other. The spines have a peripheral thickening. The open postis anterior is interpreted as a sign of insufficent ossification.

In embryonic and neonatal bones, the postis anterior is often missing, and the round window chamber is open ventrally down to the tube funnel. It may be that in the last intrauterine months, the sustentaculum does not develop either, because the insufficent osteogenesis is unable to produce an osseous capsule for the inferior tympanic artery.

Postis Anterior Plexiformis (8%).   The upper insertion of the postis is a regular cylinder, but downwards it branches, and the branches form a plexus. The trabecules are not parallel. They are inserted on the fundus with a wide base, and the plexus is constituted by a meshwork of partially fused, partially separated trabecules. It is mostly seen in younger individuals and is accompanied by a similar structure at other sites of the tympanic cavity.

The area concamerata of the hypotympanum is either trabeculocellular or lamellocellular, so that closer to the jugular wall either cellules (more cranially), plates, or trabecules occur. It is well areolated. The lower part of the promontory, sustentaculum, protectum, and sacellus—as well as the promontorial and infundibular areas of the hypotympanum are abundantly structured. The promontory has a thick periosteal layer. (Fig. 255).

The plexiform postis anterior develops when the periosteal layer of the promontory is thick, the jugular fossa is not bulging high into the tympanic cavity, and the hypotympanum contains osteophytes. The osseous structures of the hypotympanum are delicate.

Postis Anterior Sigmoideus (7.2%).   Between the caudal angle of the tegmen and ventral aspect of the styloid prominence, an S-shaped trabecule is found with a backward curvature on its promontorial and a forward curvature on its lateral third (Fig. 256). This trabecule is the isolated

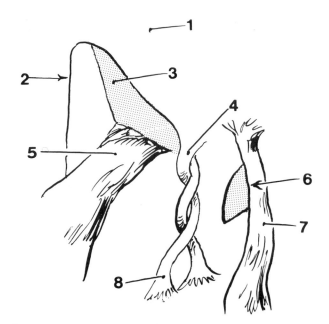

Figure 255.   Postis anterior plexiformis. 1, Promontory. 2, Postis posterior. 3, Secondary tympanic membrane. 4, Postis anterior. 5, Fustis. 6, Tunnel promontorii. 7, Sustentaculum promontorii. 8, Widening base of the postis anterior.

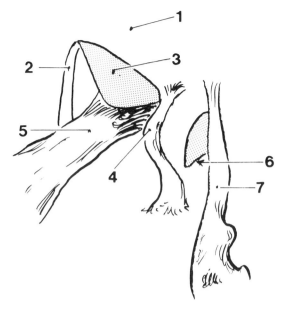

Figure 256. Postis anterior sigmoideus. 1, Promontory. 2, Postis posterior. 3, Secondary tympanic membrane. 4, S-shaped postis anterior. 5, Fustis. 6, Tunnel of the promontory. 7, Sustentaculum promontorii.

column of the postis anterior, which is found coupled to a narrow chamber entrance with a deep cavity directed towards the fossa jugularis between the postis and fustis. The cavity can be followed to the tuba funnel under the caudal plate of the scala tympani, and above the plate separating the promontory from the hypotympanum. The postis posterior is separated from the sinus tympani by a high dentated bone plate—the *styloid brachium.* On the styloid prominence, ventrodorsal wrinkles are visible. The area concamerata of the hypotympanum is under the tunnel entrance of the lamellocellular structure. This structure continues on the territory of the sustentaculum.

The S-shaped postis anterior develops when the styloid prominence bulges towards the promontory approaching it, and when the jugular fossa is far from the floor of the tympanic cavity (a thick jugular wall). Enhanced mesenchymal activity produces a lamellocellular area on the hypotympanum and isolate postis anterior from the lower promontorial wall. The periosteal layer of the promontory is thick, accentuating the lateral thickness of the chamber frame. However, curvature of the postis anterior points to an important developmental mechanism. The periosteal layer formed between the promontory and the hypotympanum is near the styloid prominence; when this later bulges into the tympanic cavity, it not only reaches the insertion of the chamber frame, but also displaces it ventrally. This is likely to bring about the S-shaped curvature of the postis anterior under the pressure of the styloid prominence. It seems that the osteoblastic and osteoclastic activity that induces bone transformation cannot keep pace with the dynamics of development.

Postis Anterior Gracilis (6.8%). It is seen mostly in square or rectangular round window chambers. The promontory is linked to the fundus either by a slender trabecule, well demarcated from the sustentaculum (postis anterior trabecularis), or by a plate that can vary in size. Usually, the sustentaculum has an oblique course. It is canaliculized, while the promontory is smooth or bumpy. Jacobson's canals are shallow; the fustis is low and wide. The area concamerata is a lamellocellular structure (Fig. 257).

The development of this variant is explained by the areolated, well-structured area concamerata. The jugular fossa does not bulge high into the tympanic cavity. Thus, the jugular wall is thick, giving room for lamellocellular structures under the effect of increased vascularization of the area concamerata.

In front of the round window chamber, the perivascularly accumulated embryonic mesenchyme and tubotympanic epithelium initially form a bone protrusion between the sustentaculum and chamber floor. The protrusion is connected with the sustentaculum by a mucosa duplicature—the *membrana sustentaculo postica,* which serves as a guide for ossification. Under circumstances of reduced blood supply and/or osteogenic factors, a slender postis anterior develops.

The inframicroscopic morphology of the postis anterior can also be modified by formation of pneumatic cellules. The starting point of tympanic cavity pneumatization is the tympanic sinus, from which the biological process rapidly reaches the postis anterior, which is *a priori* thinner and looser in structure than the postis posterior. This is the reason why variations in the postis anterior structure occur on a wider scale than those in the postis posterior structure.

Thus, mesenchymal activity is effectively operational in

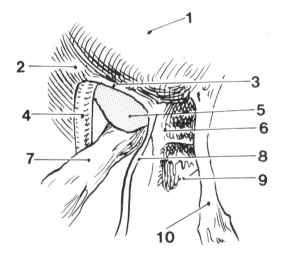

Figure 257. Postis anterior gracilis. 1, Promontory. 2, Subiculum promontorii. 3, Tegmen of the round window niche. 4, Postis posterior. 5, Secondary tympanic membrane. 6, Lamella sustentaculopostica. 7, Fustis. 8, Slender postis anterior. 9, Tunnel of the promontory. 10, Sustentaculum promontorii.

the area between the pavimentum pyramidis and labyrinth capsule, causing an increased bone destruction around the postis anterior, but sparing the postis anterior itself in the form of an isolated trabecule or plate.

Variant of the Fustis

The bony trabecule running transversely on the fundus of the round window chamber was termed the *fustis* because of its resemblance to a widening stick. Generally, it links the basal turn of the cochlea with the styloid prominence. It has a horizontal course and is located closer to the postis posterior. When the chamber entrance and dorsal edge of the promontory lean ventrally up to down, it forms an acute angle with the plane of the chamber entrance so that this acute angle is ventrally open between the chamber segment of the fustis and the ventral part of the entrance. Its surface is consistently smooth inside the chamber, whereas towards the styloid prominence, it is mostly uneven, dentated, lamellar, or cellular. The medial and lateral edges of the incumbent semicylinder are usually well demarcated towards their surroundings; and, occasionally, a cavity is found at its sides, penetrating into the covering bone layer of the jugular wall. The fustis may be present in rudimentary or well-developed forms. It may be quite rudimentary when it is seen in the chamber as a vaguely limited low hillock, and in the area concamerata as a few spines. In other cases, it may be a conspicuous emerging bone formation narrowing the chamber lumen.

As to the embryology of the fustis, which was briefly described previously, it has to be emphasized that it develops in close connection with the structures of the rear part of the tympanic cavity. In the *four-month-old fetus* the hypotympanum is still poorly developed. The tympanic bone, resembling an open ring, adheres to the osseous capsule of the sacculocochlear part of the inner ear. The covering bone substance of the subiculum has no continuation towards the facial canal, but bends with a wide covering cylinder into the round window chamber. At this stage, the chamber is still filled with abundant masses of embryonic mesenchyme.

In the *five-month-old fetus,* the fustis has not yet developed because the chamber is almost filled with the recurrent bone cylinder of the postis posterior. This bone cylinder does not start thinning out before the sixth month. It supports, as the recurrent trabecule of the postis posterior, beneath the initial part of the osseous spiral lamina the scala tympani of the cochlea. The thinning of the bone cylinder takes place via a longitudinal partition resulting from tympanic cavity enlargement. The upper medial part of the partitioned cylinder remains connected to the postis posterior. The lower lateral part is resorbed, and only a few crestae or bone tubercules remain. This resorption results in widening of the round window chamber, with a concomitant accumulation of covering bone on the chamber frame during the *seventh month* of gestation.

The widening of the chamber in the *eight-month-old fetus* reaches a degree where instead of its former round shape, it acquires a rectangular or rhomboid form. Simultaneously, in the thickened covering bone of the fundus, the fustis is definitely formed and isolated as a result of pneumatization of its neighborhood. Covering bone increases in the *nine-month-old fetus,* and continues to grow even postnatally until puberty. The fustis becomes connected with the posterior part of the tympanic cavity by various bone formations most often with the styloid prominence.

About the time of birth, this bone column moves dorsally and often bridges the posterior part of the tympanic cavity, or it may fuse with the postis posterior. The bone column terminates dorsally in the chamber entrance; from there it continues on the slightly thicker floor of the tympanic cavity only up to the lower posterior edge of the tympanic ring. The postis posterior forms dorsally a crista sharply separating the tympanic sinus from the area concamerata of the hypotympanum. This dorsal process of the postis posterior fuses with the partly developed lamellar osseous capsule of the styloid prominence. Postnatally, the dorsal crista of the postis posterior is resorbed in relation to the expansion of the sinus tympani. Cranially, it is attacked by the subepithelial-connecting tissue, which is widening the sinus tympani below. The crista is replaced by cellules. A trabeculocellular structure also develops at the dorsal continuation of the fustis. However, these trabecules are soon stabilized and arranged in parallel rows between the fustis and the developing styloid prominence. Later, they multiply vertically and stand out from their surrounding as the intrachamber continuation of the fustis. Then they thicken, solidify, and establish a continuous connection between the fustis and styloid prominence. At this stage, the fustis is found immediately under the postis posterior.

Particularly in the chamber entrance, the fustis indicates the rear edge of the pavimentum pyramidis. This is an independently developing covering bone plate that constitutes the osseous cover towards the tympanic cavity of two large vessels, and adheres to the labyrinth block and pars tympanica. However, in the line of adhesion to the covering bone of the pars petrosa at the posterior part of the tympanic cavity, there appears to be an overproduction of covering bone. This is analogous to the supporting trabecule at the joining of the pars petrosa and pars squamosa at the tegmen antri and aditus. Nevertheless, on the tegmen, antri bone overproduction occurs on the upper part of the os petrosum; while on the tympanic cavity floor, this takes place on the lower part of it. This trabecule, particularly when extremely large in size, serves static purposes on both the tegmen and the area concamerata.

Fustis Trabeculo-Cellularis (37.4%). The ventral (promontorial) end of the fustis terminates in two, fork-like slender trabecules and is inserted on the cochlea (Fig. 258). Within the chamber, its course is parallel to the promontorial wall of the oval window; that is, it crosses the chamber entrance obliquely (Fig. 258). Inside the chamber, it narrows ventrally to dorsally with the narrowest being its midportion falling in the plane of the chamber entrance. Here it forms

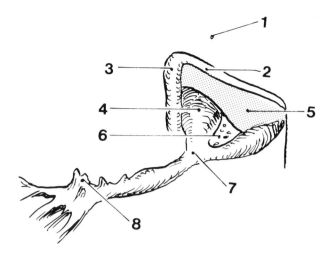

Figure 258. Fustis trabeculocellularis. Trabecules appear mostly on the rear part of the fustis. The fustis bifurcates in the chamber. 1, Promontory. 2, Tegmen of the round window niche. 3, Postis posterior. 4, Medial branch of the fustis inside the chamber. 5, Secondary tympanic membrane. 6, Pneumatic cellules in the fundus of the round window niche between the two branches of the fustis. 7, Fustis. 8, Trabecules and spines emerging cranially.

an angle, broadens towards the styloid prominence, and is divided into trabecules running partly parallel or crossing each other. They stand out cranially, and their upper edge is constituted by protrusions and trabecules. They make a further caudal turn back to the styloid prominence because this structure is situated on the floor, rather than on the posterior wall of the tympanic cavity. Occasionally, it occupies the place of the sinus hypotympanicus.

The trabeculocellular fustis is accompanied by similar structures in the infundibular area of the hypotympanum, vallecula, and even the aditus. The sacellus and sustentaculum are also trabecular. The periosteal layer of the promontory is thick, with deep canalicules and fissures. The vessel-free surface of the promontory is also uneven, and is impressed by numerous excavations and fissures. The sinus tympani is well developed and deep, and penetrates downwards to behind the styloid prominence, forming a deep pouch behind the thick body of the pyramidal eminence.

This variant is part of the trabeculocellular structure of the whole tympanic cavity. The fustis is broken in the plane of the chamber entrance. It turns downwards because, on the lower back part of the tympanic cavity, it is located in the area concamerata connecting it with the round window chamber. The jugular fossa is located deeply under the floor of the tympanic cavity. Thus, the jugular wall is thick, and an abundant trabeculocellular structure has been excavated on it by the subepithelial mesenchyme. However, excavations are not too deep, and do not form either thin lobulated plates or extensive cellules. On the other hand, the tympanic sinus is large and deep, especially caudally with smooth walls.

Fustis Dentatus (12.8%)   The promontorial segment of the fustis is doubled in the full length of the chamber. The two parts run parallel in the horizontal direction. The dorsal border of the cranial branch is the sinus tympani process towards the chamber. The cavity of the sinus cuts the bone cylinder vertically at this point. This, in fact, is the genuine fustis as, more caudally, the pars anterior of the fundus bulges in a cylindrical fashion into the chamber causing a structure similar to the fustis. The two fuse in the chamber entrance, and the lower cylinder continues dorsally into the area comcamerata; but instead of inserting into the styloid prominence, it is inserted on the inferior wall of the tympanic ring. The fustis proper is cranially dentated. The postis posterior is a wide, convex column bifurcating on the fundus. One branch turns to the chamber, while the other turns towards the pyramidal eminence. The promontorial process of the sinus tympani cuts between the two, while in its ventral continuation, the free cut edge of the fustis proper is found. The fustis proper is invisible from the meatus (Fig. 259).

Pseudofustis Dentatus.   The plate well isolated from the parallel to the real fustis is termed the *pseudofustis.* It is located caudally to the fustis proper. If its edge is dentated, it is called the *pseudofustis dentatus.*

The pseudofustis is a derivative of the covering bone of the hypotympanic area concamerata built up partly under the guidance of mucosa duplicatures, and partly in the covering bone lamelles of the posterior tympanic artery crossing the hypotympanum from the facial canal. When it develops in intrauterine life, the spines are already supplied with arterioles from either laterally or the fustis proper. This bone formation, therefore, is most likely to be a product of primary angiogenic ossification. On the bony column lying horizontally in the chamber and looking in the absence of any similar structure in the chamber entrance like the fustis, small sharp spines emerge cranially. This bony column differs from the fustis by the similarity of

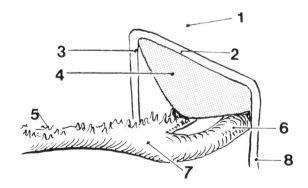

Figure 259. Fustis dentatus. 1, Promontory. 2, Tegmen of the round window niche. 3, Postis posterior. 4, Secondary tympanic membrane. 5, Protrusions on the fustis. 6, Later branch of the fustis inside the chamber. 7, Fustis. 8, Postis anterior. The fustis bifurcating in the chamber is covered by bony protrusions at its stem and medial branch.

spines on both its intrachamber and promontorial, while in the case of the fustis proper, the former site is consistently smooth.

On the entire surface of the tympanic cavity, mostly in the promontorial and infundibular areas of the hypotympanum, sharp spines occur. The jugular wall is of medium thickness, and the sacellus is small, thinly lamellar, and finely dentated at its free edge. The protectum is also constituted by a thin dentated plate. This is found in the vallecula, on the wall of the multicompartmented sinus tympani, on the tympanic cavity surface of the styloid prominence, in the retrotympanic sinus, in the fossa incudis at the basal lamina, on the lamelle edges of the hamulus, and even along the tympanic portion of the facial canal. The promontory is uneven and bumpy, while the subiculum contains a row of bony spines towards the facial brachium.

The pseudofustis dentatus is seen when the sinus tympani has an extension into the round window chamber separating the postis posterior and brachium pyramidale. The part of the fustis outside the chamber is sharply cut off at the base of the above structures. In these cases, the fustis does not continue in the area concamerata. Still, a fustis—a similar but less prominent bony cylinder—may be present running down from the chamber entrance, because the lower segment of the fundus is due to absence of the fustis. In this region, the pavimentum pyramidis fixed on the labyrinthine capsule bulges into the chamber in the direction of the tegmen. The pseudocharacter is underlined by the fact that the pseudofustis adheres with a downward turn to the tympanic ring, and not to the styloid prominence.

Extension of the sinus tympani results in an inverted chamber entrance. The angle between the fundus and postis posterior is acute, while that between the fundus and postis anterior is either a right angle or obtuse (fossula fenestrae rotundae inversa). The missing fustis at the anterior part of the fundus gives room for an insertion of the postis in a right angle. The wide chamber entrance may be narrowed here by the periosteal layer of the promontory. However, the extension of the deep sinus tympani interposed and widened between the postis posterior and brachium pyramidale brings about the situation in the chamber entrance that, from the acoustic meatus, only the cranially compressed trabecule of the brachium pyramidale is visible, forming an acute angle with the chamber floor.

Formation of the pseudofustis is facilitated by the fact that the suture line of the pavimentum pyramidis with the covering bone is usually the ventral edge of the genuine fustis. Thus, the fustis proper originates from the covering bone of the petrosa, while the rest of the hypotympanum and the area concamerata is derived from the pavimentum pyramidis leaning with fine processes on the labyrinth capsule. Virtually another variant is the double fustis, which is double only on its posterior part; in the chamber, only a single fustis is present. However, short of its joining to the styloid prominence, it gives off a recurrent branch towards the chamber. This branch is thinner and more dentated than the fustis proper. It runs closely under (along) the fustis, but in the chamber entrance, it is smaller and deviates towards the postis anterior. The secondary fustis can be regarded as the lower, isolated remnant of the postis anterior that has reached the arch of the fustis due to the horizontal growth of the tympanum.

The pseudofustis dentatus may also be the result of a pathologic process. It may develop after acute or chronic ear inflammations in the richly structured area concamerata of the round window niche. The stylomastoid, posterior, and anterior tympanic arteries are anastomosing abundantly. Along these anastomoses—under favorable trophic, hormonal, vitamin-metabolic, and vascular conditions of the bone—tissue-pronounced trabecules and lamellas develop. Diseases of the tympanum may destroy these structures. Either rows of tubercles are left behind, or the tubercles are formed by the osteogenic infection itself. The resulting strange bone structures may mimic the genuine fustis not only in its course, but also in its inframicroscopic morphology. Its occurrence is along the vascular anastomoses.

Fustis Latus (12.6%). The fustis may reach a width by which it occupies almost the whole chamber entrance. Its course within the chamber is short due to its immediate adhesion to the labyrinth capsule and the scala tympani of the basal turn of the cochlea. Similarly short is its dorsal part outside the chamber, because the styloid prominence is quite near to the promontory, which gives a place dorsally, on the place of the retrofenestral sinus, for a narrow sinus tympani. The wide fustis is thus short as well as wide, and narrows the frame of the round window. It forms a smooth osseous wall starting from its insertion to the cochlea. This wall also corresponds to the medial wall of the tunnel. The part of the fustis latus outside the chamber is uneven or trabecular. In the latter case, the chamber may also show a trabecular structure or ramification; but the surface of this region is smoother than that of the tympanic region, and it is always found closer to the postis posterior. Rarely, in the plane of the chamber entrance, the fustis is narrowed by grooves, lacunes, and cellules at both of its sides. In these cases, a similar cellularization is seen on and around the dorsal part of the fustis. The fustis inserts on the cranial end of the styloid prominence by thick trabecules. These thick trabecules form an intricate network of bone structures with cellules located between them. The fustis and this trabecular network constitute the floor of the sinus tympani, deepening cranially above the styloid prominence while its lower segment continues without transition into the hypotympanum, where the randomly located, pronounced trabecules yield a characteristic pattern (Fig. 260).

Along with the fustis latus, a narrow, long sinus tympani is observed with an uneven styloid prominence extending deep into the tympanic cavity, a thick solid sustentaculum, and a similarly thick periosteal layer on the promontory. From the promontorial apex, a spine often emerges in the direction of the nearby styloid prominence.

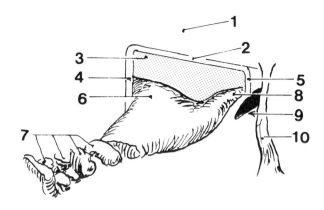

Figure 260. Fustis latus. 1, Promontory. 2, Tegmen of the round window niche. 3, Secondary tympanic membrane. 4, Postis posterior. 5, Postis anterior. 6, Medial branch of the fustis in the chamber. 7, Parts of the fustis. 8, Lateral branch of the fustis inside the chamber. 9, Tunnel of the promontory. 10, Sustentaculum promontorii.

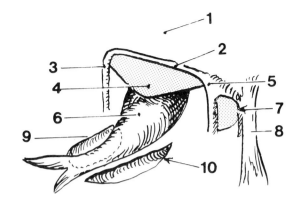

Figure 261. Fustis pisciformis. 1, Promontory. 2, Tegmen of the round window niche. 3, Postis posterior. 4, Secondary tympanic membrane. 5, Postis anterior. 6, Fustis. 7, Tunnel of the promontory. 8, Sustentaculum promontorii. 9, Elongated medial sinus concameratus. 10, Elongated lateral sinus concameratus.

The fustis latus is due to the moderate opening of the tympanic cavity in the horizontal direction. The covering bone substance of the tympanum is thicker than usual. The bulky trabecules of the fustis, styloid prominence, and hypotympanum are a product of specific subepithelial mesenchymal and osteoblastic activities.

Fustis Pisciformis (11.8%). This adult variant resembles the former one. The fustis is wide in the chamber, and narrows gradually dorsally and shortly to the styloid prominence. It takes the form of a fish tail by ramifying into trabecules with which it joins to the bumpy, moderately developed styloid prominence. From the postis posterior, united trabecules run to the pyramidal eminence. This plate may occasionally be perforated at the trabecule adhesions. It separates the retrofenestral sinus from the sinus tympani. Under the trabecular plate, between it and the tympanic segement of the fustis, a deep groove is found that causes the thinning of the base of the fish tail formation. A similar sulcus is located in the sinus tympani, which continues caudally without transition into the area concamerata (Fig 261).

The postis anterior is open and sends a thin dentated plate to the chamber entrance. The sustentaculum is low and short. The promontory has an uneven surface. Apart from the fustis, the area concamerata is a smooth bone surface, but the promontorial and infundibular areas are packed with plates and trabecules. Their structures are trabeculocellular. This is a feature of the aditus, as well where the fossa of the incus is covered by a meshwork of ventral trabecules. The basement lamina is doubled—trabecular with well-developed cellules. A large, deep, basally trabecular infrabasal sinus and a similar retropyramidal sinus are present. The hamuli are also trabecular. The jugular fossa bulges high into the tympanic cavity. The jugluar wall is the thinnest at its part underlying the fustis. This gives a different character to the different areas.

The fustis may be fish-shaped when the sinus tympani fuses with the hypotympanum and the jugular fossa bulges into the tympanic cavity, so that its cranial-most part appears in the area concamerata. The tympanic end of the fustis is narrowed by two grooves, and its dorsal end is connected to the styloid prominence with diverging trabecules. Should this *tail* not contain an isolated narrow portion, more structures would appear around the fustis in the deep area concamerata. The trabecular nature of the dorsal end of the fustis is a general trend in the tympanic cavity, as it is found throughout from the aditus to the tube funnel. It seems that a certain abundance of tissue requires a proportional subepithelial mesenchymal activity (osteoblast and osteoclast function) to produce the generally moderate trabecular appearance of the tympanum.

Fustis Triangularis (6.6%). The triangular fustis is positioned in the round window chamber, with one angle leaning onto the labyrinth capsule at the lower posterior apex of the scala. From here, an initially slender trabecule begins, widening gradually by leaving the chamber for the fundus. The upper angle of the triangle is between the postis posterior and brachium pyramidale, while the lower is on the fundus at the level of the postis anterior. Both dorsal angles give rise to an irregular, slender trabecule running to the styloid prominence. The edges of the triangular fustis are rounded off, and its lateral surface is also convex and smooth. The sides of the triangle are demarcated from its surrounding by deep grooves. The deepest one is the sulcus limiting the lower ventral wall, because it slightly undermines the fustis and continues into the tunnel, which is narrow but deep and lamellar. The shallowest one is the sulcus above the cranial side where the fustis approaches the ventral process of the postis posterior.

The postis posterior is the thickest one towards the fundus of the chamber, narrowing cranially. This groove continues from behind the postis down to the fundus, forming a short incisure above the ventral process of the postis. Thus, in the chamber, not only the fustis, but also the postis anterior, appears isolated from its surrounding. Between the zig-zag trabecules leading from the two dorsal angles of the triangle to the styloid prominence, a sharp-edged excavation is found permeated towards the styloid prominence by irregular plates and trabecules. The postis anterior meets the fundus in a right angle. Dorsal to it, a dentated lamelle extends to the tympanic ring. The sustentaculum is caudally a full canal, but it opens upwards. From its cranial edge, a slender dentated plate runs parallel with the plate of the postis anterior to the tympanic ring (Fig. 262).

Accompanying the triangular fustis, not only the chamber structures and area concamerata, but also the other parts of the tympanic cavity, are compartmentalized. This rare appearance of the tympanic cavity is seen mostly in childhood (the preparation shown is derived from an eight-year-old child). The jugular fossa does not bulge high into the tympanic cavity; all three hypotympanic areas are densely packed with trabecular and irregular thin lamelles. The sinus tympani is small, reaching deeply below the pyramidal eminence, but it ends short of the dorsal plate of postis posterior. The promontory is dorsally elongated, the sacellus is bordered by wide, thin plates, and the protectum is formed by slender trabecules. The vallecula has a cellular structure.

The triangular fustis is seen in childhood because, at this time, the hypotympanum is rich in structures and the whole tympanic cavity is in a state of dynamic changes. The subepithelial mesenchyme actively shapes the covering bone of the tympanic cavity. The position of the labyrinth capsule relative to its surrounding is not yet finalized. The

jugular wall is also in development; the jugular fossa has not yet reached its final configuration. Enhanced osteoclastic activity demarcates the fustis from its neighborhood. This extraordinary compartmentalization does not necessarily disappear by adulthood. The size and course of structures and grooves and angles between them modify until a lesser degree of compartmentalization is attained. Accordingly, the triangular fustis may also occur in adults, but in a more elongated and less isolated, irregular form.

Fustis Arcuatus (6%).   The labyrinthine and tympanic portions of the fustis, instead of meeting in an angle, bend in a downward arch from the chamber entrance caudodorsally to the styloid prominence. The fustis is lower inside the chamber. Peripherally, the fustis gradually becomes higher, reaching its highest point at the promontorial insertion. The chamber is low, and the styloid prominence is rudimentary. Its surface is smooth. The limit of the fustis is indicated by a shallow groove. The body of the pyramidal eminence is connected to the promontory be a similarly arcuate plate—the *ponticulus lamellosus.* Above it, a retrofenestral sinus, under a deep, smooth sinus tympani, is encountered.

Downward, the sinus tympani is limited by the styloid prominence and fustis. The sinus extends deeply behind the prominence and the pyramidal eminence. From the insertion of the fustis to the styloid prominence, a plate runs to the lower insertion of the postis anterior. The plate has a dentated edge and gradually lowers towards the promontory, delimiting together with the fustis and chamber entrance a triangular area of the area concamerata. The triangle continues towards the labyrinth in the chamber entrance and constitutes the fundus of the chamber (Fig. 263).

The jugular wall has a thin, smooth, bony surface. Trabecules and small plates are found only in the concamerata and infundibular areas. From the dorsal aspect of the postis anterior, a protrusion having a wide base stands out towards the styloid prominece. The sustentaculum is canaliculized, but it does not emerge above the level of its surrounding. The canalicules of the promontory are deeply engraved, and the edge of the grooves are obtuse.

The arcuate fustis develops when the pavimentum pyramidis also joins in an arch to the posteriorly covering bone of the tympanic cavity. The cranial segment of the styloid prominence starts to develop later than the lower segment, and the dynamics of development dislocate the peripheral insertion of the fustis caudoventrally. The promontory is covered by a rich periosteal layer. The jugular fossa bulges deeply, causing a thin jugular wall. Therefore, the hypotympanum is poor in bone structures. The cranial edge of the fustis is isolated by the intrachamber extension of the sinus tympani.

Fustis Cristatus (5.6%).   In the wide chamber, the fustis runs a horizontal course, turns sharply at the level of the chamber, and bends in an arch to its insertion on the styloid prominence. The intratympanic portion of the fus-

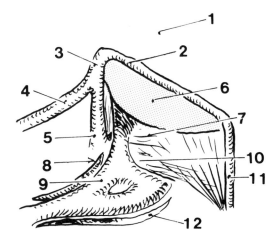

Figure 262.   Fustis triangularis. 1, Promontory. 2, Tegmen of the round window niche. 3, Postis posterior. 4, Pyramidal arm. 5 and 7, Arciform plate of the fundus of the round window niche under and above the fustis. 6, Secondary tympanic membrane. 9, Triangular fustis with a central excavation. 10, Cranioventral edge of the widening fustis. 11, Postis anterior. 8 and 12, Grooves at the edge of the fustis in the area concamerata.

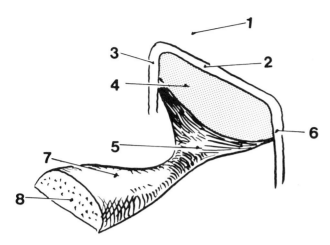

Figure 263. Fustis arcuatus. 1, Promontory. 2, Tegmen of the round window niche. 3, Postis posterior. 4, Secondary tympanic membrane. 5, Cranially arcuate part of the fustis. 6, Postis anterior. 7, Stem of the fustis. 8, Cross-sectioned fustis.

tis is a narrow, high plate forming an upwards open acute angle with the tympanic cavity floor. The free edge of the plate is regularly dentated. The cristiform fustis and styloid prominence constitute the inferior edge of the sinus tympani. Directed towards the highest protrusion of the crest, a spine emerges from the promontory edge. The upper part of the fundus is deepened by the extension of the sinus tympani, while the lower part is wide, and well demarcated from the fustis. This is the reason why the fustis is emerging high into the tympanic cavity and on the area of the fundus. It is widened and flattened inside the chamber. Beneath the tympanic segment of the fustis, the area concamerata is occasionally packed with minor plates and crests.

A well-discernible groove separates the fustis from the styloid prominence, but its insertion to the prominence widens so that it forms a separate part—the *pars concamerata* of the prominence. The high crest formation may be explained by the accumulation of osseous substance at the joint line between the upper bony cover of the tympanic cavity and pavimentum pyramidis. At the free cranial edge, the protrusions are brought about either by blood supply or by osteogenetic factors. The role of the latter is supported by the similar morphologies of the area infundibularis, sacellus, and protectum.

Fustis Duplex (4.6%). On the chamber floor, two genuine fustes are found. One of them joins the angle of the scala tympani and vestibuli of the cochlea, while the other joins the lower lateral wall of the scala tympani. The upper fustis is higher and wider at its ventral end; the lower fustis flattens ventrally and does not extend to the plate of the scala tympani, but forms a sharp angle with it. In the plane of the chamber, the two fustes are of equal size. They are almost fused towards the styloid prominence, but separate again dorsally from there. The upper fustis runs a course towards the body of the pyramidal eminence and, when reaching it,

turns sharply downwards, where it widens and adheres to the rudimentary styloid prominence. The lower fustis is a continuation of the pars labyrinthine. It is flattened when it meets the styloid prominence.

In between the peripheral ends of the two fustes, a major cavity is found. The upper fustis forms the marked edge of the short, doubled sinus tympani, penetrating to behind the upper part of the pyramidal eminence. The sinus has an extension into the upper part of the chamber. The aditus contains irregular trabecular structures. The protectum consists of a row of protrusions. The sacellus is bordered by a small, ventrally bending plate. The vallecula is flat. Spines emerge towards the promontory from the carotid wall. The jugular wall is a thin plate. The sustentaculum is wide, pronounced, canaliculized, and fused with the postis anterior. The latter is indicated on the fundus by a small spine emerging from insertion of the sustentaculum towards the chamber.

The sustentaculum and lower fustis are connected with an uneven plate; thus, there is no room for tunnel formation at this site. However, the tunnel can be found ventrally to the sustentaculum, where it begins with a narrow opening, runs deep to the basal turn of the cochlea, and is covered towards the area promontorialis of the hypotympanum by an irregular plate strengthened at some places with trabecules (Fig. 264).

From the developmental point of view, the double fustis is explained by the development of a wide fustis in a wide round window chamber. The covering bony plate of the pavimentum pyramidis leaning upon the sacculocochlear part of the labyrinth joins the covering bone of the petrosa, so that in the suture line, a covering bony substance is accumulated. The wide fustis in the wide chamber entrance later thins out due to formation of pneumatic cellules

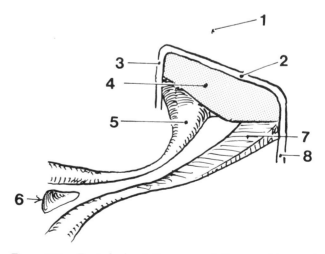

Figure 264. Fustis duplex. 1, Promontory. 2, Tegmen of the round window niche. 3, Postis posterior. 4, Secondary tympanic membrane. 5, Fustis running to the postis posterior. 6, Large pneumatic cavity between the dorsally separated fustis-partis. 7, Fustis running to the postis anterior. 8, Postis anterior.

beginning from the sinus tympani. Thus, on the fustis, a shallow longitudinal sulcus results. Subephithelial mesenchymal activity is lower in the chamber entrance; therefore, the two fustis components join tightly together, whereas dorsally the fustis widens due to the osteogenic effect of arterioles arising from the stylomastoid artery, which produces a hollow cavity in the fustis and divides it into two definite parts. The medial fustis joins the bony capsule of the pyramidal eminence as its closest structure. Later, however, the two are separated by the caudal expansion of the sinus tympani.

The abundant periosteal layer of the promontory forms a tunnel ventrally to the sustentaculum, because the sustentaculum is connected to the labyrinth capsule by a continuous plate that the tunnel cannot penetrate under the promontory. Nevertheless, it is the abundant periosteal bone connecting the labyrinth to the hypotympanum that allows room for the subepithelial mesenchyme to excavate a well-developed tunnel ventrally to the sustentaculum. This variant suggests that tunnel formation is marked between the labyrinth capsule and hypotympanum. In this process, a role is attributed to the distribution of the periosteal layer, to the depth of the floor of the tympanic cavity (i.e., the position of the jugular fossa), and to mesenchymal activity.

Fustis Lamellosus (2.6%). The promontorial end of the fustis may occasionally bifurcate in a fork-like fashion and adhere to the cochlea. Its intrachamber part is wide, smooth surfaced and turns sharply in the plane of the chamber entrance or slightly dorsally to it, bending laterally to run in an arch to the styloid prominence. The part outside the chamber differs markedly from the intrachamber portion. From the turn, it is thinning dorsally; and by reaching the area concamerata, it is a perpendicular plate with a trabecular structure at its midportion. Holes between trabecules are round or ellipsoid. The plate forms a cranially open angle with the styloid prominence, and covers its ventromedial aspect. Cranially towards the sinus tympani and area concamerata, respectively, trabecules of different length ramify from it that are, at some places, curved and surround cellules on the tympanic floor (Fig. 265).

Similar to its previous variant, the sinus tympani is large, extending deeply behind and under the styloid prominence and pyramidal eminence. However, the wall of the sinus is more uneven. Also uneven is the surface of the styloid prominence, with major cellules and plates. The structure of the area infundibularis of the hypotympanum is lamellar. In the area promontorialis, plates are found parallel to the fundus. They are directed dorsally; their prominent free edge is dentated, with small cellules underneath communicating through narrow openings with the tympanic cavity.

The postis anterior is also lamellar. The sustentaculum is an open canal, the protectum is dentated, and the saccellus is deep and bordered ventrally by a thin plate, the free edge of which is dentated. In the vallecula, parallel plates are seen perpendicularly to the walls and bridging the space between the two bony surfaces. The pyramidal eminence

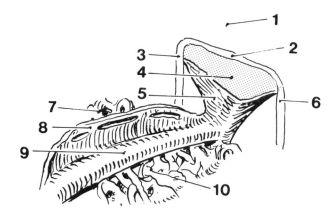

Figure 265. Fustis lamellosus. 1, Promontory. 2, Tegmen of the round window niche. 3, Postis posterior. 4, Secondary tympanic membrane. 5, Round window frame in the continuation of the fustis. 6, Postis anterior. 7, Pneumatic cavities surrounded by trabecules above the fustis. 8, Perforated plate extending cranially from the fustis. 9, Fustis. 10, Pneumatic cavities surrounded by trabecules under the fustis.

is connected to the subiculum by a cranially curved, thin ponticulus. The jugular fossa is deep, and the jugular wall is thick. Thus, also at other tympanic cavity sites, we find similar situations as on the fustis. The turn of the fustis is also caused by the bulging into the tympanic cavity of the styloid prominence. The approaching to the promontory of the posterior tympanic wall may have happened in a developmental stage, when such a process had resulted not in bone resorption, but in the bending of structures. This is supported by the cranial curvature of the ponticulus and the lamellar part of the fustis.

Mucosa Duplicatures

Mucosa formations in the round window chamber show a wide range of variations. These are classified according to localization and extent as follows:

1. The round window chamber is lined throughout with a single layer of mucosa. No duplicatures occur.

The simple duplicature-free mucosal lining of the chamber entrance is a state characteristic of puberty and adulthood. In embryonic and infant chambers, duplicatures surrounding the mesenchyme that are accumulated perivascularly are seen rather frequently. Mucosa duplicatures are common, particularly in the sixth or seventh intrauterine month, when the tympanic cavity is formed and the tubotympanic epithelium has shaped the aditus and antrum. At this gestational age, most frequent are mucosa duplicatures that bridge both the round window chamber and the sinus tympani. They are occasionally parallel to the fundus, but run more often in an oblique direction. In such cases, the lateral edge of the wide mucosa duplicatures is a twig forming an anastomosis between the stylomastoid and inferior tympanic arteries, and connecting the tegmen of the round window niche to the styloid prominence.

From here, the duplicature runs obliquely to the facial brachium or ponticulus medialis. Around the blood vessel, angiogenic ossification is induced that later degenerates. The isolated trabecules between the chamber roof and fustis or postis anterior are formed in a similar fashion. In adults, mucosa duplicatures are met with the following embryonic remnants (mucosal duplicatures):

2. *Minor mucosa duplicatures connecting the angles in various directions.*

3. *Mucosal duplicatures that cover the chamber entrance longitudinally.* On these obliterating mucosa duplicatures always present are smaller, round, ellipsoid, or semilunar holes.

4. *Mucosa duplicatures that cross the chamber transversely.* These duplicatures originate either on the convexity or on the lower uneven portions of the fustis and run to the tegmen.

5. *Narrow duplicatures between the postes and the posterior wall of the tympanic cavity.* These narrow further towards the styloid prominence. Spines and protrusions inside the duplicature may elongate and emit from the edge of the promontory along trabecules resembling the ponticulus.

6. *A frequently observed duplicature type found at the lower part of the chamber entrance in the angle between the postis anterior and fundus.* These duplicatures connect protrusions.

7. *Mucosal duplicatures covering partly or totally the tunnel entrance into the chamber.* The tunnel of the promontory is known to be open not only towards the chamber, but also towards the infundibular area and promontory. Thus, the ventilation of the tunnel is ensured in cases when its entrance in the round window chamber is covered by a mucosa duplicature.

8. *Plexiform, irregular mucosa duplicatures inside the round window chamber.* Mucosa duplicatures and plates connect not only osseous structures to each other, but also form mucosa-to-mucosa links. Thus, they may also be secondary. In some cases, the abundant plexus, with its labyrinthine appearance, almost covers the chamber entrance.

In fresh preparations, blood vessels are easily seen through the mucosa duplicature. As judged by their arrangement, the duplicatures receive twigs mainly from the stylomastoid and inferior tympanic arteries. However, twigs are met coming from the promontory, tegmen of the chamber, postis posterior, anterior tympanic, and pyramidial arteries.

Blood Supply

The round window niche receives twigs mainly from the stylomastoid, inferior tympanic, and anterior tympanic arteries.

From the stylomastoid artery, three groups of arterioles run to the round window chamber. Most of them leave the facial canal on the body and aperture of the pyramidal eminence through various perforating holes. Twigs pass through the sinus tympani; some turn to the postis pos-terior and others to the chamber floor, where they supply the medial aspect of the fustis and medial sinus concameratus. Twigs ascending on the postis posterior also supply the tegmen of the round window niche as they run parallel to its edge and enter the chamber. The posterior tympanic artery originates from the stylomastoid artery through the external aperture of the chordal canalicule, and runs to the postis anterior. From there, it passes to the tegmen of the round window niche, where it anastomoses with the inferior tympanic artery. However, the chamber receives direct twigs from the stylomastoid via perforations in the facial canal.

From the inferior tympanic artery, twigs reach the round window chamber from two directions. One group is found on the sustentaculum, and comes from the hypotympanum to reach the postis anterior of the chamber. The other leaves the vascular trunk at the promontorial apex and mainly supplies the tegmen of the round window niche. They also give off branches that cross the tegmen and enter the chamber.

Small branches of the tympanic artery supply the chamber roof, where they anastomose with the branches of the stylomastoid and inferior tympanic arteries. Some minor twigs contribute to the supply of the postis posterior.

The functional anatomy of osseous elements of the fenestra rotunda are summarized as follows:

1. The window chamber protects the labyrinth window. This protective effect is ensured partly by accessory structures and partly by the own elements of the chamber forming an excavation containing in its depth the secondary tympanic membrane.

2. The postes anterior and posterior ensure the height of the chamber. The size and shape of the round window chamber depends primarily on the dimensions, mainly height, of these structures. If the postes are low, the chamber is elongated. High postes, particularly if located near to each other, elongate cranially the chamber entrance.

3. The postis posterior is built together with the subiculum; thus, in addition to the chamber, it also participates in support of the pars sacculocochlearis.

4. The ventral process of the postis posterior connects the basal turn of the cochlea to the pavimentum pyramidis and the covering bone of the pars petrosa.

5. The posterior process of the postis posterior sends a strengthening plate to the fundus of the sinus tympani. This covering bone process adheres usually to the pyramidis eminence or facial canal, and its long trabecule supports statically the back portion of the tympanic cavity.

6. The fossa triangularis—a frequently occurrent excavation between the postis posterior and fustis—forms shallow pneumatic cavities around structures of static function thereby decreasing the weight of the bone.

7. The fustis is one of the most important trabecules of the posterior tympanum. It supports the promontory by fastening it to the covering bone structures of the posterior tympanum or styloid prominence.

8. The frame of the fenestra is not fully vertical, but it stands obliquely from up to down and ventrally. This posi-

tion is particularly pronounced in the infant and young children. This ensures that sound energy reaching the round window is smaller than that reaching the stapes foot plate since the pressure difference between the two improves sound perception.

9.   The postis anterior is more unstable than the postis posterior, since its function in supporting the cochlea is greatly overtaken by a nearby pronounced bone structure—the *sustentaculum*.

10.   The role of the medial and lateral sinus concamerata is to decrease bone weight under balanced statics and well-developed postes and fustis. The role played by these larger cellules of the tympanic cavity, which at the inframicroscopic level appear as sinuses in the resonance of the tympanic cavity, is still obscure.

11.   The tegmen fossulae fenstrae rotundae is a ridge of varying width of the promontorial periosteal layer that hides and protects the round window. The wider the periosteal layer of the promontory, the more hidden and protected is the secondary tympanic membrane.

12.   The distance between the postes and the opening of the covering bone of the chamber also serves to protect the secondary tympanic membrane. In neonates and infants the opening is larger, as well as the relative distance between the postes; thus, the chamber entrance is wider compared to that in the adult. The position of the window frame is also more oblique. The oblique postion of the window frame in neonates and infants also serves to protect the secondary tympanic membrane. In adults, the window chamber is more exposed, as the secondary tympanic membrane stands more obliquely; nevertheless, protection is achieved by a narrower entrance.

Pathology

Despite ontogenic situations, the position and structures of the round window chamber favor pathologic processes.

1.   The chamber is a deep excavation of the posterior tympanum that is suitable for storing exudate. The influx of exudate into the chamber is facilatated by the nearby sinus tympani, often forming a cavity that is common with the chamber.

2.   The round window chamber is, under certain conditions, a favorable background for the formation of abundant granulation tissue. During our procedures, we have observed that when the posterior part of the tympanic cavity (i.e., the sinus tympani, sinus retrofenestralis, and area concamerata) is filled with chronic inflammatory or granulation tissue, tissues of similar type fill in and obliterate the round window chamber.

3.   In inflammations accompanied by bone softening or necrosis, these can be readily diagnosed on the covering bone substance of the promontory and in the hypotympanum after adequate exposure via steromicroscopic examination reveals bone softening and/or destruction on the postes, fustis, and ridge of the chamber tegmen.

4.   In chronic, progressive inflammations, pseudomembrane formation occurs at the posterior edge of the chamber that can be mistaken for the secondary tympanic membrane. Between the pseudomembrane covering the chamber and the secondary tympanic membrane, granulation tissue is found; the exudate is drained towards the tympanic cavity through a pinhole-sized opening.

5.   As a residue to tympanic cavity inflammations, connective tissue bundles may be formed between the fustis and tegmen and between the postes and tegmen. These bundles do not fully separate the round window chamber from the tympanic cavity; however, granulation tissue develops behind them.

6.   In chronic cholesteatomas the pathologic tissue filling the sinus tympani often invades the chamber of the round window. The destructive process widens and deepens the chamber. Similar bone destructions were often found before the advent of chemotherapy and antibiotics. They were particularly frequent in scarlatina otitis that destroyed the chamber walls, thereby widening the chamber.

7.   Before the era of modern pharmaceuticals bone necrosis—coupled to severe acute diseases and cholesteatomatous chronic infections—was often seen to destroy even the window frame, thus opening the scala tympani and causing deafness.

8.   After the cessation of inflammation, similar to other covering bone structures, the covering bone substance of the round window chamber shows osteogenesis. Newly formed osseous structures, however, never perfectly replace the destroyed covering bone. To osteogenetic infections, the inframicroscopic bone elements of the round window chamber respond as follows:

a.   The postis posterior thickens and fuses with surrounding structures such as the subiculum, chamber fundus, and sinus tympani. However, as a result of osteogenesis, the orignally smooth surface of the postis posterior becomes uneven.

b.   In the postis anterior, osteogenesis takes place on a minor scale compared to the postis posterior. Destroyed covering bone substance of this territory regenerates only moderately, and the earlier inflammation is earmarked by lacerated bone protrusions and randomly distributed bone tubercles. Much less frequent is the situation in which osteogenesis narrows from the direction of the postis anterior both the chamber and tunnel entrance. The blood supply of the postis anterior is usually better than that of the postis posterior. There is circumstantial evidence for the destruction of vessels provided by the moderate osteogenetic reaction of the postis anterior to infections.

c.   After inflammatory bone destructions, the fustis may be lacerated, irregular, sharply dentated, or tuberous. The latter is explained by the better blood supply of the structure.

d.   In response to osteogenetic infection, a row of bone tubercles is found on the fundus. It seems that at this site, a trabecule or plate used to be present earlier, and the row of tubercles is formed by osteogenesis following destruction of the original structures.

e.   The morphology of tegmen may also change. After the cessation of the inflammatory process, the tegmen becomes narrower, and its surface is dentated and uneven.

f.   Cords of cicatrix formed after inflammation may ossify, resulting in curved trabecules or irregularly dentated plates that narrow the chamber.

9. Osteogensis following the inflammatory process may deform the entire chamber. As a consequence, the entrance of the chamber becomes narrow.

10. In tympanoscleroses, the calcified or ossified cicatrix filling in the sinus tympani invades the chamber, forming a cast of it to the edges by a pseudomembrane.

11. In otosclerosis, the newly formed otospongiosis starting from the enchondral layer of the otic capsule may partly or totally fill the chamber.

Diagnostics

In the case of the round window chamber, which is similar to the stapes chamber, a thorough chamber diagnostic examination should always be performed when possible. A good survey of the chamber is facilitated by a wide promontoriofacial recess and obliquely positioned chamber.

Chamber diagnostics should cover the following points:

1. *Chamber structure.* In an obliquely positioned round window chamber, structures of the postes, tegmen, and fundus can readily be diagnosed.

The height, width, and trabecular or cellular build-up of the postis posterior can be inspected. Observable is the structure, openings, and plates of the postis anterior, as well as its relationship with the sustentaculum and fustis. The relationship between the fustis and postes, cavities of the fundus, medial and lateral sinus concamerata can all be checked. The latter are especially of surgical importance.

2. *Pathologic alterations of chamber structures.* When surveying the bone structures, the shape and extent of destruction, the advance of osteogenesis, and its morphology are to be diagnosed. From the prognostic point of view, the morphology, localization, and extent of osseous stubstance filling the chamber should be checked so that the progress of the process can be assessed. Destruction of the postis anterior is indicated by uneven, irregular surfaces, sharp plate edges, and acute protrusions. The appearance of smooth-surfaced tubercles and obtuse edges, suggests that the process came to a standstill and the reparative osteogenesis has just begun. The completion of osteogenesis is shown by the lack of edges and a row of tubercles replacing the destroyed bone. Intense covering bone hypertrophy narrows or even fills in the chamber, altering its shape and normal morphology of constituent structures.

3. *Chamber diagnostics should also include the observation of pathologic soft tissues in the chamber.* Transparent, small, spheroid granulation tissue pieces are indicative of an active process. Thin pseudomembranes that connect structure and abridge cavities suggest the resting phase of a subacute inflammation. Sclerotic cicatrix and solid connective tissue outgrowth occur mostly in tympanosclerosis, progressive inflammations, and torpid processes, when (as suggested by our experience) signs of periodically recurrent or exacerbating inflammations can be seen at other sites of the inner ear. In tympanosclerosis, white, granulated plaques filling the ex-

cavations of the chamber and the medial and lateral sinus concamerata were often seen. The plaque was fixed elastically to its environment, and was easily removable from the floor of the sinus. Calcified plaques were also observed. A similar type of sclerosis was encountered in the membrane sustentaculopostica of a 72-year-old man. In the elderly, nonsclerotic, transparent, well-vascularized membranes connecting covering bone elements are quite common at other tympanic cavity sites; for example, in the area infundibularis, it is presumed that mucosa duplicatures remaining from embryronic life may—when blood supply is adequate—cicatrize and show sclerotic appostions without a total destruction.

In a destroyed round window chamber, cholesteatoma is often observed. This pathologic proliferation of epithelium starts in the stapes chamber, from which it invades first the sinus tympani, and then the fenestra rotunda chamber. Cholesteatomas destroying the secondary tympanic membrane were not encountered. In chronic ear diseases, osteogenesis narrowing the chamber protects the perilymphatic space and valuable ectodermal neuroepithelium of the cochlea. A frequently seen surgical artifact is the coagualte filling the chamber. This can readily be sucked out.

4. *A diagnostic test of paramount importance is the examination of the round window chamber reflex, which is a condition sine qua non of functional diagnostics.* The stapes is left *in situ,* and the vestibulum is closed; that is prior to any decision as to the way (of tympanoplastics) in which the stapedovestibular articulation is gently moved with a probe, while the scar and granulation tissue and coagulate filling in the round window chamber are watched under a surgical stereomicroscope. In the case of a positive chamber reflex, the smallest movement in the fenestra vestibuli alters the light refexion of soft tissues in the chamber and causes a characteristic glitter. If so, any procedure inside the stapes chamber, from the simplest placing of cartialge columella to a stapedectomy or vestibulum covering, may be performed with hope of success. On the contrary, when a chamber reflex cannot be evoked, any kind of function-restoring tympanoplastic surgery is useless.

Surgery in the Round Window Chamber

Prior to surgery planned in the round window chamber, visibility must be ensured. No insight into the round window chamber is obtained if the osseous sound-conducting wall is left intact. Exceptional are the cases where the posterior wall of the sound conductor has a straight course and the promontory is ventrally far from the sound conductor. The visibility is better if the chamber is oblique and widens, while it is difficult if the chamber is vertical and narrow. In conservative tympanoplastics, one of the important steps of surgery is ensuring visibility in the direction of the stapes and round window chambers.

Diagnostic and surgical aspects of the round window chamber are dealt with separately, because despite their close correlation, surgery must always be preceded by a careful chamber diagnostics examination.

The understanding of inframicroscopic surgical principles of the round window chamber facilitates the decision regarding minor procedures within the chamber. As is well known, the secondary tympanic membrane does not fully occupy the chamber; caudally, from the chamber fundus, it is slightly elevated. The explanation for this elevation and the kidney-shaped frame is the formation of the lower edge of the window frame by the upward convex ridges of the postis posterior and fustis. The two ridges meet in an angle in the five-month-old fetus. Later, the postis posterior is dislocated dorsomedially, the angle between the two ridges is filled in with covering bone, and most of the window frame is occupied by the plate of the fustis, widening in a fan-like fashion. The window is thus protected because:

1. From the fundus, the window frame extends cranially; therefore, the secondary tympanic membrane approaches the tegmen of the fossula fenestrae rotundae.
2. The tegmen has a posteriorly directed ridge that often hampers the approaching and surveying of the membrane.
3. The position of the chamber does not favor surgical introduction of an instrument into the chamber, which is not easy from the tympanic cavity or the aditus.
4. The chamber entrance is narrowed by the various sizes of the fustis to an extent that even an aspirator often cannot be introduced. With a fine tympanic cavity aspirator, the fustis can be avoided, but this is not used in and around the chamber. A thin, elastic aspirator can be forced into the chamber; and through the thin membrane, the scala tympani of the perilymphatic space can be reached.
5. The chamber may be narrowed by osteogenesis, especially in chronic ear diseases and otosclerosis, which may fill the whole chamber and cause either alone or together with the osteosclerotic focus of the stapes chamber a conduction-type decay of hearing.

When choosing from the most frequently used instruments, the secondary tympanic membrane may be pierced with the above-mentioned fine tympanic aspirator, tympano-plastic hook, curved raspatory 000-curette, No. 2 to 4 spheric drill, or curved fine tympanic forceps. The hazard of the fine tympanic cavity aspirator is that it not only pierces, but also aspirates.

Procedures inside the chamber can be considered in two groups.

Procedures on Soft Tissues.   Under this point, we note the removal of physiologically and/or pathologically formed soft tissues. The chamber must be freed of excess soft tissue, even if there is no destruction or obliteration. Structures to be removed are:

1. Mucosa duplicatures between bone elements, because they may be the starting sites of recidivistic inflammation. The membrana sustentaculopostica is removed together with its osseous frame by a drill; then the chamber is rinsed with physiologic saline solution and aspirated.

2. Full or partial pseudomembranes running parallel to the secondary tympanic membrane must be removed with great caution from the chamber entrance, because they insert—particularly at the dorsomedial portion of the chamber—near the membrane. Behind the large obliterating pseudomembranes—between them and the secondary tympanic membrane—usually chronic inflammatory granulation tissue and serous exudate are found. For removal, a tympanic raspatory is recommended.
3. Most difficult is the removal of adhesive scars. These may occur randomly and abridge the chamber from all directions. They can be removed from their adhesions by hooks.
4. Thin granulation tissue plates covered with tympanic cavity epithelium are to be freed from their osseous frames with fine dissectors, hooks, and raspatory, and then removed by a forceps.
5. Edematous inflammatory sprouts can usually be removed by aspiration. From their insertion, they can be lifted away with a fine tympanic forceps.
6. Sclerotic plaques fixed peripherally with soft tissue are readily removable with fine-needle dissectors, and can be lifted out with a tympanic cavity forceps.

Bone Surgery.   Osseous substance of the round window chamber requires resection if: (1) it serves for insertion of pathologic soft elements; (2) active bone process can be verified; and (3) accumulated bone obliterates totally or partially the chamber. *Beware of the secondary tympanic membrane.* Here, also, caution has to be exercised mainly on the territory of the postis posterior, as the window frame is in the proximity of this structure.

The hazard of damage to the secondary tympanic membrane is much less at the territories of:

1. The postis anterior.
2. The tunnel entrance.
3. The sustentaculum.
4. The posterior part of the fustis (pars tympanica); that is, outside the chamber. Covering bone structures need resection if they are destroyed or form cavities surrounding pathologic soft tissue, as is the case with the sinus concamerata medialis and lateralis. In the case of the pronounced, bulky pavimentum pyramidis, the pneumatic cavities of the fundus are surrounded and/or filled by bleeding soft tissue sprouts. Their walls must be resected and their contents removed.

In cholesteatomatous processes, the pathologic accumulation of epithelia filling the fossa fenestrae rotundae is hidden in the fossa triangularis, the recess under the tegmen, and the angle between the postes and secondary tympanic membrane. This pathologic aggregate can generally be removed by an aspirator without major difficulties. Also in these cases, attention should be given to the lacerated, softened, or necrotic surfaces and pathologic bone formations, to cellules or trabecules of the postis anterior, to the tunnel entrance, and to the fossa triangularis.

Summary

On the posterior surface of the promontory, towards the sinus tympani, an excavation of varying size and shape is found from which a well-defined cavity—the chamber of the fenestra rotunda—extends under the promontory. The craniocaudal part of this cavity contains the round window, with its covering secondary tympanic membrane.

The chamber of the round window resembles, in most cases, an entrance of a real cave, and is found between the sustentaculum promontorii and subiculum. Since the introduction of tympanoplastics, the classic anatomic description of the chamber has been complemented with functional data.

It is well established that during ossification of the otic capsule, the closure of the fenestra rotunda is prevented by a cartilage ring that differentiates in the third month, and transforms desmally to give room to the secondary tympanic membrane.

Our own observations were carried out in dried embryo preparations from the fourth fetal month until newborn and infant ages. In the *four-month-old fetus*, after removal of the mesenchyma, a *large round chamber* was found on the lower back portion of the promontory in which the *bean shape of the secondary tympanic membrane* is ensured by a *thick semicylinder turning from the subiculum into the chamber*. This semicylinder is gradually transformed *in the fifth month; its medial part gives rise to the postis posterior, while its lateral part* gives rise a few months later *to the fustis*. At six to seven months, the periosteal layer increases further. In addition to the above-mentioned fustis, *the postis anterior and the tunnel develop. In the eight-month-old fetus* the postis anterior fuses partially or totally with the sustentaculum, the tunnel becomes deeper, and—in the *last intrauterine month*—a *sinus concameratus* forms under and above the fustis, indicating the development of pneumatic cavities.

During intrauterine life and about the time of birth, the fossula of the fenestra rotunda is *relatively larger* than in adult ages. In neonates and infants, the round window chamber is nearly vertical and lyre-shaped with rounded off angles. *Its tegmen shows a stratification between protrusions of the postis anterior mucosa duplicature; in the area of the postis posterior, secondary cellule formation occurs. The fustis is usually relatively wide.*

Recent descriptions enlarge on the structure of the round window, so that more inframicroscopic details are considered. *We have carried out the inframicroscopic classification of the chamber because, based on our own preparations, we have thought it feasible, and because our surgical material showed pathologic alterations relevant to the different structural patterns.* On this basis, we distinguish in the chamber a *fundus, tegmen, and postes anterior and posterior.* The fundus is composed of three developmentally distinct parts: (1) medial or superior; (2) lateral or inferior; and (3) middle or fustis. The tegmen of the round window chamber corresponds to the thinned periosteal process towards the posterior tympanic wall of the labyrinth capsule, forming the basal turn of cochlea.

The postis anterior connects, on the territory of the scala tympani and the basal turn of the cochlea, to the jugular wall of the tympanic cavity; whereas the postis posterior constitutes the upper back edge of the fenestra entrance.

According to the position of the walls and fustis, their shape, size, connections, and relationships to each other and to their surrounding the entrance of the fenestra and its constituent structures show a wide range of variability. The inframicroscopic variants are described as follows:

1. According to its *direction, the apertura fossulae fenestrae rotundae verticalis, horizontalis, and dorsalis* are distinguished.
2. According to *size*, the following variants were seen: (a) *fossula fenestrae rotundae lata*, found in deep, wide tympanic cavities; and (b) *fossula fenestrae rotundae alta*, coupled to the narrow tympanum containing a fustis close to the postis anterior rather than to the postis posterior.
3. On the basis of *shape*, the following variants were described: *fossula rotundae fenestrae rotundae, fossula fenestrae rotundae ovalis, and semilunaris*, and as its subtypes, the *lyre-shaped* and *semilunar chambers, triangular, quadrate, rhomboid, trapezoid, lateral, dentate, and spinous.*

Of the internal structures, the fossula fenestra rotunda postes and the fustis were separately dealt with, as these can be readily distinguished from the embryologic, functional anatomic, inframicroscopic anatomic, pathologic, and surgical points of view.

Variants of the postis posterior are partly due to its developmental circumstances and partly to its relationship to its surroundings. Accordingly, we distinguished *double, tuberous, lamellar, and cellular types of postes posterior.* In a similar vein, the *gracile, lamellar, sigmoid, plexiform, and disjunct variants of postes anterior* were described.

The chamber mucosa shows a variety of formations that, according to appearance, localization, and extent, were classified in the following groups:

1. The round window chamber lined throughout with a single layer or mucosa with no duplicatures at all. This is a state typical from puberty onwards.
2. Mucosa duplicatures connecting the angles in various directions.
3. Duplicatures covering the chamber entrance longitudinally.
4. Duplicatures crossing the chamber transversely.
5. Duplicatures between the postes and posterior tympanic wall.
6. Duplicatures between protrusions of the tegmen and styloid prominence.
7. Duplicatures in the angle between the postis anterior and fundus.
8. Duplicatures covering the tunnel entrance in the chamber.
9. Plexiform, irregular, folded duplicatures.

The function of the round window chamber has been

dealt with extensively, particularly since the introduction of tympanoplastics. Its role is summarized as follows:

1. It ensures a protection to the round window.
2. The postes determine the height of the chamber.
3. The postis posterior fuses with the subiculum and participates in supporting the pars sacculocochlearis.
4. The ventral process of the postis posterior connects the basal turn of the cochlea to the pavimentum pyramidis.
5. Its posterior extension strengthens the fundus of the sinus tympani.
6. The pneumatic fossa triangularis located between the postis posterior and fustis reduces the weight of the bone.
7. The fustis supports the promontory.
8. The plane of the window frame differs from that of the oval window, producing a pressure difference.
9. The postis anterior is rather unstable; its supporting role is mostly overtaken by the sustentaculum.
10. The medial and lateral concamerata supposedly participate in tympanic cavity resonance and also reduce bone weight.
11. The tegmen fossulae fenestrae rotundae ensures the protection of the round window chamber.
12. The distance between the postes and the opening of the covering bone of the chamber are also protecting the secondary tympanic membrane.

Despite the protecting role of round window chamber structures, under pathologic conditions, they may have a pathogenic effect. The chamber is a preferential site for pathologic processes as a deep cavity storing exudate and nursing granulation tissue. Bone diseases affecting the promontory and hypotympanum can, by adequate exposure, be observed in the chamber; and the pseudomembrane formed can be mistaken for the secondary tympanic membrane. Exudate is drained to the tympanic cavity through a pinhole-sized opening, in contrast to chronic situations when connective tissue cords close the chamber only partially. A cholesteatoma filling the sinus tympani spreads preferentially into the chamber, widening and excavating it. After the disease, as at other tympanic cavity sites, osteogenesis may be induced, thickening the postes, lacerating the fustis, and producing a row of tubercles on the fundus. The tegmen become narrower, with an uneven surface.

As in the case of the stapes chamber, in the round window chamber, a diagnostic survey of structures also is essential prior to interferences. If possible, the examination should include inspection of chamber structures, pathologic alterations, and excess soft tissues, and the observation of the round window chamber reflex.

Prior to surgery inside the fenestra rotunda, visibility must be maximally ensured. This is greatly facilitated by *posterior tympanotomy;* that is, a better insight into the chamber is obtained if, in addition to a marked thinning of acoustic meatus, the threshold cellules are resected. Instruments can be introduced into the chamber, exploiting the presence of structures protecting the secondary tympanic membrane. Interferences are divided into two groups: (1) *soft tissue procedures,* under which the removal of remnants of mucosa duplicatures, pseudomembranes, adhesive scars, epithelium remnants, edematous sprouts, and sclerotic plaques are meant; and (2) the *bone procedures,* involving the constituent structures of the chamber affected by acute processes. Caution has to be exercised with manipulations on the territory of the postis posterior, which is the nearest structure to the secondary tympanic membrane.

10 *Accessory Conduits*

Under this term, we consider the vestibular aqueduct, cochlear aqueduct, and internal auditory canal. These three conduits present a common characteristic, which is they put the labyrinth in relation with the posterior cranial fossa (see Fig. 69).

The Vestibular Aqueduct

The vestibular aqueduct is a very straight bony conduit in which one can barely pass a hair. It contains the endolymphatic canal, which is the extension of the endolymphatic spaces of the membranous labyrinth. It arises in the vestibule. It follows the sulciform groove, which is located on the internal wall of the vestibule, a little below the anterior border of the orifice of the common crus of the superior and posterior canals (see Fig. 200). It rises first in the thick internal wall of the vestibule (see Fig. 205), and is separated from the vestibular cavity by 0.1 0.2 mm. It then ascends in the inner wall of the common crus of the superior and posterior semicircular canals, while inclining toward the cerebellar fossa (see Fig. 131).

When it arrives at the top of the common crus, it leaves the otic capsule to penetrate into the retrolabyrinthine space. It next makes a bend, runs horizontally, and proceeds posteriorly towards the cerebellar fossa and externally towards the lateral sinus (see Fig. 131). It traverses the petrosal cortex, enlarging like an estuary while doing so to form a bony cleft called the *endolymphatic meatus* (see Fig. 131) (apertura external aqueductus vestibuli; fossette ungueale). This opening (4 to 14 mm) faces externally and inferiorly. It contains the endolymphatic sac.

The superior lip of the endolymphatic meatus is sometimes enlarged by air cells of the retrolabyrinthine group. The location of the endolymphatic meatus is very variable. Normally, the meatus is in the middle of the posterior petrosal wall, equidistant from the crest to the posterior lacerated foramen, and from the lateral sinus to the internal auditory meatus. At times, the opening is very low—2 to 3 mm from the posterior-lacerated foramen and 15 mm from the petrosal crest. At other times, the inverse occurs, and

one finds it nearer the crest. Similar variations occur in the horizontal direction. At times, one finds the endolymphatic meatus opening into the edge of the sigmoid fossa; and at other times, it is found 18 mm from the same internal edge of the sigmoid fossa and (as a consequence) a short distance (8 mm) from the internal auditory meatus.

These considerable variations are due to the great variety of forms that the petrous pyramid can take. On a small nonpneumatic petrosa, the vestibular aqueducts are short (6 mm), and the endolymphatic meatus would be far back from the lateral sinus. On a large and well-pneumatized petrosa, the aqueduct would be long (12 mm), and the meatus approaches the sigmoid groove.

Despite all variations, there is a precise landmark for localizing the endolymphatic meatus. It is the posterior semicircular canal. The meatus is normally found in the area corresponding to the bow of the posterior canal, and most often in the inferior part of this space.

The Cochlear Aqueduct

The cochlear aqueduct (ductus perilymphaticus) connects the perilymphatic spaces of the cochlea (scala tympani) with the subarachnoid space of the cerebellar fossa. It is a bony conduit that is narrower than the vestibular aqueduct. Occasionally, it is large, so that if the stapes foot plate is removed during surgery for otosclerosis, there may be a large flow (gushes) of perilymph out of the oval window. A large cochlear duct will permit the free flow of cerebrospinal fluid into the labyrinth. It arises on the posterior wall of the scala tympani by a small orifice (see Figs. 193, 219) situated in front of the crest, which stands out from the inferoexternal edge of the round window in order to proceed under the spiral lamina. From there, it is directed backwards, outwards, and inferiorly. It passes under the ampullary arm of the posterior semicircular canal, which it crosses (see Figs. 202, 203). It then proceeds into the petrosa, nearly parallel to the internal auditory canal, and empties into the posterior fossa at the level of the inferior border of the petrosa by a wide orifice—the pyramidal fossa, which is found 4 to 5 mm below the internal auditory meatus (see Figs. 131, 203). It is 10 to 12 mm long. It is surrounded by a thick cushion of compact bone, which bars the route to the petrous apex and often from the cellular sublabyrinthine tract (see Fig. 69). The cochlear aqueduct transmits a small vein.

The Internal Auditory Canal

The internal auditory canal is a nerve conduit. It gives passage to the auditory nerve, the facial nerve, and the intermediate nerve of Wrisberg. The dura mater accompanies the nerves to the depth of the internal auditory meatus. It opens onto the posterior surface of the petrosa at the junction of its internal and middle thirds by an oval orifice called the *internal auditory meatus*, whose diameter varies between 3 to 7 mm. From there, it is directed outward, penetrating deeply into the interior of the petrosa in a direction that makes an angle of 45° with the longitudinal direction of the temporal bone. After a course varying from 5 to 12 mm, it ends as a passage at the internal wall of the vestible.

The depth of the internal auditory canal is a sort of cul-de-sac pierced by a large number of foramina—some are large like those that allow passage to the facial nerve and to the inferior ampullary nerve; the others are much smaller, grouped in the fossettes and allowing passage to the terminal branches of the cochlear and vestibular nerves (see Figs. 128, 132).

The cul-de-sac terminating the internal auditory canal is divided horizontally into two parts by a prominent crest—the *falciform crest* (crista transversa). It projects on the far end of the canal, and also anteriorly on the lateral wall (see Fig. 127). Above the transverse or falciform crest, one finds the orifice of the Fallopian aqueduct (facial canal) anteriorly and the superior vestibular recess posteriorly. Below the transverse crest, one finds the inferior vestibular recess, the spiral sieve of the modiolus with the cochlear recess, and the foramen singulare of Morgagni.

Orifice of the Facial Canal (fovea facialis, orifice of the Fallopian aqueduct, facial fossette)

The facial nerve, with the intermediate nerve of Wrisberg, occupies the anterosuperior region of the internal auditory canal, which is grooved to accommodate it. It is limited above by the superior wall of the canal and below by the falciform crest, which extends onto the anterior wall of the canal. Upon arriving at the bottom of the canal, 1.5 mm from the vestibule, it deviates anteriorly and enters a tunnel 1 mm in size into the petrosa. This is the origin of the facial canal (see Figs. 127, 128, 202). The origin of the facial canal is then found in the fundus of the internal auditory canal and entirely above the anterior wall.

Superior Vestibular Area (superior vestibular fossette, superior fossa, cribriform fossette, fossette utriculare).

It is situated adjacent to the facial canal, from which it is separated only by a vertical crest (Bill's bar). It appears in the depth of the internal auditory canal (its terminal wall), where one sees it very high and in front (see Fig. 192). In the depth of the superior vestibular area are two orifices—one superimposed on the other. The inferior orifice allows access to the utricular nerve via a short canal, which breaks up into fine canaliculi that empty by small openings onto the vestibular pyramid and around it, forming the cribriform utricular plate (see Fig. 204).

The superior orifice allows passage for the superior and horizontal ampullary nerves. It enters a canal that divides immediately into two groups of canaliculi which empty into the cribriform plate of the superior semicircular canal ampulla and into the cribriform plate of the horizontal canal (see Figs. 194, 202).

Inferior Vestibular Area (inferior vestibular fossette, inferior fossa, fossette sacculare)

The inferior vestibular area lies in the bottom half of the meatal fundus just below the posterior half of the transverse crest. It is pierced by numerous orifices, which are in relation with the saccular cribriform plate. At this spot, the bottom of the internal auditory canal is separated from the vestibule by only a thin lamella of bone, which corresponds to the saccular recess in the vestibule, and is found directly opposite the oval window (see Fig. 194).

Spiral Foraminous Tract (spiral cribriform of the modiolus, cochlear area, cochlear fossette)

Below the inferior vestibular area and a little behind it, at the junction of the fundus and floor of the auditory canal, one finds the initial portion of the spiral foraminous tract—from which point small fibers leave to enter the vestibule and reach the subvestibular portion of the osseous spiral lamina (see Fig. 194).

The spiral foraminous tract, in the form of a ribbon 1 mm wide and formed by porous bone, begins at the junction of the floor and the vestibular wall of the auditory canal, extending for about 3 mm on the floor, passing onto the anterior wall, and penetrating into a little circular recess called the *cochlear fossette*. There, it makes a spiral turn and a half. The porous bone constituting the fossette is pierced by a large number of fine holes—the origin of small canals, which are directed toward the periphery of the modiolus, where they open into a common canal called the *spiral canal of Rosenthal.*

Foramen Singulare of Morgagni (singular foramen)

On the posterior wall of the auditory canal, at a point 1 mm from the fundus of the canal and 2 mm above its floor, is located the *singular foramen.* This orifice, 0.3 mm in diameter, is the origin of a canal 3 to 4 mm long that proceeds to the cribriform plate of the ampulla of the posterior semicircular canal. It carries the posterior ampullary branch of the vestibular nerve (see Figs. 127, 128).

The internal auditory meatus is one of the routes of propagation of labyrinthine infections toward the meninges. The surgeon seeks to reach the fundus directly across the labyrinth or via the cerebellar fossa and the posterior wall of the petrosa. The internal auditory meatus is difficult to reach due to its depth of 38 to 46 mm from a cortical mastoidectomy. The very firm adherence of the dura mater at this level increases the difficulties. The current approach to this area for removal of acoustic tumors may be undertaken via the translabyrinthine, middle fossa, or posterior fossa.

The Internal Auditory Meatus

The internal auditory meatus is a space that first becomes apparent in a 7 mm fetus. The mesenchyme then gradually changes into the cartilaginous anlage, the growth pressures of which cause the cochlea to develop in front of the acousticofacial bundle, while the vestibular apparatus grows toward the back. By the 30 mm stage, there is a growth spurt of the inner ear part of the inner ear structures compared with the other elements of the skull and face.

The growth of the skull during intrauterine life displaces the inner ear from the midline to its final position. The motor root of the facial nerve and the parasympathetic components to the lacrimal and nasal apparatus have now appeared. The facial nerve is the most anterior, making its way transversely toward the geniculate ganglion, which is situated outside the capsule from the beginning.

The nervus intermedius appears as a satellite of the vestibular nerve. Its point of exit is much closer to the vestibular nerve than to the motor root of the facial nerve. This close relationship persists as the nerves take a common course towards the future geniculate ganglion. It is during this part of its course that the nervous intermedius gives off fibers joining the vestibular nerve. These fibers come from the same bundle that is destined to form the chorda tympani[96] therefore, it is reasonable to consider these as parasympathetic fibers, and to conclude that this constitutes the first sign of an acousticofacial anastomosis.

This makes the nervous intermedius the true autonomic nerve of the inner ear.

General Anatomy

The variations in shape and size of the bony internal auditory canal are, in large part, due to the size of the petrosa, and to the degree of pneumatization. Its orientation is not simply transverse, but also slightly oblique anterolaterally. It is almost cylindrical, and makes an angle of about 45° with the longitudinal axis of the petrous pyramid. Since this, in turn, is directed at an angle of 53° to the sagittal plane, the general axis of the internal auditory meatus makes an angle of 8° with the transverse biauricular plane (Fig. 266).

In general terms, the internal auditory canal is a cylinder 4 mm in diameter and 8 mm in length; but these measurements are variable. The *porus,* or inlet of the internal auditory meatus, is an orifice opening onto the posterior intracranial surface of the petrosa at the junction of its inner and middle thirds. It is closer to its superior than inferior margin. The plane of the intracranial surface of the petrous bone is set at an angle in the general direction of the internal auditory canal, which explains its ovoid shape (about 5 mm high and 8 mm wide). It also explains why the lateral lip of the *porus,* which borders it laterally and posteriorly, is sharp and concave, whereas the medial border is continued inwards as a sort of gutter; this appears to extend the canal medially and superiorly towards the petrous apex onto its posterior intracranial surface. In reality, at the level of the *porus,* this gutter is empty and does not allow passage to any nerve fibers (see Fig. 7).

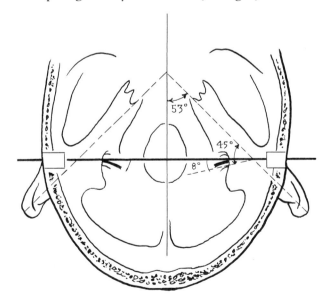

Figure 266.   The internal auditory canal makes an angle of about 45° with the longitudinal axis of the petrous pyramid. Since this, in turn, is directed at an angle of 53° to the sagittal plane, the general axis of the internal auditory meatus makes an angle of 8° with the transverse binaural plane.[99]

A few millimeters above and posterior to the internal auditory meatus, and very close to the superior border of the petrosa, is a narrow impression called the *subarcuate fossa;* in its depths lies the anterior end of the petromastoid canal, which reaches the mastoid by passing beneath the arch of the superior semicircular canal and opens into the antrum above the lateral canal. It sometimes contains a vessel that may be encountered when the internal auditory meatus is approached surgically by the middle fossa route, or during a translabyrinthine route as the bone is being drilled in the plane of the superior canal.[93]

Papangelou[97] reported his findings in 121 pairs of temporal bones, and his results may be summarized in the following paragraphs.

1. The vertical diameter varied from 2 to 7 mm, with a mean of 4.6 mm. There was a difference of 1 to 3 mm between the two sides in 54 cases; but in 67 cases, the vertical diameter was the same on the two sides.
2. The horizontal diameter was rather similar, and varied between 3 and 7 mm, with a mean of 4.5 mm. There was less variation between the two sides, with only 1 to 3 mm difference in 51 cases and no difference in 70 cases.
3. The length of the anterior wall—as measured from the fundus of the canal to the point where this wall widens out into the posterior surface of the temporal bone—varied between wide limits; that is, 9 to 19 mm, with a mean of 14.9 mm. The difference between the two sides was 1 to 5 mm in 90 cases; and in 31 cases, the length of the anterior walls on the two sides were the same.
4. The length of the posterior wall from the most concave part of the *porus* to the fundus of the canal varied from 6 to 14 mm, with a mean of 9.2 mm. The difference between the two sides was 1 to 5 mm in 73 cases, and the length was the same in 48 cases.
5. The length of the roof, measured from the highest point of the *porus* to the fundus of the canal, varied between 8 and 17 mm, with a mean of 11.5 mm. The difference between the two sides varied from 1 to 5 mm in 82 cases, and the length was the same in 39 cases.
6. The length of the floor, measured from the lowest point on the *porous* to the fundus of the meatus, varied between 8 and 16 mm, with a mean of 11.8 mm. The difference between the two sides was 1 to 6 mm in 79 cases, and the lengths of the floor were the same in 42 cases.

   There is a contrast between the fairly constant diameters of this cylindrical canal and the great variations in length. This contrast reflects the fact that the volume of the neurovascular content is always about the same, whereas the degree of pneumatization of the bone—and therefore the distance between the labyrinth and the posterior cranial fossa—is very variable.
7. There can be variations of 1 to 2 mm in the horizontal and vertical diameters, depending on whether they are measured at the fundus, the *porus,* or the middle of the canal. The vertical diameter is constant in 35% of cases.

The canal seems to be oval vertically in 13.5% of cases, narrowed at the medial end in 9.5% to present a waist-like central narrowing in 0.4%, and narrowed at the lateral end in 41%. The shape was the same on the two sides in 40% and differed in 60% of cases.

Variations of the same order have been found in the horizontal diameter, and only 7% of the meatus was truly cylindrical about a horizontal axis. None were oval, and none were narrowed at their medial extremity; 0.8% were narrowed in the center, and 92.2% were narrowed at their lateral end at the point of contact with the vestibule. The shape was the same on the two sides in 42% of cases, and differed in 58%. It must therefore be concluded that in the great majority of cases, as far as the horizontal plane is concerned, the internal meatus is a cylinder that is slightly narrowed at its lateral end.

The dura mater accompanies the acoustic and facial nerves to the depth of the meatus. The internal auditory canal opens on the posterior surface of the petrosa at the union of its internal and middle thirds by an oval orifice whose diameter varies between 3 and 7 mm. From there, it is directed outward, penetrating deeply into the interior of the petrosa, following a direction forming an angle of about 45° with the longitudinal axis of this bone; after a course varying from 5 to 12 mm, it ends as a passage at the internal wall of the vestibule.

The far end of the internal auditory canal is a type of cul-de-sac pierced by a large number of foramina. Some are large, like those allowing passage to the facial nerve and the inferior ampullary nerve, the others are much smaller and grouped in the fossettes, allowing passage to the terminal branches of the cochlear and vestibular nerves (see Figs. 127, 128).

A strongly projecting crest (falciform crest, transverse crest) divides the cul-de-sac horizontally into two layers. The crest extends onto the lateral wall of the internal auditory canal (see Fig. 130).

At the superior level, one sees the orifice of the facial canal and the superior vestibular area (fossette); at the inferior level, one see the inferior vestibular area (fossette), the spiral tract of the foramina with the cochlear fossette or recess, and the foramen singular of Morgagni (see Fig. 132).

Facial Fossette or Origin of the Facial Canal

The facial nerve with the intermediate nerve of Wrisberg occupies the anterosuperior region of the internal auditory canal. The facial canal origin is limited above by the superior wall of the internal auditory canal, and below by the transverse crest, which is more or less prolonged onto the anterior wall of the canal. The orifice of the facial canal is 1.5 mm from the vestibule, and is only 1 mm in size (see Figs. 232, 233). It lies entirely above the anterior wall.

The Superior Vestibular Area (superior vestibular fossette, fossa utriculare, superior fossa)

This is situated adjacent to the origin of the facial canal, from which it is separated only by a vertical crest (Bill's bar), (see Figs. 132, 202). It appears at the depth of the internal auditory canal at its terminal wall, where one sees it very high and in front.

Its depression carries two superimposed orifices. The inferior orifice allows access to the utricular nerve—a short canal that breaks up into fine canaliculi emptying by small openings onto the vestibular pyramid and around it forming the cribriform utricular plate (see Figs. 192, 206). The superior orifice allows passage for the superior and horizontal ampullary nerves; it allows access in a canal that divides immediately into two groups of canaliculi that empty into the cribriform plate of the superior semicircular canal ampulla and the cribriform plate of the horizontal canal (see Fig. 128).

The Inferior Vestibular Area

At the inferior level below the transverse crest, one finds the inferior vestibular area, which is pierced by several orifices in relation with the saccular cribriform plate (macula cribrosa media). At this spot, the bottom of the internal auditory canal is separated from the vestibule by only a thin lamella of bone that corresponds to the hemispherical or saccular recess in the vestibuli, and is found opposite the oval window (see Fig. 192). It is only 3 mm deep to the medial aspect of the stapes foot plate.

Spiral Cribriform of the Modiolus (spiral tract of the foramina)

Below the inferior vestibular fossette and a little behind the union of the depth and floor of the internal auditory canal, one finds the initial portion of the spiral cribriform of the modiolus, from which small nerve filaments leave, forming the vestibular origin and subvestibular portion of the spiral lamina (see Fig. 202).

The spiral cribriform, in the shape of a ribbon 1 mm wide formed of porous bone, begins at the union of the floor and the terminal or vestibular wall of the canal, extending for about 3 mm on the floor and passing onto the anterior wall while penetrating into a little circular fossette—the cochlear fossa; there it describes a spiral of a turn and a half. The porous bone that constitutes it is pierced by a large number of fine holes (origin of the small canals), which are directed towards the periphery of the modiolus, where they open into a common canal called the spiral canal of the modiolus (spiral canal of Rosenthal) described earlier.

Foramen Singulare of Morgagni

Finally, on the posterior wall of the internal auditory canal, 1 mm from the bottom and 2 mm above the floor, there exists an isolated orifice—the foramen singulare of Morgagni. This orifice, 0.3 mm in diameter, is the origin of a canal (3 to 4 mm long) that proceeds to the cribriform plate of the ampulla of the posterior semicircular canal. It is occupied in the living by the posterior ampullary branch of the acoustic nerve (see Fig. 127).

The internal auditory canal may be the site of an acoustic neurinoma. It is one of the routes of propagation of labyrinthine infections towards the meninges. The surgeon seeks to reach the fundus directly across the labyrinth via the cerebellar fossa and the posterior wall of the petrosa, or via the middle fossa approach.

Contents

In the internal auditory canal, we find the meninges with their associated spaces and certain nerves and blood vessels.

The Meninges

The meninges of the posterior fossa continue into the internal auditory meatus. The dura is firmly adherent around the porus, as well as to all of the walls of the meatus. It is thicker medially than towards the outer part of the meatus. At the fundus of the meatus, the dura is extremely thin. It is continuous with the thin periosteal layer of the first part of the facial canal.

The pia mater forms a covering over the various neurovascular structures. Physiologic tags of pia connect the neurovascular structures with the dural walls of the meatus. The spaces contain cerebrospinal fluid and represent an extension of the cysterna magna, with which the meatus is in communication. Therefore, opening the meatus may well drain the cysterna magna.

The Nerves

The general direction of the acousticofacial bundle is more anterior than that of the internal auditory canal, which by comparison appears to lie more transversely. Both structures run anterolaterally. As it enters the porus, the bundle is closer to the outer angled border of the canal than to the inner smooth border when viewed from the surgical position. The slightly funnelled shape of the bony meatus (which accounts for the obliquity of the porus) corrects these relationships, so that at the lateral end of the canal, its walls are parallel to the nerves within it. If the middle fossa approach to the canal is made too small (for fear of injury to the cochlea or superior semicircular canal), and at the same time very medial (to avoid the superior petrosal sinus), it is not uncommon to find a cavity that apparently contains no nerves. If this happens, the opening into the meatus must be widened posterolaterally—when the first nerve to appear will be the facial as it takes an oblique course anterolaterally. The vestibular nerve is in close relationship with it, and is next seen lying in a more posterior position.[93]

The components of the acousticofacial bundle move apart from each other as they run laterally. The only exception is the intermediate nerve, which is separated from the facial nerve in the posterior fossa and moves gradually towards it, so that by the time they enter the internal auditory meatus, the two nerves are invested with the same covering of pia mater. They come to have a progressively closer relationship until, by the time that they enter the facial canal, the two nerves are fused as one.

Just before it enters the *porus,* the vestibulocochlear nerve (which is the largest of the three) forms a gutter with its concavity directed anterosuperiorly; the posterior ring of this gutter is thinner than the anterior one. The nerve then divides into a larger anterior portion, made up of the anterior two thirds, that forms the cochlear nerve and a smaller posterior portion that becomes the vestibular nerve. The separation into these two nerves is rarely visible macroscopically before the *porus.*

The Facial Nerve.   The facial nerve is the most superiorly placed of the nerves. It enters the internal meatus near its lateral rim. Its direction, however, is more anterior than that of the meatus; therefore, it crosses over to gain the anterior wall, and slides into the hollow of the bony gutter resulting from the anterior prolongation of the transverse crest. This gutter leads directly towards the first portion of the facial canal. By taking a transverse line with a slight obliquity upwards forwards and outwards, it seems as if, in this part of its course, the nerve is already embarking upon the curved course (concave anteromedially) of the first part of the facial canal. The intermediate nerve of Wrisberg lies beneath and behind the facial nerve. At this point, it receives a sympathetic twig from the artery.

The Vestibulocochlear Nerve.   On entering the meatus, the vestibulocochlear nerve divides into an anterior cochlear branch and a thinner vestibular branch. The cochlear nerve is flattened and shaped into a gutter with its concavity directed upwards; the motor and sensory roots of the facial nerve rest in this. The nerve travels outwards and slightly forwards to reach the cochlear recess, which is a depression hollowed out of the osseous spiral lamina. Here it spirals around itself, making two complete turns in the same direction as the bony contours—that is, from before backward, and from medial to lateral. The fibers pass through the foramina in the cochlear recess, which are arranged in two tiers in the depths of the rectangular foramina.[93]

The Vestibular Nerve.   The vestibular nerve is smaller than the cochlear nerve and approaches the fundus of the internal auditory meatus, where it presents a fairly large swelling, the vestibular, or Scarpa's ganglion. The ganglion becomes progressively thinner as it proceeds laterally.

Fibers from the utricular macula and from the ampullae of the superior and lateral semicircular canals are grouped together as the superior vestibular nerve as they pass into the ganglion (Fig. 127). Filaments from the saccule take the same course as the cochlear nerve and their proximity increases as they travel medially. The nerve from the ampulla of the posterior semicircular canal is much thinner and passes through the foramen singular of Morgagni.

The Acousticofacial Anastomoses.   The acousticofacial anastomoses make their connection between the posterolateral aspect of the intermediate nerve and the anterior border of the superior vestibular nerve. They consist of a network of two or more bundles which arise in the intermediate nerve and join the vestibular nerve at its anterior edge. The tight network which they form are small and can be quite difficult to divide during the course of a neurectomy. At this point, the close proximity of the facial and superior vestibular nerves allows them to have a common sheath of pia mater.

The Sheaths of Pia Mater.   The nerve to the saccule has its own sheath of pia mater right to the point where it passes beneath the transverse or falciform crest; more medially, however, it is associated more and more closely with the nerve to the utricle and in the medial part of the internal auditory meatus the two nerves join as the vestibular nerve which is itself already beginning to fuse with the cochlear nerve. When during the course of a vestibular neurectomy the superior vestibular nerve has been sectioned distally below Scarpa's ganglion, and the medial part of the nerve to the utricle is identified medially and superiorly, the line of demarcation between it and the nerve to the saccule (which was so clear laterally) becomes increasingly difficult to make out as the dissection proceeds medially; it sometimes seems that the dissection is being done within the very substance of the nerve trunk itself. At the same time there is an equally close relationship anteriorly between the cochlear nerve and the nerve to the saccule. So the proximal dissection, which precedes the resection of the nerve to the saccule, is sometimes carried out in direct contact with the cochlear fibers. It is easy to appreciate how these close relationships can give rise to difficulties during the operation (Portmann et al.).[93]

Relations of the Internal Auditory Meatus

There is a variable degree of obliquity of the internal auditory meatus. In wide temporal bones it lies almost transversely whereas in narrow bones it lies more anteroposteriorly. Because of this obliquity, most of the walls of this cylindrical canal may be approached according to the two directions in which they face. For example, the posterior wall is related at first to the posterior cranial fossa, which lies behind it. Laterally, it is in relation to the mastoid cortex, permitting one surgical approach to it. The superior wall is related to the temporal lobe, but it also bears an oblique relationship with the squamosa, which permits a means of surgical access.

In highly pneumatized bones, the system of perilabyrinthine cell tracts (see Figs. 69, 123) have an important relationship.

Sublabyrinthine cell tract. This is the most constant cell tract. It runs beneath the labyrinth, behind the carotid canal, and above the jugular bulb. When the bulb is not too high, a few cells may be found beneath the floor of the internal auditory meatus.

Precochlear cell tract. This is also known as the anteroinferior or intercarotico-cochlear cell tract.

Posterosuperior cell tracts. These are divided into:

1. A prelabyrinthine cell tract that passes in front of the superior canal and lies by the superior wall of the meatus.
2. An occasional translabyrinthine cell tract that passes beneath the arch of the superior canal to rejoin the prelabyrinthine cell tract above the internal auditory meatus.
3. A petrous crest chain that passes between the posterior and superior canal to rejoin the others above the roof of the meatus.
4. A superior retrolabyrinthine cell tract that passes between the posterior canal and the posterior fossa plate. Instead of passing beneath the internal auditory meatus, which would be the shortest route, it encircles the meatus by passing above it, and then joins the other cell tracts above the roof of the meatus.

Inferior Wall

The inferior wall of the internal auditory meatus is related to the inferior surface of the petrosa. It may be separated from it slightly in its lateral part by the jugular bulb when this is sufficiently well developed. Sometimes the bulb may form the floor of the meatus. Cases have been described where there is a bony dehiscence, and the dura of the bulb is in direct contact with the nerves. Most often, the jugular fossa and the meatus are separated posteriorly by the sublabyrinthine cell tract. This begins lateral to the hypotympanic and retrofacial cells, passes beneath the cochlea behind the upper part of the horizontal section of the carotid canal, and meets the internal auditory meatus at an oblique angle. When the jugular fossa is not well defined, this cell tract is very obvious; on the other hand, when there is a well- developed jugular fossa, there is less room, and this region is closed by compact bone. In these cases, the sublabyrinthine cell tract ends in a cul-de-sac very close to the meatus. More posteriorly, and only if the bone is wide, a small tract of inferior labyrinthine cells will be found passing behind the posterior semicircular canal and beneath the vestibular aqueduct before reaching the petrous apex by traversing the medial part of the inferior wall of the meatus. The vestibular aqueduct lies along the posterior aspect of the inferior wall of the meatus; this ends in a triangular depression on the posterior intracranial surface of the petrous bone 4 or 5 mm below the *porus* (see Fig. 7). Finally, at the extreme lateral end of the meatus, near the fundus, the inferior wall is related to the begin-

ning of the cochlea, which extends slightly more medially than the medial surface of the vestibule.

Superior Wall

A thick layer of bone separates the internal auditory meatus from the sharp angle made by the junction of the anterior and posterior surfaces of the petrosa. This bone consists of a thick cortex and underlying air cells, which are the medial ends of the four superior labyrinthine cell tracts.

This description is true if the petrous bone is considered in the classic anatomic position. In the surgical position, however, the superior surface of the meatus corresponds to the anterior intracranial surface, or roof, of the petrous bone, which borders the middle cranial fossa. Therefore, on passing through this layer of bone, less air cells are found than might be expected from the classic descriptions. The reason is that this approach misses the most posteriorly placed of the superior labyrinthine cells. In bones that are only moderately well pneumatized, it is not uncommon to work through the entire thickness of the bone roofing the meatus without coming across a single cell.

Medial to the arcuate eminence, the superior surface of the petrosa presents a smooth and slightly depressed meatal area; this area is triangular, with its apex facing medially, and is in marked contrast with what is the most undulating part of the superior surface immediately lateral to it. Thus, in the course of a surgical approach from the squamosa, the roof of the petrosa is followed medially. Thus, one encouters, in turn, the roof of the tegmen, the irregular projections of the arcuate eminence and geniculate area, and finally the flattened meatal area, which is easily identifiable by its plateau-like appearance. The dura mater of the middle cranial fossa can be dissected easily until the meatal area is reached. It is only there that it becomes closely adherent posteriorly along the superior border of the petrosa (where the superior petrosal sinus runs) and anteromedially over the region of the Gasserian ganglion and carotid canal. Quite often, some small vessels from the dura penetrate the bone after they have run on its surface for a few millimeters in channels of varying depths.

Posterior Wall

The posterior wall of the meatus is in the anatomic position in relation to both the posterior cranial fossa and the posterior extracranial surface of the temporal bone, which means essentially the jugular bulb. Surgically, however, the main relation of this wall is to the posterior intracranial surface of the petrous pyramid, and thus the posterior cranial fossa. The cortex over this surface is separated from the posterior meatal wall by cell tracts that have already been described. The petromastoid canal crosses transversely from the depression in the petrosa towards the mastoid antrum.

Because of its obliquity, the posterior wall also has lateral relations, which are encountered during the translabyrinthine approach. It is separated from the mastoid cortex by the superior and posterior semicircular canals, by the vestibular aqueduct, and more laterally by the lateral semicircular and facial canals anteriorly and lateral sinus posteriorly. The surgical route to the posterior wall of the internal auditory meatus passes between these two structures—the facial nerve and the lateral sinus—and then crosses, in turn, the posterior part of the lateral semicircular canal, the superior and posterior semicircular canals, and the vestibular aqueduct. The posterior wall of the internal auditory meatus is found by opening the posterior wall of the vestibule. It can be followed right to the *porus,* and the access can be widened if necessary by resecting the posterior wall of the petrosa. In the surgical position, since the line of approach across the mastoid is very posterior, a very direct view of this wall of the internal auditory meatus is possible.

Anterior Wall

The anterior wall of the internal auditory meatus is related to the basal turn of the cochlea. The first part of the basal turn, which is situated below the vestibule and the internal auditory meatus, continues forward in company with the anterior wall of the meatus (Figs. 136, 206). Medial to the geniculate ganglion and immediately posterior to the hiatus for the petrosal nerves, the cupula is adherent by its upper surface to the cortex of the anterior surface of the petrosa; and at this point, it is very unusual to encounter any cells.

No part of the cochlea ever passes medial to a sagittal line drawn 28 mm from the internal surface of the squamosa. Medial to this line, no vital structure lies anterior to the anterior wall of the meatus, with the exception of the horizontal limb of the carotid canal, which is some distance away and well inferior. In wide petrosas, this is the area where the precochlear cells are found. In narrow bones, the meatus is closer to the carotid, but always superior to it.

The collection of cells at the petrous apex, which is the focal point of the various cell tracts, lies anterior and a little above and medial to the internal auditory meatus.

The Fundus

The fundus faces laterally and anteriorly. It is in contact with the medial wall of the vestibule and the base of the cochlea (see Figs. 192, 194). The floor of the vestibule is at the same level as the floor of the internal auditory meatus. The common wall separating these two cavities has, on the external face, the medial wall of the vestibule and, on the internal face, the fundus of the meatus. Each of these faces is divided into two levels by a bony ridge—the vestibular crest on the external face and the transverse or falciform crest on the internal face. These two ridges are at the same height on the party wall. At the lower level on the vestibular side is situated the saccular recess, and on the other side is the inferior vestibular area, which transmits filaments to the saccule. The upper area lodges the utricular recess, which corresponds with the superior vestibular area on the

side of the internal auditory meatus. Anterolaterally, the inferior saccular area corresponds with the oval window. The party wall between the vestibule and the fundus of the meatus is very thin at the sites of the maculae cribrosae, but is more than 1 mm thick at the transverse crest and at the periphery.

The tractus spiralis foraminosus of the fundus of the meatus corresponds with the base of the cochlea, the basal turn, which is not curved at first, runs an almost horizontal line beneath the vestibule, and then passes beneath the angle formed by the inferior wall and the fundus of the internal auditory meatus. It then continues in front of the outer part of its anterior wall, where it joins the fundus to reach the region of the geniculate ganglion.

The tractus spiralis foraminosus faces more anteriorly than the rest of the fundus of the meatus. This orientation corresponds to the ending of the cochlear nerve, which fans out anterolaterally. It also explains the relationship of the cochlear duct with the anterior wall of the meatus. It allows for orientation of the osseous spiral lamina, which is at right angles to it.

The anterosuperior part of the fundus contains the opening of the facial canal. The curved line of the first part of the facial canal, with its concavity facing anteromedially, is continued in the petrosal nerves. The cortex that covers the facial canal is thick medially, but it becomes increasingly thinner laterally so that it may be dehiscent at the level of the geniculate ganglion. This first part of the canal is overhung posteriorly by the superior semicircular canal as it lies in the gulley between the vestibule and the cochlea. The canal is almost parallel to it, but angled posteriorly and medially. The line of the superior canal, which is directed externally and forwards, makes an angle of about 60° with the general line of the internal auditory meatus.

The Porus

The porus, facing posteromedially, is in direct relation to the cerebellopontine angles and its boundaries. These boundaries are the cerebellum posterolaterally, the brainstem (especially the pons) medially, and the posterosuperior surface of the petrosa with its dural covering in front and laterally. It is bounded above by the tentorium cerebelli. The outer border of the tentorium, which contains the superior petrosal sinus, is attached to the superior border of the petrosa.

Within the porus, the acousticofacial bundle is the main feature. The VIII cranial nerve is the largest component and the most inferiorly placed. It is directed forwards, outwards, and slightly upwards. It forms a concave gutter upwards, and its posterior rim is higher than its anterior rim. It divides into an anterior portion (forming about two thirds of its bulk), which is the cochlear nerve, and a posterior vestibular portion. The whole nerve spirals so that in the surgical position for the posterior fossa approach, the vestibular fibers are at first situated posterosuperiorly; then, as the nerve progresses laterally, they come to lie posteriorly and posteroinferiorly to the cochlear fibers.

The facial nerve takes the same course, but is directed

slightly more laterally; whereas it is first placed anteromedially to the VIII cranial nerve, it then appears above its medial border and comes to lie finally above the anterior cochlear part of the nerve. The more slender intermediate nerve begins behind the facial nerve and then slides between it and the VIII cranial nerve.

In summary, the mutual disposition of these three nerves is as follows:

1. Medially, in the depths of the cerebellopontine angle, the vestibular nerve lies posterosuperiorly, the vestibular nerve lies anteroinferiorly, and the facial and intermediate nerves lie above the cochlear nerve. They are in the same horizontal plane as the vestibular nerve; when viewed from above, they hide the cochlear nerve almost completely.
2. Midway between the cerebellum and the petrosa, the vestibular nerve lies posteriorly and tends to sink inferiorly. The cochlear nerve is anterior and tends to rise. The facial nerve lies above the cochlear nerve.
3. Laterally, near the petrous bone, the vestibular nerve is posteroinferior, the cochlear nerve is anterosuperior, and the facial nerve lies above both of them. It must be noted that these relationships have been described when the posterior fossa approach is used. The various arterial and venous vessels of this area will be described later. The cerebellar artery describes a loop near the internal auditory meatus. This loop is a constant finding, but may penetrate within the meatus. The vein of Dandy is more medially placed.

The lateral cerebellopontine cistern is a pool of cerebrospinal fluid that connects below with the lateral medullary cistern and the cisterna magna, into which the foramen of Magendi opens. Medially, this cistern opens into the pontine and interpeduncular cisterns.

Below, and at some distance from the porus, is the posterior inferior cerebellar artery, which arises from the basilar trunk and passes backwards, downwards, and outwards beneath the acousticofacial bundle, (which it crosses almost at right angles). This vessel may form a wide loop in this area, with its convexity outwards. The inferior petrosal sinus follows the petrooccipital suture to reach the jugular foramen.

The last cranial nerves, which run almost horizontally, are more laterally placed and lie on the sloping surface of the jugular tubercle before they reach the jugular foramen (see Figs. 6, 21).

The endolymphatic sac is found more laterally, below the porus. It rests in a depression on the posterior surface of the petrosa. It separates the porus from the lateral sinus, which runs a sinuous course with its concavity medially.

The motor and sensory roots of the trigeminal nerve are above and in front of the porus.

Blood Vessels

The arterial supply can be studied in three groupings.

1. The *cerebellar arteries,* from which the blood supply of the internal auditory meatus originates and among which the anterior inferior cerebellar artery plays the most important part.
2. The *arteries of the internal auditory meatus*—the labyrinthine (or internal auditory) artery and its branches, which supply the walls and contents of the canal.
3. *The subarcuate artery.* A loop, usually supplied by the anterior inferior cerebellar artery or by its accessory companion, lies either inside (40%) or at the orifice of the internal auditory canal (27%), or in contact with the VII and VIII cranial nerves in the cerebellopontine angle and close to the canal (33%).

The arterial loop is the main trunk or a branch of (1) the anterior inferior cerebellar artery in 80% of cases; (2) the accessory anterior inferior cerebellary artery in 17% of cases; and (3) a branch of the posterior inferior cerebellar artery in 3% of cases.

From the arterial loop (meatal loop) arises the internal auditory and subarcuate arteries and, in almost one half of cases, a cerebellosubarcuate artery. An independent origin of the internal auditory artery from the basilar artery, although possible, is rare.

The meatal loop, as an artery looping into or close to the internal auditory canal, is a constant feature. It is, however, exceedingly variable as to its size and relationship to the VII and VIII cranial nerves. Its variations may be grouped in a number of basic patterns, the most common of which shows the loop either intermediately or inferiorly to the nerves.

The internal auditory artery, which is double in one half of cases, has a rather constant course either on the anterior and then superior side of the VII cranial nerve or on the inferior posterior side of the same nerve.

The subarcuate fossa is, in a lateral surgical approach, an area of critical importance, since in one third of cases—besides the small subarcuate artery—the larger cerebellosubarcuate artery or recurrent limb of the meatal loop lie either adherent or very close to the dura of the fossa.

The subarcuate artery is the second vessel connecting the cerebellar loop to the temporal bone. It arises either directly from the cerebellar loop or from a collateral of the loop—or, in a minority of cases, from the loop having a common trunk with the internal auditory artery.

After entering into important relationships with the VII and VIII cranial nerves, the subarcuate artery usually enters the dura at the subarcuate fossa's depression; but, occasionally, it enters at any point between the fossa and lateral border of the porus acousticus, or at the posterior wall of the proximal portion of the internal auditory canal.

For more detail on the blood supply to the internal auditory meatus one can consult the studies by Mazzoni[98,99,100] and the text by Portman et al.[93]

Veins

The vein of the cochlear aqueduct drains the cochlea and about half of the vestibule. The vein of the vestibular aqueduct drains the remainder of the vestibule and the semicircular canals. The internal auditory vein drains only the meninges of the meatus and the acousticofacial bundle. A particularly large venous branch arises near the superior vestibular area, and travels on the sheath of the facial nerve and superior vestibular nerve (anterior vestibular vein). This vein, which usually enlarges in size towards the porus, may be referred to as the *internal auditory vein*. It may have one to three channels of communication, with branches of the posterior spiral vein at the base of the cochlea.

Boussens et al.[101] had 11 cases with a single internal auditory vein. Of these, four emptied into the trunk of the superior petrosal vein, five emptied into the vein of the lateral recess of the fourth ventricle, one emptied into one of the veins arising from the cerebellomedullary fissure, and one emptied into one of the veins from the inferior surface of the cerebellum. They also showed that the superior petrosal vein (vein of Dandy) may vary in length between 5 and 10 mm. The point at which it empties into the superior petrosal sinus is very variable, and can be anywhere between the trigeminal nerve and acousticofacial bundle.

Lymph is dissipated directly into the subarachnoid space. The first lymphatics are found at the level of the jugular bulb.

11 Vasculature of the Temporal Bone

The External Carotid Artery

The external carotid artery arises from the common carotid artery at about the level of the upper border of the thyroid cartilage. Then it is directed upward and slightly backward towards the angle of the jaw, where it enters the substance of the parotid gland (Figs. 170, 172, 177) and continues upward in that structure to just below the root of the zygoma. Here it gives rise to a large branch—the *internal maxillary artery*—and then continues upward over the root of the zygoma upon the side of the skull; this terminal portion of it is called the superficial temporal artery.

Branches

The following arise from below and upward from the anterior surface of the carotid artery: (1) the superior thyroid; (2) the lingual; (3) the facial; and (4) the internal maxillary arteries. From the carotid artery's posterior surface, in the same order of succession, arise: (1) the ascending pharyngeal; (2) the sternomastoid; (3) the occipital; and (4) the posterior auricular arteries. We will consider the arterial supply to the ear.

From the *facial artery*, a branch (*ascending palatine*) terminates by sending twigs to the soft palate, tonsils, and eustachian tube.

The Internal Maxillary Artery

The internal maxillary artery is a large branch arising from the anterior surface of the external carotid artery, opposite the neck of the mandible. It passes forward with a flexuous course, lying at first between the neck of the mandible and the sphenomandibular ligament, and then passing either between the two pterygoid muscles (in which case it crosses the inferior dental and lingual nerves) or over the external surface of the external pterygoid between that muscle and the temporal. It then passes between the two heads of the external pterygoid—in one case passing from below upward and in the other from without inward—and enters the sphenomaxillary fossa, where it is directed upward and inward towards the sphenopalatine foramen, which it transverses as the *sphenopalatine artery.*

Branch

For convenience in description, it is customary to regard the internal maxillary artery as consisting of three portions:

1. The *mandibular portion* lies internal to the neck of the mandible.
2. The *pterygoid portion* traverses the zygomatic fossa, and is in relation with the pterygoid muscles.
3. The *sphenomaxillary portion* extends between the two heads of the external pterygoid muscle to its entrance into the sphenopalatine foramen.

Of the 16 identified branches arising from the internal maxillary artery, five arise from the first portion, five from the second, and six from the third.

From the first or mandibular portion arise: (1) the *deep auricular;* (2) the *tympanic;* (3) the *middle meningeal;* (4) the *small meningeal;* and (5) the *inferior dental* arteries.

The *deep auricular artery* is a small branch that passes behind the temporomandibular articulation, to which it sends branches, and perforates the anterior wall of the external auditory meatus to supply the skin lining that passage and the outer surface of the tympanic membrane.

The *tympanic artery* (anterior tympanic artery), also a small branch, passes upward, giving off branches to the temporomandibular joint and entering the Glaserian fissure. Then it traverses the iter chordae anticus along with the chorda tympani, and reaches the middle ear—to whose mucous membrane it is distributed, anastomosing with the tympanic branches of the stylomastoid artery.

207

The *middle meningeal artery* is the largest of all the branches. It ascends vertically towards the base of the skull and enters the cranium by the foramen spinosum. After passing outward and upward for a short distance upon the great wing of the spenoid, it divides into anterior and posterior terminal branches, which ramify over the surface of the dural and supply nearly all of its lateral and superior surfaces, making abundant anastomoses with the vessel of the opposite side. The *anterior branch,* the larger of the two terminal branches, passes obliquely forward over the greater wing of the spenoid. It then crosses the anterior inferior angle of the parietal bone, and ascends along the anterior border of that bone almost to the superior longitudinal sinus, sending off numerous branches. The *posterior branch* passes backward and upward over the squamous portion of the temporal bone; it then passes over the posterior part of the parietal bone, giving off numerous branches that pass upward as far as the superior longitudinal sinus and backward as far as the lateral sinus. In addition to these terminal branches, the main stem within the cranium also gives origin to the following arteries.

The *superficial petrosal artery,* which enters the hiatus Fallopii and anastomoses with the terminal portion of the stylomastoid arteries.

The *Gasserian branches*—minute twigs that pass to the Gasserian ganglion and the fifth nerve.

The *superior tympanic artery,* which descends through the petrosquamous suture to the mucous membrane of the middle ear and the mastoid cells.

The *orbital branch.* A small vessel that passes into the orbit through the outermost portion of the sphenoidal fissure and anastomoses with the lachrymal branch of the ophthalmic.

The *small meningeal artery* (accessory meningeal) is an inconstant branch, sometimes arising from the middle meningeal. It passes upward along the mandibular division of the fifth nerve, and enters the cranium through the foramen ovale to be distributed to the Gasserian ganglion and the dura mater in its neighborhood.

The *inferior dental artery* (inferior alveolar artery) is given off from the lower surface of the artery and descends along with the inferior dental nerve to the mandibular foramen.

From the second, or pterygoid portion arise branches distributed chiefly to the adjacent muscles; they are the: (1) *masseteric;* (2) the *deep temporal;* (3) the *internal pterygoid;* (4) the *external pterygoid;* and (5) the *buccal* artery.

The *masseteric* branch passes with the corresponding nerve through the sigmoid notch of the mandible to enter the deep surface of the masseter.

The *deep temporal branches* are two in number, the anterior and the posterior. The *posterior branch* arises close to or in common with the masseteric, while the *anterior* one is given off near the termination of the pterygoid portion of the artery. They both pass upward between the temporal muscle and the bone, supplying the muscle and anas-

tomosing with the middle temporal branch of the temporal artery.

The *internal* and *external pterygoid* branches are short and variable in number. They pass directly into the muscles of the same names.

The *buccal branch* passes downward and forward along the anterior border of the tendon of the temporal muscle, and supplies the buccinator muscle and the mucous membrane of the mouth.

From the third or sphenomaxillary portion arise: (1) the *alveolar;* (2) the *infraorbital;* (3) the *descending palatine;* (4) the *Vidian;* (5) the *pterygopalatine;* and (6) the *sphenopalatine.*

The *alveolar branch* (superior posterior alveolar artery) descends upon the tuberosity of the maxilla and breaks up to distribute to the molar and premolar teeth and to the mucous membrane lining the maxillary sinus.

The *infraorbital artery* passes forward and upward through the sphenomaxillary fossa and sphenomaxillary foramen to traverse the infraorbital groove and canal along with the infraorbital nerve.

The *descending palatine artery* passes through the posterior palatine canal to emerge from the posterior palatine foramen. It divides into an anterior and a posterior branch. The former passes forward beneath the mucous membrane of the hard palate and at the anterior palatine foramen anastomoses with the sphenopalatine artery. The latter passes backward to supply the soft palate and the tonsil.

The *Vidian artery* (artery of the pterygoid canal) is a small branch which passes backward through the Vidian canal and sends branches to the roof of the pharynx and to the eustachian tube.

The *pterygopalatine artery* passes backward through the pterygopalatine foramen along the pharyngeal nerve from the sphenopalatine ganglion, and supplies the roof of the pharynx, the eustachian tube, and the mucous membrane lining the sphenoidal cells.

In the early stages of development the main portion of the internal maxillary is represented by a stem which arises from the internal carotid. This is known as the *stapedial artery,* since it traverses the middle ears, passing through the foramen of the stapes. It makes its exit from the middle ear by the Gasserian fissure and divides into two stems, one of which passes through the foramen spinosum and is distributed to the supraorbital region—while the other divides into two branches, which from their distribution are termed the *infraorbital* and the *mandibular* branches. A branch arises from the external carotid artery and anastomoses with the lower stem, where it divides into the two branches just mentioned. The main stem of the stapedius disappears, except in its distal portion, which persists as the tympanic branch of the internal maxillary artery. Thus, the adult internal maxillary artery is formed, with the supraorbital branch becoming the middle meningeal and the mandibular branch the inferior dental, while the infraorbital branch becomes the main stem of the artery from which the remaining branches gradually develop.

The Ascending Pharyngeal Artery

The *ascending pharyngeal artery* differs from all the other branches of the external carotid artery by its vertical course. This comparatively small artery arises close to the origin of the external carotid and passes upward—at first between that vessel and the internal carotid artery, and later between the internal carotid artery and internal jugular vein.

Branches

A *prevertebral branch* supplies the prevertebral muscles of the neck.

The *pharyngeal branches*, two or three in number, supply the constrictor muscles and mucous membranes of the pharynx.

The *meningeal branches* are a number of small twigs into which the artery breaks up as it approaches the base of the skull, passing through the jugular and anterior condyloid foramina to supply the dura mater of the posterior fossa of the skull, and through the cartilage of the middle lacerated foramen to supply the dura of the middle fossa.

The Occipital Artery

The *occipital artery* arises from the posterior surface of the carotid artery, opposite or a little below the facial artery. It passes upward and backward, and is at first partly covered by the posterior belly of the digastric and stylohyoid muscles, the parotid gland, and the temporomaxillary vein. It crosses in succession, from before backward, the hypoglossal nerve, vagus nerve, internal jugular vein, and spinal accessory nerve. It then passes more deeply in a groove on the posterior surface of the mastoid process and beneath the origin of the posterior belly of the digastric, sternocleidomastoid, and splenius capitus. Emerging from beneath these muscles, it reappears in the upper part of the occipital triangle, and then ascends in a tortuous course over the back of the skull. Sometimes it perforates the trapezius near its origin, and breaks up into numerous branches anastomosing with branches from the artery of the opposite side and those of the posterior auricular and superficial temporal arteries. In this last part of its course, it is superficial, lying beneath the skin upon the aponeurosis of the occipitofrontalis. The artery pierces the deeper structures, accompanied by the great occipital nerve a short distance lateral to and a little below the external occipital protuberance.

Branches

The *superior sternomastoid branch*. The *posterior meningeal branches* consist of one or more vessels that

pass upward along the internal jugular vein, enter the skull by the jugular foramen, and are supplied to the dura mater of the posterior fossa.[10,102,103]

The *auricular branch* passes upward over the mastoid process to supply the pinna of the ear.

The *mastoid branch* enters the skull by the mastoid foramen and supplies the mucous membrane lining the mastoid cells, diploe, and dura mater.

The *arteria princeps cervicis* descends the neck supplying the adjacent muscles and anastomosing with the superficial cervical branch of the transversalis colli and the profunda cervicis from the superior intercostal.

Anastomoses

The occipital artery makes abundant anastomoses in the scalp with the stylomastoid and temporal arteries.

Variations

The occipital artery occasionally passes superficially to the sternomastoid muscle instead of beneath it. It frequently gives origin to the ascending pharyngeal or stylomastoid arteries.

Practical Considerations

The occipital artery is rarely formally ligated. The *cervical portion* may be reached through an incision along the anterior border of the sternomastoid, beginning midway between the ramus of the mandible and the lobe of the ear and extending downward 2.5 inches. The deep fascia at the upper angle of the incision (parotid fascia) is spared on account of the risk of salivary fistula. At the lower angle, it is divided; also, the parotid and sternomastoid are separated, and the diagastric and stylohyoid muscles are identified and retracted upward. The occipital artery, near its origin, will then be seen crossing the internal carotid artery and internal jugular vein, and in contact with the curve of the hypoglossal nerve where it turns to cross the neck. The *occipital portion* is approached through an almost horizontal incision 2 inches in length, beginning at the tip of the mastoid and extending backward and a little upward. The outer fibers of the sternomastoid, its aponeurotic expansion, and the splenius must then be divided, and the pulsation of the artery must be looked for in the space between the mastoid and the transverse process of the atlas; from there, the vessel may be traced outward. If it is isolated near to the mastoid, great care must be taken not to injure the important mastoid venous tributaries of the occipital vein, which in this region connect it with the lateral sinus.

The Posterior Auricular Artery

This arises from the external carotid artery after it has passed beneath the posterior belly of the digastric. It passes upward and backward and is covered at first by the parotid gland, which it supplies, and divides in the angle between the pinna and the mastoid process into terminal branches. Some of these supply the pinna, while others anastomose with branches from the occipital and superficial temporal arteries.

Branches

In addition to branches leading to the parotid gland and neighboring muscles, the posterior auricular artery gives rise to the *stylomastoid artery*. This vessel enters the stylomastoid foramen and traverses the facial canal (aqueduct of Fallopius) as far as the point at which the hiatus Fallopii passes off from it. During its course through the canal, it gives off branches to the mucous membrane lining the mastoid cells, the stapedius muscle, and the mucous membrane of the middle ear; those twigs pass to the inner surface of the tympanic membrane, anastomosing with the tympanic branch of the internal maxillary artery. Arriving at the hiatus Fallopii, the artery accompanies the great superficial petrosal nerve through that canal and enters the cranium, supplying the dura mater and anastomosing with branches of the middle meningeal artery.

Variations

The stylomastoid artery may arise from the occipital artery, or its place may be taken by the petrosal branch of the middle meningeal, with which the stylomastoid normally anastomoses.

The Superficial Temporal Artery

This artery is the continuation of the external carotid artery after it has given off the internal maxillary artery. At its origin, it is embedded in the substance of the parotid gland, and is directed upward over the roof of the zygoma and immediately in front of the pinna. After ascending a short distance (usually about 2 cm) upon the aponeurosis covering the temporal muscle, it divides into anterior and posterior branches, which (diverging and branching repeatedly) pass upward over the temporal and occipitofrontal aponeuroses almost to the vertex of the skull. From there, they anastomose with the supraorbital branches of the opthalmic branch of the internal carotid artery, with the posterior auricular and occipital branches of the external carotid artery and the artery of the opposite side.

Branches

The *parotid branches* are small branches leading to the parotid gland.

The *articular branches* lead to the temporomandibular joint.

The *muscular branches* lead to the masseter muscle.

The *anterior auricular branches* supply the outer surface of the pinna and the outer portion of the external auditory meatus.

The *transverse facial artery* arises just below the mainstream of the artery, crosses the zygoma, and is directed forward parallel with the zygoma and between it and the parotid duct. It gives off branches to neighboring muscles and the skin of the cheek. This artery anastomoses with the masseteric branches of the facial artery and with the buccal, alveolar, and infraorbital branches of the internal maxillary artery.

The *middle deep temporal artery* arises just above the zygoma. After perforating the temporal aponeurosis and muscle, it ascends upon the surface of the skull to anastomose with the deep temporal branches of the internal maxillary artery.

The *orbital branch* runs forward along the upper border of the zygoma, supplying the orbicularis palpebrum and sending branches into the cavity of the orbit.

Anastomoses

The superficial temporal artery makes extensive anastomoses in the scalp with its counterpart of the opposite side, with the occipital and posterior auricular branches of the external carotid artery, and with the supraorbital branch of the opthalmic artery.

The Vertebral Artery

The vertebral artery—the first and largest branch of the subclavian artery—chiefly supplies the spinal cord and the brain, joining with the internal carotid arteries to form the intracranial anastomotic circle of Willis.

At the posterior border of the pons, the vertebral artery unites with its counterpart of the opposite side to form the basilar artery. The internal auditory arteries, one on each side, are given off the anterior inferior cerebellar artery and accompany the auditory nerve through the internal auditory meatus to supply the internal ear.

The Internal Carotid Artery

The internal carotid artery is the second terminal branch of the common carotid, from which it arises on a level with the upper border of the thyroid cartilage. In the *first* or *cervical portion* of its course, it lies upon the outer side of the external carotid artery; but as it passed upward, it comes to lie behind and internal to that vessel. It passes almost vertically up the neck to the entrance of the carotid canal, resting posteriorly on the prevertebral fascia. On its medial side is the wall of the pharynx, and laterally is the internal jugular vein. The vagus nerve lies between it and the artery, and is on a plane slightly posterior to both. It is also in relation, in the upper part of this cervical portion of its course, with the glossopharyngeal nerve, which lies at first behind it, but crosses its external surface lower down as it bends forward towards the tongue and with the superior sympathetic ganglion, whose cardiac branch descends along its internal surface. The pharyngeal branches cross it and the carotid branch ascends with the artery to the carotid canal, in which it breaks up to form the carotid plexus.

In the *second* or *petrosal portion* of its course, the internal carotid artery traverses the carotid canal, conforming to its direction and passing at first vertically upward and then bending forward and inward to enter the cranial cavity at the foramen lacerum medium.

It then enters upon the *third* or *intracranial portion* of its course, ascending at first towards the posterior clinoid process. Then it bends forward and enters the outer wall of the cavernous sinus. It passes forward, accompanied by the VI cranial nerve (abducens); at the level of the anterior clinoid process, it bends upward, pierces the dura mater, and quickly divides into its terminal branches.

Branches

Throughout its cervical portion, the internal carotid artery normally gives off no branches; in its petrosal portion, in addition to some small twigs to the periosteal lining of the carotid canal, it gives origin to a *tympanic branch.* In its intracranial portion—in addition to small branches to the walls of the cavernous sinus and the related cranial nerves to the Gasserian ganglion—and to the pituitary body, there arise (1) *anterior meningeal;* (2) the *ophthalmic;* (3) *posterior communicating;* (4) and *anterior choroid arteries.* And finally, these cause its terminal branches; (5) the *middle* and *anterior cerebral arteries.*

Variations

In its cervical portion, the internal carotid artery occasionally takes a sinuous course; and in its upper part it may make a pronounced horseshoe-shaped curve. It may give rise to branches that normally spring from the external carotid artery; for example, the ascending pharyngeal and the lingual. Accessory branches may arise from its intracranial portion.

The Tympanic Artery

This is a small vessel arising from the petrous portion of the internal carotid artery. It passes through a foramen in the wall of the carotid canal to supply the mucous membrane of the middle ear, anastomosing with the tympanic branches of the stylomastoid and internal maxillary arteries.

Sinuses of the Dura Mater

The sinuses of the dura mater (Fig. 267) form a series of channels, often of considerable size, that occupy clefts in the substance of the dura mater. They receive the cerebral, meningeal, and diploic veins. They also communicate with the extracranial veins by numerous connecting veins called *emissary veins,*—the largest and most important of which are the ophthalmic veins. Drainage of these veins is mostly by the internal jugular vein.[102]

The dural sinuses are lined by an endothelium similar to and continuous with that of the extracranial veins, but they lack any extensive development of elastic fibers in their walls, which are formed by the dura. They possess no valves; but in certain ones, as in the superior longitudinal and cavernous sinuses, the lumen is traversed by irregular trabeculae of fibrous tissue. These are especially well developed and almost tendinous in character in the superior longitudinal sinus. In the cavernous sinus, they are softer; from them and the walls of the sinus, fringe-like prolongations 0.5 to 2 mm in length project freely into the lumen. Connected with certain of these sinuses and developed from certain of the smaller veins opening into them are so-called *blood lakes* (lacunae)—cavities or plexuses in the dura mater, lined with endothelium, connecting either directly or by means of a short canal with an adjacent sinus. They are usually situated more or less symmetrically with reference to the sinus with which they are connected, and some are very constant in occurrence. Thus, a certain number usually occur on either side of the superior longitudinal sinus; others occur in the middle fossa of the skull along the course of the meningeal vessels, and in the vicinity of the straight sinus. They occasionally reach a considerable size, bulging the dura outward, which encloses them. They also excavate by absorption irregular depressions upon the inner surfaces of the skull. Occasionally, this absorption of the cranial bones proceeds so far that bulging of the outer table of the skull over a lake takes place. In the case of those occurring along the course of the superior longitudinal sinus, Pacchionian bodies developed from the subjacent arachnoid tissue may invade them, pushing before them the attenuated floor of the lakes.

The Lateral Sinus

The lateral sinus (transverse sinus) has its origin opposite the internal occipital protuberance, at which point there is a meeting of five sinuses: two lateral, superior longitudinal,

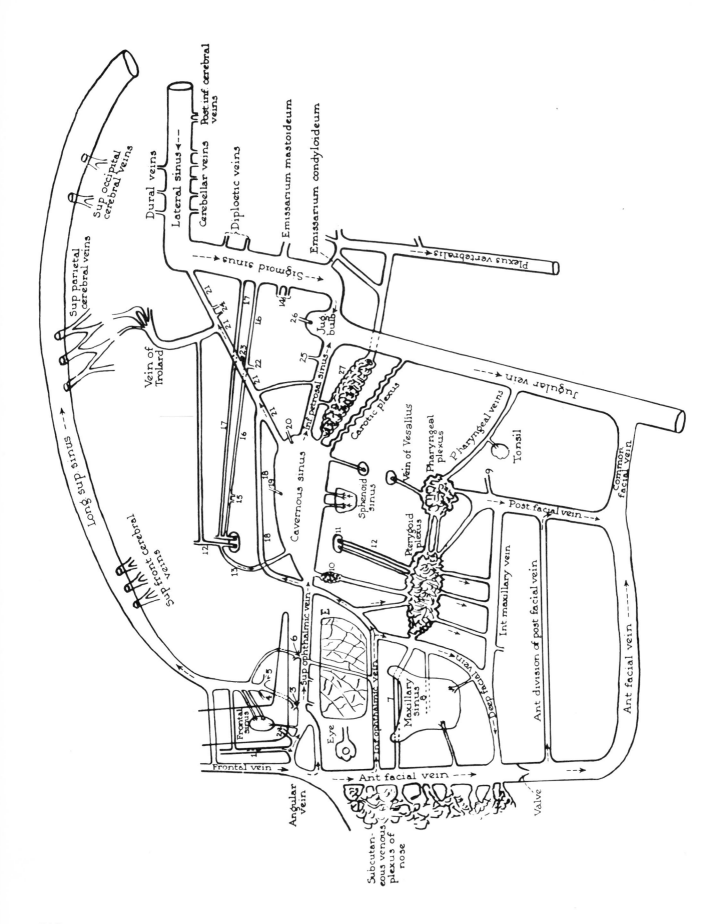

Sup parietal cerebral veins

Sup occipital cerebral veins

Post inf cerebral veins

Dural veins

Lateral sinus

Cerebellar veins

Diploetic veins

Emissarium mastoideum

Emissarium condyloideum

Plexus vertebralis

Sigmoid sinus

Vein of Trolard

Long sup. sinus

Jug. bulb

Jugular vein

Inf petrosal sinus

Carotic plexus

Sup front cerebral veins

Vein of Vesalius

Pharyngeal plexus

Pharyngeal veins

Tonsil

Cavernous sinus

Sphenoid sinus

Pterygoid plexus

Post facial vein

Sup ophthalmic vein

Deep facial vein

Common facial vein

E

Int maxillary vein

Eye

Inf ophthalmic vein

Maxillary sinus

Ant division of post facial vein

Frontal sinus

Ant facial vein

Frontal vein

Ant facial vein

Valve

Angular vein

Subcutaneous venous plexus of nose

212

Figure 267. Principal veins of the brain and face and their anastomoses with dural sinuses. 1, Supraorbital vein. 2, Frontal diploic vein. 3, Anterior ethmoid vein. 4, Vein from the olfactory bulb. 5, Veins from the dura. 6, Posterior ethmoid vein. 7, Infraorbital vein. 8, Sphenopalatine vein from the nasal mucosa to the pterygoid plexus. 9, Superficial temporal vein. 10, Rete foraminis ovalis. 11, Foramen spinosum. 12, Middle meningeal vein. 13, Sphenoparietal sinus. 14, Veins from the tympanic cavity, antrum, and mastoid. 15, Veins from the tympanic cavity. 16, Petrosquamous sinus. 17, Vein of Labbe. 18, Ophthalmopetrosal sinus. 19, Middle and inferior cerebral veins. 20, Veins from the tentorium. 21, Superior petrosal sinus. 22, Vena fossae subarcuatae. 23, Vena aquaductus vestibuli. 24, Veins from the tympanic cavity. 25, Vena auditiva interna. 26, Vena aquaductus cochleae. 27, Plexus basilaris; E. ethmoid.[109]

213

straight, and occipital. From this junction, which is called the *torcular Herophili,* each lateral sinus passes outward over the squamous portion of the occipital bone along the line of attachment of the tentorium cerebelli. Passing over the posterior inferior angle of the parietal, each is continued inward upon the inner surface of the mastoid portion of the temporal and the jugular process of the occipital to reach the jugular foramen, where it opens into the internal jugular vein. As each passes the mastoid portion of the temporal, it leaves the line of attachment of the tentorium cerebelli, passing somewhat downward as well as inward and following the line of junction of the petrous and mastoid portions of the bone in a somewhat S-shaped course; this portion is frequently called the *sigmoid sinus.*

A difference in size is usually noticeable in sinuses of the opposite sides. The sinus of the right side is usually larger. This difference is due to the mode in which the various sinuses meet at the torcular Herophili. Most frequently, the superior longitudinal sinus communicates mainly with the right lateral sinus, while the straight sinus opens principally into the left so that the greater amount of blood is carried by the superior longitudinal one (compared with that transmitted by the straight sinus, resulting in the larger size of the right lateral sinus). In some cases, the right lateral sinus is practically the direct continuation of the superior longitudinal and left lateral of the straight sinus; the two laterals are connected only by a short and relatively small connecting arm, which represents the torcular Herophili. Throughout that portion of their courses, in which the lateral sinuses lie in the line of attachment of the tentorium cerebelli, they are triangular in cross- section; but in their mastoid (sigmoid) portion, they are semicircular. The right sinus has a diameter of 9 to 12 mm, while the left sinus is 3 to 5 mm. At the jugular foramen, each sinus makes a sudden bend and opens either directly into the summit of the superior jugular bulb, or else at a varying distance downward upon the anterior surface of the bulb. The upper extremity then forms a dome-shaped structure projecting upward into the jugular foramen.

Tributaries

The lateral sinuses, in addition to the sinuses that communicate with them at the torcular Herophili, receive the following tributaries:

1. The *posterior inferior cerebral veins,* which pass backward from the temporosphenoidal region of the cerebral hemispheres.
2. Some of the *inferior cerebellar veins.*
3. The *superior petrosal sinus,* which communicates just where it leaves the line of attachment of the tentorium cerebelli.
4. The *internal auditory veins* emptying into the sigmoid portion.
5. The *mastoid emissory vein.*
6. Some of the veins of the medulla oblongata and pons.

Variations

Considerable variation exists in the relative sizes of the right and left lateral sinuses due to the superior longitudinal sinus opening more or less directly into one or the other. The tendency is for the superior longitudinal sinus to open into the right lateral. Quite often, however, it opens into the left sinus; occasionally, it may communicate equally with both. In 100 cranial specimens, Ruedinger found that the right lateral sinus was the larger in 70 cases, the left in 27, and the two laterals were equal in size in only three cases.

The horizontal portion of the left sinus has been observed to be lacking or reduced to an exceedingly fine channel. One or both of the sinuses have been observed passing through a greatly enlarged mastoid foramen, opening into the posterior auricular vein; the sigmoid sinus is represented only by a very small channel.

In a considerable number of cases, a small sinus known as the *petrosquamosal sinus* opens into the lateral sinus just as it bends downward and inward upon the mastoid portion of the temporal. This sinus passes downward over the anterior surface of the petrous portion of the temporal bone, along the line of its junction with the squamous portion. It occasionally passes through a foramen—the *foramen jugulare spurium*—which opens to the exterior just behind the articular eminence of the zygomatic process. The sinus represents the original terminal portion of the lateral sinus. The sigmoid portion of that sinus is a secondary formation and opens after its exit from the foramen jugular spurium into the internal jugular vein, although its connection in the adult is with the temporal vein.[14]

Practical Considerations

Because of its proximity to the middle ear, mastoid antrum, and cells, the sigmoid portion of the lateral sinus is more often the subject of thrombosis than any other sinus. This may arise in the following six ways:

1. Extension from chronic purulent inflammation of the middle ear.
2. Extension of acute inflammatory disease from the mouth, pharynx, and tonsils into the middle ear, antrum, and air cells.
3. Extension of thrombosis from other sinuses, especially the superior petrosal sinus.
4. Trauma, such as basal skull fractures extending through the middle ear to the sinus.
5. Pressure of tumors or discharge associated with them.
6. Infection from septic wounds of the head, neck, or mastoid region.

The Superior Longitudinal Sinus

The superior longitudinal sinus is an unpaired sinus that lies along the line of attachment of the falx cerebri to the cranial vault. It begins blindly anteriorly by a small vein-like portion that lies in the foramen caecum between the frontal and ethmoid bones; it soon becomes a true sinus that passes upward and backward in the medial line of the frontal bone beneath the sagittal suture of the parietals, and down the medial line of the squamous portion of the occipital to terminate at the internal occipital protuberance by opening into the torcular Herophili—or usually more or less directly into the right lateral sinus.

The sinus is triangular in section and increases gradually in size from front to back, measuring about 1.5 mm in diameter at the level of the apex of the crista galli and 11 mm at its termination. Its lumen is usually traversed by numerous irregular bonds of connective tissue known as *chordae Willisii,* frequently, especially in aged persons, Pacchionian bodies, which are numerous along its course, project into it.

Practical Considerations

The superior longitudinal sinus may become involved by aseptic inflammation spreading upwards from the lateral sinus, sealing off the absorption of cerebrospinal fluid into the bloodstream. This may produce increased retention of cerebrospinal fluid and produce the condition known as otitic hydrocephalus.

The Inferior Longitudinal Sinus

The inferior longitudinal sinus is an unpaired sinus that lies in the inferior or free edge of the falx cerebri. It begins at about the middle of the border of the falx and passes backward, gradually increasing in size, to the junction of the falx with the tentorium cerebelli, where it opens into the straight sinus. It receives small tributaries from the falx and occasionally from the corpus callosum.

The Straight Sinus

The straight sinus, also unpaired, lies along the line of junction of the falx cerebri with the tentorium cerebelli. It is formed at the anterior border of the tentorium by the junction of the inferior longitudinal sinus and the great cerebral vein (vein of Galen); it is directed backward to open into the torcular Herophili or, more often, into the left lateral sinus. In addition to the two trunks by whose union it is formed, it receives a number of small branches from the tentorium, the posterior portion of the medial surfaces of the cerebral hemispheres, and sometimes a medial superior cerebellar vein.

The Occipital Sinus

The occipital sinus is an unpaired or (in some cases) a paired sinus that descends from the torcular Herophili along the line of attachment of the falx cerebelli to the posterior border of the foramen magnum. There it divides into two trunks—the *marginal sinuses,* which pass forward along the margin of the foramen magnum (one on either side) to open into the bulbous superior branch of the corresponding internal jugular vein.

The occipital sinus receives as tributaries branches from the falx cerebelli and the adjacent portions of the dura, and also some veins from the inferior surface of the cerebellum. At the posterior border of the foramen magnum, where it bifurcates to form the marginal sinuses, it connects with the veins of the posterior spinal plexus.

The occipital sinus is sometimes lacking and frequently extends only as far as the posterior border of the foramen magnum, with the marginal sinuses being undeveloped. It may open above into either the right or left lateral sinus, or into the straight sinus a short distance before its termination.

The Cavernous Sinus

The cavernous sinus is a paired sinus of considerable size extending along the sides of the body of the sphenoid bone from the sphenoidal fissure in front to the apex of the petrous portion of the temporal bone. It measures about 2 cm in length, has a diameter of about 1 cm, and is almost quadrilateral in cross-section. Its external diameter does not, however, represent the actual capacity of its lumen since this is greatly reduced in size:

1. By being traversed by numerous trabeculae from which fringe-like prolongations hang freely into the blood current.
2. By the fact that the internal carotid artery and the VI cranial nerve traverse it, while certain other of the cranial nerves are embedded in its outer wall. These nerves are the oculomotor, pathetic (trochlear), and ophthalmic and maxillary divisions of the trigeminus, which lie in that order from above downward.

Tributaries

At the sphenoidal fissure, the cavernous sinus receives the ophthalmic vein and, further back, occasionally the basilar vein. In addition, it receives veins from the neighboring portions of the dura mater, and connects with the sphenoparietal and *intercavernous sinuses.* These latter are transverse sinuses that pass across between the two cavernous sinuses—the *anterior intercavernous sinus* passes in front of the sella turcica and the *posterior intercavernous sinus* passes behind that cavity, and they receive branches from the dura mater and pituitary body. The two sinuses, together with the portion of the cavernous sinus between their terminations on each side, form what is usually called the *circular sinus.*

Besides the vessels that are truly tributaries, the cavernous sinus is also connected to certain vessels that are emissary in function, leading blood away from it. The two petrosal sinuses in which it terminates are of this nature. In addition, veins pass from its under surface:

1. Through the foramen ovale, along with the mandibular division of the trigeminal nerve, to communicate with the pterygoid plexus.
2. Through the fibrous tissue, which closes the foramen lacerum medium.
3. Through the foramen of Vesalius, when this exists.
4. Occasionally through the foramen rotundum with the maxillary division of the trigeminal nerve.

Where the internal carotid artery enters the cavernous sinus at the internal orifice of the carotid canal, the sinus projects downward around the artery in a funnel-shaped manner. From it arises a close network of veins (the *carotid plexus* or *carotid sinus*) that completely invests the artery through its course through the carotid canal, at the lower opening of which it continues into one or two veins opening into the internal jugular vein.

Practical Considerations

The cavernous sinus may become infected from foci apparently far removed through the extraorbital communications of the ophthalmic veins. Thus, carbuncles of the face, empyema of the maxillary antrum, osteomyelitis of the frontal diploic tissue may each be followed by cavernous sinus thrombosis. In the presence of thrombosis, there are two groups of pressure symptoms.

1. Venous symptoms, causing exophthalmos, edema of the eyelids and the corresponding side of the root of the nose, and some chemosis.
2. Nervous symptoms, causing ptosis, strabismus, variations in the pupil, pain, etc.

An arteriovenous aneurysm between this sinus and the internal carotid artery, in addition to symptoms of venous obstruction, often causes paralyses in the distribution of the third, fourth, and ophthalmic divisions of the V cranial nerves (which lie in the dura mater on the outer wall of the sinus) and the VI cranial nerve (which is in close relation to the internal carotid artery).

The bulk of the blood in the anterior and lower portions of the skull empties into the cavernous sinus. The remaining portion—including the greater part of the cerebrum, cerebellum, pons, and cerebral peduncles—empties chiefly into the tributaries of the lateral sinus. The two sinuses through the superior petrosal sinus and other venous channels have free anastomotic connections that effectively equalize or distribute venous blood pressure.

The communication between the two cavernous sinuses through the basilar sinus or plexus and the circular sinus is an important portion of the mechanism by which the venous blood pressure within the skull is equalized. However, this same communication may, in an arterio-venous aneurysm, bring about involvement of the orbit on the other side. The blood from the aneurysm enters the opposite sinus by way of these intercommunicating sinuses, or infection may follow the same channel.

The Sphenoparietal Sinus

The sphenoparietal sinus arises at the outer extremity of the lesser wing of the sphenoid from one of the meningeal veins, and passes horizontally inward under cover of the posterior border of the lesser wing to reach the cavernous sinus near its anterior extremity. It receives dural, diploic, and some anterior cerebral veins.

The Superior Petrosal Sinus

The superior petrosal sinus is the smaller of the two sinuses into which the cavernous divides at the apex of the petrosa. It passes outward and backward along the superior border of the petrous bone, and opens into the lateral sinus just at the point where it leaves the line of attachment of the tentorium cerebelli to become the sigmoid sinus. The superior petrosal sinuses receive some small tympanic vessels and some branches from the cerebellum and cerebrum.

The Inferior Petrosal Sinus

The inferior petrosal sinus is the larger terminal branch of the cavernous sinus, and extends from the posterior extremity of that sinus, at the apex of the petrosa, along the petrooccipital suture to the jugular foramen; there it opens into the superior bulb of the jugular vein or frequently into the vein below the bulb.

In addition to small branches from the neighboring portions of the dura and the cerebellum, pons, and medulla oblongata, the inferior petrosal sinus receives some internal auditory veins and an *anterior condyloid vein,* which arises from a plexus surrounding the hypoglossal nerve in its course through the anterior condyloid foramen. In its anterior portion, the sinus is also in communication with the basilar sinus.

The Basilar Sinus

The basilar sinus, also called the *transverse sinus,* is usually a plexus of sinuses rather than a single distinct sinus. It occupies the dura mater that covers the basilar process of the occipital bone, and it communicates with the inferior petrosal and posterior intercavernous sinuses in front and behind the anterior border of the foramen magnum with the anterior spinal plexus. It receives branches from the medulla oblongata and the diploe.

Practical Considerations

Fracture of the base of the skull through the posterior fossa may involve the basilar plexus of sinuses, and be followed by an intracranial hemorrhage that slowly oozes through the line of fracture. Following the lines of vessels or nerves, this hemorrhage ultimately causes swelling and ecchymosis of the skin of the neck. The latter is likely to first show anteriorly to the mastoid tip; in this region, the blood is conducted by the cellular tissue around the auricular artery. It spreads upward and backward in a curved line.

The superior and (particularly) inferior petrosal sinuses have to be dealt with in skull base surgery, in which the temporal bone with its apex is removed.

The Diploic Veins

The spaces of the diploe are traversed by a rich plexus of veins characterized by the thinness of their walls. They open by numerous small communicating branches either into the veins of the scalp, middle meningeal veins, or cranial sinuses. Some larger, although rather inconsistant, stems also arise from the plexus and form what are termed the *diploic veins.* Of these, four are usually recognized:

1. *Anterior diploic vein.* This descends in the diploe of the frontal bone. At the level of the supraorbital notch, it opens either into the supraorbital or ophthalmic vein. It communicates with the anterior temporal diploic vein, and also with the frontal veins and superior longitudinal sinus.
2. *Anterior temporal diploic vein.* This passes downward and forward in the diploe of the anterior portion of the parietal bone, and opens either into a deep temporal vein or into the sphenoparietal sinus.
3. *Posterior temporal diploic vein.* This passes downward in the diploe of the posterior part of the parietal bone, and usually opens into the mastoid emissary vein, thus communicating with the lateral sinus. It also communicates with the posterior auricular vein and may open into it.
4. *Occipital diploic vein.* This passes downward in the squamous portion of the occipital bone, not far from the median line. It opens either into the occipital vein or into the occipital emissary vein, by which it communicates with the torcular Herophili of the lateral sinus.

Practical Considerations

The diploic veins are incapable of effective contraction, and bleed freely and persistently. They are often a source of embarrassment during surgery on the skull. Through their communications with the veins of the scalp and the endocranial sinuses and meningeal vessels, they may (as in some cases of compound fractures) convey infections from the surface to the diploe causing osteomyelitis—or within the cranium, causing septic meningitis or sinus thrombosis. Diploic infection introduced from outside the cranium (hematogenous as in tuberculosis[94]) is likely to spread rapidly within the diploic tissue itself.

The Emissary Veins

The term *emissary vein* is applied to those branches placing the sinuses of the dura mater in communication with veins external to the cranial cavity. Using the term in its broadest sense, the emissary veins are very numerous, since both the diploic and meningeal veins might be regarded as such, as well as the carotid plexus and the ophthalmic vein. All make connections with the sinuses and the extracranial veins. It is customary, however, to limit the term to certain veins that traverse special foramina in the cranail walls; a few, however, pass through the foramina, whose principal content is one of the cranial nerves.

The *parietal emissary vein,* rather variable in size, traverses the correspondingly variable parietal foramen, placing the superior longitudinal sinus in communication with the veins of the scalp.

The *occipital emissary vein* traverses the occipital protuberance, and places the torcular Herophili or one or the other lateral sinuses in communication with the occipital veins. Its size is variable; it usually receives the occipital diploic vein, and may perforate only the external or internal table of the occipital bone, representing the terminal portion of the diploic vein rather than a true emissary.

The *mastoid emissary vein* passes through the mastoid foramen and places the lateral sinus in communication with either the occipital or posterior auricular veins. It is occasionally lacking and may be so large that it appears to be the continuation of the lateral sinus. The terminal portion of that vessel between the mastoid and jugular foramina is greatly reduced in size.

The *posterior condyloid emissary vein* is very inconstant. When present, it traverses the posterior condyloid foramen, extending between the lateral sinus near its termination and the vertebral veins.

The *anterior condyloid emissary vein* is a network that surrounds the hypoglossal nerve in its course through the anterior condyloid foramen. From the plexus, two veins arise, one of which passes to the inferior petrosal sinus and the other to the vertebral veins.

The *emissaries of the foramen ovale* are formed by two veins that communicate above with cavernous sinus and pass to the foramen ovale, where they form a plexus surrounding the mandibular division of the trigeminal nerve and communicate with the pterygoid plexus of veins. Occasionally, a similar plexus accompanies the maxillary division of the trigeminal nerve through the foramen rotundum.

The *emissary vein of the foramen of Vesalius* is inconstant, like the foramen, occurring only about once in three cases. It extends between the cavernous sinus and the pterygoid plexus of veins.

Finally, a variable number of small veins pass through the connective tissue and close the foramen lacerum medium, placing the cavernous sinus in communication with the pterygoid plexus.

Practical Considerations

The relations of the emissary veins explain many cases of the spread of extracranial infection to the meninges and sinuses. The largest of these veins is usually the mastoid—the communication between the lateral sinus and the occipital or posterior auricular vein. It may be responsible for the extensive edema behind the ear and around the mastoid region often seen in lateral sinus thrombosis. The escape of pus via the mastoid foramen indicates extradural pus in the cerebellar fossa around the sigmoid groove.

In suppurative sigmoid sinus disease, the posterior condyloid vein may convey infection to the cellular tissue in the upper part of the posterior cervical triangle, causing an abscess beneath the deep fascia. The emissary veins are important pathways for equalization of intracranial pressure.

References

1. Proctor B, Nielsen E, Proctor C: Petrosquamosal suture and lamina. Otolaryngol Head Neck Surg 1981;89:482-495.

2. Proctor B: Embryology and anatomy of the eustachian tube. Arch Otolaryngol 1967;86:503-514.

3. Proctor B: Anatomy of the eustachian tube. Arch Otolaryngol 1971;97:2-8.

4. Proctor B: The development of the middle ear spaces and their surgical significance. J Laryngol Otol 1964;78:631-648.

5. Proctor B: Surgical anatomy of the posterior tympanum. Ann Otol Rhinol Laryngol 1969;78:1026-1041.

6. Proctor B, Nager GT: The facial canal: Normal anatomy, variations and anomalies. Ann Otol Rhinol Laryngol 1982;97 (Suppl 97):33-61.

7. Cheatle AH: *Surgical Anatomy of the Temporal Bone.* London: J & A Churchill Ltd, 1907.

8. Anson B, Donaldson J: *Surgical Anatomy of the Temporal Bone and Ear,* ed. 2. Philadelphia: WB Saunders Co, 1973, p 190.

9. Politzer A: *Diseases of the Ear,* ed. 5. London: Bailliere, Tindall and Cox, 1909, pp 30-37.

10. Anson B, Bast T: *The temporal Bone and the Ear.* Springfield: Charles O Thomas, 1949, p 203.

11. Bellocq P: *L'os Temporal.* Paris: Masson et Cie, 1924.

12. Schulman A, Rock EH: Koerner's (petrosquamous) septum in otology. Arch Otolaryngol 1972;96:124-129.

13. Wigand ME, Trillsch K: Surgical anatomy of the sinus epitympani. Ann Otol Rhinol Laryngol 1973;82:378-384.

14. Piersol GA: *Human Anatomy.* Philadelphia: JB Lippincott Co, 1930, pp 733-745.

15. Lindsay JR: Pneumatization of the petrous pyramid Ann Otol Rhinol Laryngol 1941;50:1109-1113.

16. Anson BJ, Bast TH, Richany SF: The fetal and early postnatal development of the tympanic ring and related structures in man. Ann Otol Rhinol Laryngol 1955;64:802-824.

17. Proctor B: Attic-aditus block and the tympanic diaphragm. Ann Otol Rhinol Laryngol 1971;80:371-375.

18. Hawke M, Farkashidy J, Jahn AJ: Non-lamellar new bone formation in the anterior attic recess. Arch Otolaryngol 1975; 101:117-119.

19. Gacek RR: Surgical landmark for the facial nerve in the epitympanum. Ann Otol Rhinol Laryngol 1980;89:249-250.

20. Spector GJ, Ge X: Development of the hypotympanum in the human fetus and neonate. Ann Otol Rhinol Laryngol 1981; 90 (Suppl):88.

21. Hammar JA: Studien ueber die Entwicklung des Vorderdarms und einiger angrenzender Organe. Arch Mikrosk Anat 1902; 59:471-628.

22. Fraser JE: The nomenclature of diseased states caused by certain vestigial structures in the neck. Brit J Surg 1923;11:131-136.

23. Eichel BS, Hallberg OE: Hamartoma of the middle ear and eustachian tube. Laryngoscope 1966;76:1810-1815.

24. Jacobson AG: Inductive processes in embryonic development. Science 1966;152:25-34.

25. Zollner F: *Ohrtrompete.* Berlin: Springer-Verlag, 1942.

26. Terracol J, Corone A, Guerrier Y: *La Trompe d'Eustache.* Paris: Masson et Cie, 1949.

27. Weber (quoted by Terracol J, Corone A, Guerrier Y): *La Trompe d'Eustache.* Paris: Masson et Cie, 1949.

28. Zukerkandl E: Zur Anatomie und Physiologie der Tuba Eustachiana. Mschr Ohrenheilk 1873;7:146, 1874;8:126.

29. Bezold F: *Textbook of Otology.* Chicago: EH Colgrove Co, 1908,p 189 (translated by J Holinger).

30. Wolff D: Microscopic anatomy of the eustachian tube. Ann Otol 1931;40:1055-1067.

31. Farrior JB: Histopathological considerations in treatment of the eustachian tube. Arch Otolaryngol 1943;37:609- 621.

32. Hamberger CA, Marcuson G, Wersall J: Blood vessels of the ossicular chain. Acta Otolaryngol 1963;183(Supp):66-70.

33. Richardson GS: Aditus block. Ann Otol 1963;72:223-236.

34. Allam AF: Pneumatization of the temporal bone. Ann Otol Rhinol Laryngol 1969;78:49- 64.

35. Girard L: Atlas d'anatomie et de médecine opératoire du labyrinthe osseux. Paris: Libraire Maloine, 1939.

36. Fisch U: Surgery for Bell's palsy. Arch Otolaryngol 1981; 107:1-11.

37. Guerrier Y: Surgical anatomy, particulary vascular supply of the facial nerve. In: Fisch U (ed): *Facial Nerve Surgery.* Birmingham, AL: Aesculapius, 1977.

38. Walker AE: Attachment of dura mater over base of skull. Anat Rec 1933;55:291-295.

39. Hoshino T, Suzuki J: Anterior attic wall anatomy. Arch Otolaryngol 1978;104:588-590.

40. Litton W, Krause C, Anson B, Cohen W: Relationship of fa-

cial canal to the annular sulcus. Laryngoscope 1969;79:1584-1604.

41. Paturet G: *Traite d'anatomie Humaine,* Vols. I & IV, Paris: Masson et Cie, 1951.

42. Anson BJ, Harper DG, Warphea RI: Surgical anatomy of the facial nerve. Ann Otol Rhinol Laryngol 1963;72:713-734.

43. Baxter A: Dehiscence of the fallopian canal. J Laryngol Otol 1971;85:587-594.

44. Dietzel K: Ueber die Dehiszenzen des Facialiskanals. Z Laryngol Rhinol Otol 1961;40:366- 376.

45. Guild SR: Natural absence of part of the bony wall of the facial canal. Laryngoscope 1949;59:668-673.

46. Politzer A: In: Dalby W (ed): *A Textbook of the Diseases of the Ear and Adjacent Organs* (translated by O Dodd). Philadelphia: Lea Brothers & Co, 1894.

47. Schuknecht H: Anatomical variants and anomalies of surgical significance. J Laryngol Otol 1971;85:1238- 1241.

48. Donaldson JA, Anson BJ: Surgical anatomy of the facial nerve. Symposium on disease and injury of the facial nerve. Otolaryngol Clin North Am June 1974.

49. Jahrsdoerfer RA: The facial nerve in congenital middle ear malformations. Laryngoscope 1981;91:1217-1225.

50. Johnsson LG, Kingsley TC: Herniation of the facial nerve in the middle ear. Arch Otolaryngol 1970;91:598-602.

51. Babin RW, Fratkin J, Harker LA: Traumatic neuromas of the facial nerve. Arch Otolaryngol 1981;107:55-58.

52. Arndt HJ: Zweiteilung des Nervus facilis zwischen Ganglion geniculi und Foramen stylomastoideum. Berlin: HNO 1967; 15: 116-118.

53. Kullman GL, Dyck PJ, Cody TR: Anatomy of the mastoid portion of the facial nerve. Arch Otolaryngol 1971;93:29-33.

54. Fowler EP Jr: Variations in the temporal bone course of the facial nerve. Laryngoscope 1961;71:937-944.

55. Dworacek H: Die Anatomischen Verhaeltnisse des Mittelohres unter Operations—mikroskopischer Betrachtung. Acta Otolaryngol 1960;51:15-45.

56. Altman F: Zur Anatomie und formalen Genese der Atresia auris congenita. Monatsschr Ohrenheilkd Laryngo-Rhinol 1933; 67:765-771.

57. Miehlke A, Partsch CJ: Ohrmissbildung, Facialis und Abducenslaehmung als Syndrom der Thalidomidschaedigung. Arch Ohren Heilk Z Hals Heilk 1963;181:154-174.

58. Durcan DJ, Shea JJ, Sleeckx JP: Bifurcation of the facial nerve. Arch Otolaryngol 1967;86:619-631.

59. Marquet J: Congenital malformations and middle ear surgery. J Royal Soc Med 1981;74:119-128.

60. Butler GE: Transstapedial congenital malposition of the facial nerve. Arch Otolaryngol 1968;88:268.

61. Martin H, Martin C: Anomaly of the facial nerve pathway and congenital ankylosis of the footplate. J Fr Oto-Rhino-Laryngol Chir Maxill-Fac 1977;26:543-545.

62. Mayer TG, Crabtree JA: The facial nerve coursing inferior to the oval window. Arch Otolaryngol 1976;102:744-746.

63. Leek JF: An anomalous facial nerve; the otologist's albatross. Laryngoscope 1974;84:1535- 1544.

64. Henner R: Congenital middle ear malformation. Arch Otolaryngol 1960;71:454-458.

65. Dickinson JT, Srisomboon P, Kamerer DB: Congenital anomaly of the facial nerve. Arch Otolaryngol 1968;88:357-359.

66. Kodama A, Sando I, Myers EN, Hashida Y: Severe middle ear anomaly with underdeveloped facial nerve. Arch Otolaryngol 1982;108:93-98.

67. Bast TH, Anson BJ, Richany SF: The development of the second branchial arch, facial canal and associated structures in man. Quart Bull Northwestern U Med School 1956;30:235-250.

68. Hanson JE, Anson BJ, Strickland EM: Branchial sources of the auditory ossicles in man. Arch Otolaryngol 1962;76:200-215.

69. Kettel K: Surgery of the facial nerve. Arch Otolaryngol 1963;77:327-341.

70. Wright JW: Polytomography and congenital external and middle ear anomalies. Laryngoscope 1981;91:1806-1811.

71. Kettel K: Abnormal course of facial nerve in the fallopian canal. Arch Otolaryngol 1946;44:406-408.

72. Miehlke A: *Surgery of the Facial Nerve.* Munich: Urban und Swarzenberg Verlag, 1973; Philadelphia: WB Saunders Co, 1973.

73. Glasscock M: Unusual facial nerve problems. Laryngoscope 1971;81:669-683.

74. Pou JW: Congenital anomalies of the middle ear: Presentation of two cases. Laryngoscope 1971;81:831-839.

75. Pracy R: Surgery for congenital conductive deafness. Proc R Soc Med 1977;70:823-826.

76. Harpman JA: A congenital aural deformity and its correction. Eye Ear Nose Throat Monthly 1971;50:10-13.

77. Bellucci RJ: Congenital aural malformations, diagnoses and treatment. Otolaryngol Clin North Am 1981;95-124.

78. Hahlbrook KH: Zweiteilung des N facialis im Warzenfortsatz. Arch Ohren Nasen Kehkopfheilkd 1960;174:465-469.

79. Basek M: Anomalies of the facial nerve in normal temporal bones. Ann Otol Rhinol Laryngol 1962;71:382-390.

80. Botman JW, Jongkees LBW: Endotemporal branching of the facial nerve. Acta Otolaryngol (Stock) 1955;45:111-114.

81. Heermann J Jr: Zwei und dreigeteilter Facialis in der Pauke mit Aplasie des ovalen Fensters. Facialis neurinom unter dem Ambosschenkel. Z Laryngol Rhinol 1967;46:451-457.

82. Hawley CW: Abnormalities of the mastoid with special reference to the facial nerve. Illinois Med J 1922;41:116-120.

83. Tobeck A: Ueber den Verlauf des Facialiskanals im Roentgenbild. Arch Ohren Nasen Kehlkopfheilkd 1938;144:276.

84. Altman F: Missbilungen des Ohres. In: von Berendes J, Link R, Zoellner F (eds): *Hals Nasen Ohrenheilkunde,* Vol. III. Stuttgart: Thieme Medical Publishers 1965, p 653-654.

85. Aubry M, Pialoux P, Jost G: *Chirurgie Cervicofaciale et Otorhinolaryngologique.* Paris: Masson et Cie, 1966; pp 56-58.

86. Mouret J, Rouviere H: The petromastoid canal. Toulouse, France: L'Assoc des Anatomistes, 6th session, 1904.

87. Bast TH: Blood supply of the optic capsule of a 150 mm human fetus. Anat Rec 1931;48:141-151.

88. Lindsay JR: Osteomyelitis of the petrous pyramid of the temporal bone. Ann. Surg. 1945;122:1060-1070.

89. Lindsay JR: The petrous pyramid of the temporal bone. Arch Otolaryngol 1940;31:231-255.

90. Nager GT: Origins and relations of the internal auditory artery and the subarcuate artery. Ann Otol Rhinol Laryngol 1954; 63:51-61.

91. Nager GT, Nager M: The arteries of the human middle ear with particular regard to the blood supply of the auditory ossicles. Ann Otol Rhinol Laryngol 1953;62:923-949.

92. Rouviere H: *Anatomie Humaine,* Vol. I. Paris: Masson et Cie, 1967, p 415.

93. Portmann M, Sterkers JM, Charachon R, Chouard CH: *The Internal Auditory Meatus: Anatomy, Pathology and Surgery.* Edinburgh: Churchill Livingston, 1975.

94. Proctor B, Lindsay JR: Tuberculosis of the ear. Arch Otolaryngol 1942;35:221-249.

95. Bollobos BA: *Halloszerv Mikrochirurgiai Anatomiaja.* Budapest: Medicina Konyokiado, 1972.

96. Eyries C, Chouard CH: Les anastomoses acoustico-faciales chez l'homme. Ann Otolaryngol 1970;87:321.

97. Papangelou L: Study of the human internal auditory canal. Laryngoscope 1972;82:617-624.

98. Mazzoni A: Internal auditory artery supply to the petrous bone. Ann Otol Rhinol Laryngol 1972;81:13- 21.

99. Mazzoni A: Internal auditory canal. Arterial relations at the porous acousticus. Ann Otol Rhinol Laryngol 1969;78:794-814.

100. Mazzoni A, Hanson CC: Surgical anatomy of the arteries of the internal auditory canal. Arch Otolaryngol 1970;91:128-135.

101. Boussens J, Caille JM, Koehler R et al: A propos de la vascularisation du conduit auditif interne. Cah ORL Montpellier 1972;7:763-774.

102. Brunner H: *Intracranial Complications of Ear, Nose and Throat Infections.* Chicago: Year Book Medical Publishers, 1946, pp 2-21.

103. Bochenek A, Reicher M: *Anatomia Czlowieka Tom VII.* Warsaw: Panstwowy Zaklad Lekarskich, 1965.

Index